QUANTUM ELECTRONICS — PRINCIPLES AND APPLICATIONS

A Series of Monographs

EDITED BY

YOH-HAN PAO

Case Western Reserve University

Cleveland, Ohio

N. S. Kapany and J. J. Burke. Optical Waveguides, 1972

Dietrich Marcuse. Theory of Dielectric Optical Waveguides, 1974

Benjamin Chu. Laser Light Scattering, 1974

Bruno Crosignani, Paolo Di Porto, and Mario Bertolotti. Statistical Properties of Scattered Light, 1975

John D. Anderson, Jr. Gasdynamic Lasers: An Introduction, 1976

W. W. Duley. CO_2 Lasers: Effects and Applications, 1976

CO_2 Lasers

Effects and Applications

CO_2 Lasers

Effects and Applications

W. W. Duley

Department of Physics
York University
Downsview, Ontario, Canada

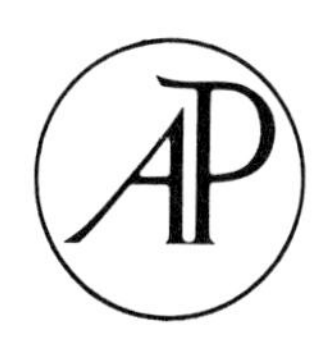

ACADEMIC PRESS New York San Francisco London 1976

A Subsidiary of Harcourt Brace Jovanovich, Publishers

ACADEMIC PRESS, INC.
111 Fifth Avenue, New York, New York 10003

United Kingdom Edition published by
ACADEMIC PRESS, INC. (LONDON) LTD.
24/28 Oval Road, London NW1

Library of Congress Cataloging in Publication Data

Duley, W W
CO_2 lasers : effects and applications.

(Quantum electronics series)
Bibliography: p.
1. Carbon dioxide lasers. I. Title.
TA1695.D84 621.36′63 75-44757
ISBN 0-12-223350-6

PRINTED IN THE UNITED STATES OF AMERICA

To Irmgardt, Nicholas, and Mark

Contents

Chapter 3 Detectors, Resonators, and Optical Components

Chapter 4 Laser Heating of Solids: Theory

Chapter 5 Drilling

Chapter 6 Welding and Machining

Preface

It is now over 10 years since the CO_2 laser was developed. During that time the CO_2 laser has become well established as a tool in the laboratory, in the shop, and in the production line. The purpose of this book is to examine and to summarize some of the more important applications of this device in physics, chemistry, and engineering. Many of these applications use the CO_2 laser simply as a controllable and highly directional source of heat. Since this is a characteristic of all types of lasers, the discussion in this book often includes a consideration of the applications of lasers in general.

Several levels of treatment of the subject matter are presented. Many sections require little in the way of a mathematical background. In other sections a knowledge of university level mathematics or some specialized knowledge of another area of physics or chemistry is assumed. It is hoped that this treatment will make the book useful to the neophyte as well as the laser scientist and to undergraduates as well as graduate students. An introduction to lasers in general is given in Chapter 1; the discussion is kept at the elementary level.

CO_2 lasers as such are discussed fully in Chapter 2, while Chapter 3 is a fairly comprehensive overview of detectors, detection methods, windows, mirrors, and other optical components for use at 10.6 μm. As many industrial applications of the CO_2 laser derive from the use of this laser as a heat source, the relevant theory for laser–surface heating effects is presented in Chapter 4. This treatment is rigorous and is supplemented by tables and graphical data on thermal constants of many materials, so that the formulas derived may be readily applied to practical problems. A summary of empirical observations on cutting, welding, drilling, and machining follows in Chapters 5 and 6.

Application of the CO_2 laser in the generation of other thermal effects is discussed in Chapter 9. Chapter 7 treats a number of applications of laser-induced evaporation including laser deposition of thin films, laser triggered switching, laser trimming of resistors, and applications in surface science.

Spectroscopy with lasers and laser photochemistry is surveyed in Chapter 8, which also includes a section on laser isotope separation.

The final chapter reviews applications of the CO_2 laser in meteorology and in communication systems.

An extensive bibliography covering the literature up to the end of 1974 is provided at the end of the book.

Acknowledgments

It is a great pleasure to acknowledge the contributions of many people in the preparation of this book. Many colleagues read over the manuscript and offered constructive criticism: I thank Dr. J. N. Gonsalves, Dr. Rita Mahon, Dr. R. W. Weeks, and Mr. W. A. Young. Professor Kurt Dressler provided the facilities for writing a large part of this book while I was on sabbatical leave at the E.T.H. in Zürich. The Defense Research Board of Canada and the National Research Council have supported my own research in this field. I also wish to thank Dr. Jacques Beaulieu for first introducing me to the study of CO_2 lasers.

I am indebted to Mrs. Doreen Myers for a superb job of typing the manuscript from handwritten copy and to Sally Lakdawala and G. R. Floyd for the preparation of the drawings.

I am most grateful to all those who freely granted permission to quote, adapt, or reproduce data from their publications.

Finally I offer special thanks to my wife and children for their encouragement and forbearance during the preparation of this work.

CO_2 Lasers

Effects and Applications

Chapter 1

Introduction

1.1 HISTORICAL BACKGROUND

Infrared laser emission from CO_2 was first reported by Patel (1964) and others in pulsed discharges through pure CO_2. By the time more complete reports of this work had been published (Patel, 1964a,c) it had already been realized (Legay and Legay-Sommaire, 1964) that a much more efficient system based on the transfer of vibrational energy from N_2 to CO_2 was possible. A CO_2 laser based on this principle had soon been developed (Patel, 1964b) and is shown in Fig. 1.1. In this system N_2 is excited in a rf discharge to produce vibrationally excited N_2 ($X^1\Sigma_g^+ v'' = 1$) molecules, which stream into an interaction region to mix with unexcited CO_2. The CO_2 is then vibrationally excited through the reaction

$$N_2\ (X^1\Sigma_g^+\ v'' = 1) + CO_2\ (00^00) \rightarrow N_2\ (v'' = 0) + CO_2\ (00^01) - 18\ \text{cm}^{-1} \quad (1)$$

which occurs efficiently since thermal energies at or near room temperature are $\simeq$200 cm^{-1}. Laser emission subsequently occurs from rotational levels of the (00^01) state to rotational levels of lower vibrational states (see Fig. 2.22 for a complete description of the appropriate energy levels). Prior to the development of the CO_2 laser Polanyi (1961, 1963) had suggested that

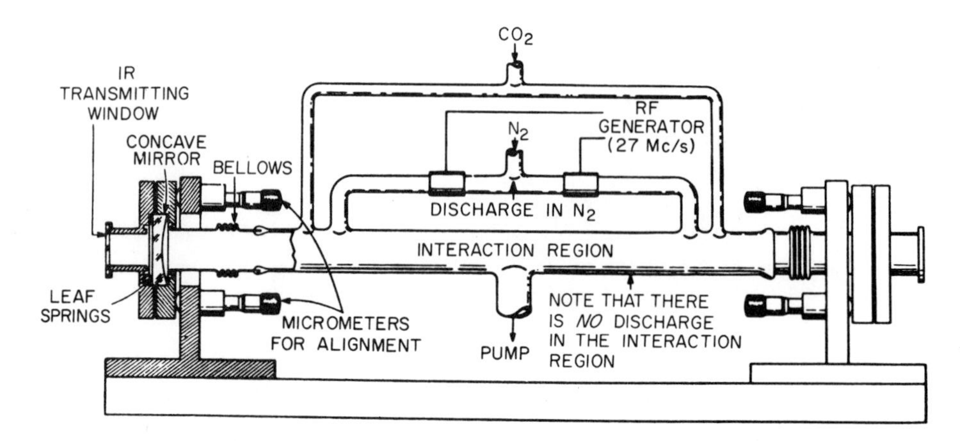

Fig. 1.1. System developed by Patel (1964b) demonstrating laser emission due to transfer of vibrational energy from N_2 to CO_2.

the type of resonant transfer of vibrational energy given in Eq. (1) might form the basis for a variety of efficient infrared lasers.

In these initial studies, continuously operating (cw) laser powers of 1 mW (Patel, 1964c) to 200 mW (Legay-Sommaire *et al.*, 1965) were obtained. The addition of N_2 was found to increase the overall efficiency from 10^{-6} (Patel, 1964c) to $\simeq 10^{-3}$ (Legay-Sommaire *et al.*, 1965; Patel, 1964b). Excitation of CO_2 in both these studies occurred as shown in Fig. 1.1. Direct excitation of a flowing mixture of N_2 and CO_2 or air and CO_2 using a dc discharge (Patel, 1965) was soon found to yield even higher cw output powers (11.91 W from a 2-m tube) and efficiencies that were $\simeq 3\%$. Cooling the gas to $-60°C$ improved the efficiency to $\simeq 5\%$ (Bridges and Patel, 1965).

Another major advance occurred soon after (Patel *et al.*, 1965), when the addition of helium was found to increase the cw power obtainable from a flowing N_2, CO_2 system to 106 W. The efficiency of this system was $>6\%$. Thus, in little over one year, the cw power obtained from the CO_2 laser had increased by a factor of 10^5 (from 1 mW to 10^2 W) and the efficiency with which this power could be generated had increased from 10^{-6} to 6×10^{-2}. Since the theoretical efficiency of the CO_2 laser operating at a wavelength of 10.6 μm is $\simeq 40\%$, while these early experiments showed that this figure could easily be approached in laboratory prototypes, the future of the CO_2 laser as an efficient converter of electrical power to infrared radiation was secure. By 1969 a 750-ft long cw CO_2 laser based on the design of Patel *et al.* (1965) had been built and operated at a power output of 8.8 kW (Horrigan *et al.*, 1969). Subsequently, the development of electric discharge convection and gas dynamic lasers (see Sections 2.3 and 2.4) has resulted in the generation of cw laser powers in excess of 100 kW.

The year 1969 marked a turning point in the development of high-power cw and pulsed CO_2 lasers. Late in 1969, Beaulieu (1970) reported that CO_2 laser emission could be obtained at atmospheric pressure and above by exciting the gas transversely so that the discharge passed perpendicular to the optical axis (Section 2.5). This has led directly to devices that rely on the creation of high densities of electronic charge using electron-beam excitation (Fenstermacher *et al.*, 1971) or volumetric photoionization (Seguin and Tulip, 1972) independent of the discharge that is used to excite laser emission. Using this approach, microsecond pulses with energies in the kilojoule range have been obtained. By way of contrast, pulse energies of 1.1 mJ were reported in the first study of a Q-switched CO_2 laser (Kovacs *et al.*, 1966).

The same year also saw the development of lasers based on convective cooling (Lavarini *et al.*, 1969; Deutsch *et al.*, 1969; Cool and Shirley, 1969) and a report was published describing the operation of a compact closed system cw laser using rapid transverse gas flow capable of generating output powers of 1 kW (Tiffany *et al.*, 1969).

The extraordinary increase in powers obtained from CO_2 lasers in the 10 years since Patel's first report has opened wide areas of application for these devices in basic and applied research and in many areas of technology. Now 10–15-kW cw CO_2 lasers can be purchased (Locke and Hella, 1974). While it is unlikely that a corresponding increase in power output will be obtained in the next 10 years, further advances can be expected.

1.2 INTERACTION OF LIGHT WITH A TWO-LEVEL SYSTEM

If we consider a system of N atoms or molecules each of which has only two electronic energy levels (Fig. 1.2), then when this system is exposed

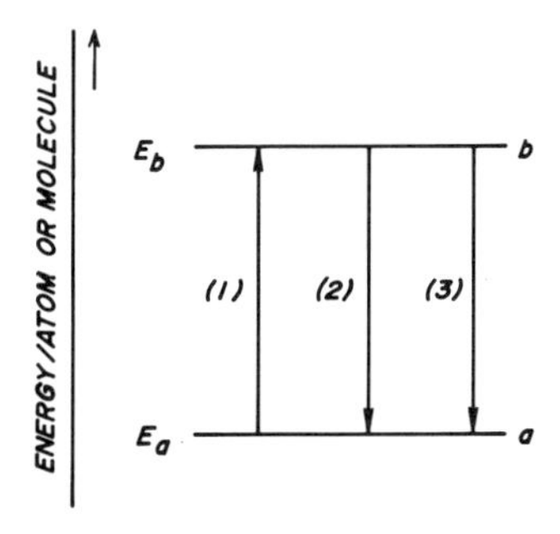

Fig. 1.2. Two-level system interacting with electromagnetic radiation of frequency ν_{ab}.

to light of frequency ν_{ab}, the electromagnetic field of the incident light will promote transitions between the two energy levels. The condition for this resonance is

$$h\nu_{ab} = E_b - E_a \tag{2}$$

where h is Planck's constant ($h = 6.626 \times 10^{-34}$ J-sec).

If this system is connected to a thermal reservoir at a temperature T (°K) and allowed to come to equilibrium, a well-known result of statistical mechanics predicts that the ratio of the number of atoms or molecules in level a to that in level b is given by

$$N_a/N_b = \exp[(E_b - E_a)/kT] \tag{3}$$

where k is Boltzmann's constant (1.38×10^{-23} J/°K). Since by definition $E_b > E_a$, N_a is always greater than N_b and at absolute zero all the atoms or molecules will be in the lowest energy level a.

Returning now to the effect of an incident radiation field at a frequency ν_{ab} we see that an atom or molecule in state a can be raised into state b by absorption of a photon of energy $h\nu_{ab}$. The rate at which this will occur is given by

$$R_1 = B_{ab}N_a\rho(\nu_{ab}) \tag{4}$$

where N_a is in m^{-3}, $\rho(\nu_{ab})$ is the energy density of the resonant frequency (J/m^3 Hz), and B_{ab} is the Einstein B coefficient, which is a measure of the strength of the $a \rightarrow b$ transition (in units of $m^3/J\text{-}sec^2$). R_1 is the rate at which atoms or molecules are transferred from level a to level b due to the incident field. However, this field can also induce the reverse transition, i.e., one in which an atom or molecule is caused to lose a quantum of energy to the radiation field while making the transition from level b to level a. The rate at which this occurs is

$$R_2 = B_{ba}N_b\rho(\nu_{ab}) \tag{5}$$

where N_b is the number of atoms or molecules in level b (per m^3). A simplification is obtained since $B_{ab} = B_{ba}$.

However, in the absence of an applied electromagnetic field, atoms or molecules in level b can spontaneously emit a quantum of energy $h\nu_{ab}$ to drop to level a. The rate at which this occurs is

$$R_3 = N_bA_{ba} \tag{6}$$

where A_{ba} (sec^{-1}) is the Einstein A coefficient and is simply the inverse of the radiative lifetime τ_{ab} of the upper level. Also

$$A_{ba} = (8\pi h\nu_{ab}^3/c^3)B_{ba} \tag{7}$$

where c is the velocity of light. Since we have only two energy levels and the atoms or molecules in the system must be in either one of the two levels we can write

$$R_1 = R_2 + R_3$$

or

$$N_a\rho(\nu_{ab})B_{ab} = N_bA_{ba} + N_b\rho(\nu_{ab})B_{ba} \tag{8}$$

Two immediate conclusions that can be obtained from this simple analysis are that, first, as $N_a > N_b$ the system will always absorb energy from the incident radiation field at a greater rate than energy is returned to the field through stimulated emission, and second, that even when $\rho(\nu_{ab})$ is made very large, the effect on the system will be only to equalize the populations in the two energy levels ($N_a = N_b$). The first effect accounts for the fact that systems at a lower temperature than the temperature of a background light source always appear to absorb incident radiation, while the second effect is responsible for the saturation that occurs in absorbing systems at very high incident light levels. A system in thermal equilibrium or any system in which $N_a > N_b$ can only act as an attenuator for incident radiation of frequency ν_{ab}. Even when $N_a = N_b$ [infinite temperature or infinite $\rho(\nu_{ab})$] the system only provides a rate of stimulated emission that exactly balances the rate at which incident radiation is removed through absorption. To obtain a system in which the stimulated emission term is larger than R_1 we must have $N_b > N_a$ or a population inversion between the two levels. To make full use of this population inversion we want to make $\rho(\nu_{ab})$ as large as possible so that R_2 can be kept large. This latter requirement is necessary only if it is desired to turn the system from an amplifier at frequency ν_{ab} to an oscillator.

Practical laser systems are always more complex than this: one never has simply two energy levels involved. However, the net result is always to produce a population inversion between pairs of energy levels so that the stimulated emission term can become dominant.

1.3 THE PRODUCTION OF POPULATION INVERSION

We have seen that in a two-level system a means by which N_b can be made greater than N_a must be found in order that the system may act as an amplifier for radiation of frequency $\nu_{ab} = (E_b - E_a)/h$. Two ways in which this can be accomplished are shown schematically in Fig. 1.3. Figure 1.3a is a representation of the energy level diagram in a typical solid state laser system in which pumping is done optically while Fig. 1.3b is a simplified schematic of the energy levels in the CO_2 laser pumped by resonant energy transfer from electrically excited N_2.

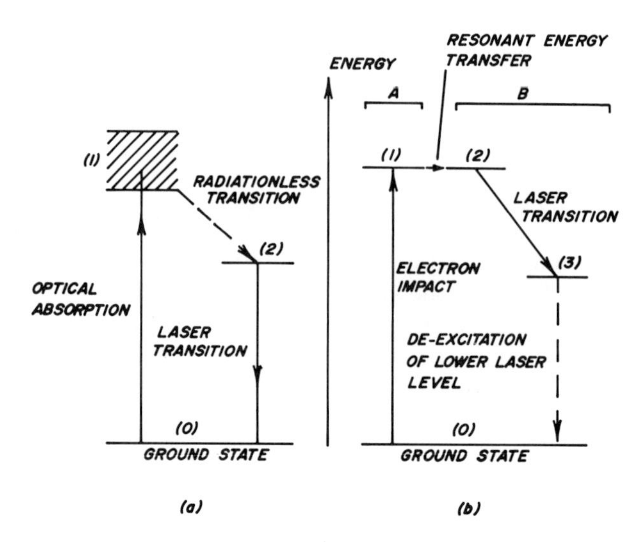

Fig. 1.3. Pumping mechanisms in two representative laser systems. (a) Solid state laser, e.g., ruby. (b) Gaseous laser, e.g., CO_2, N_2, or He. A could be N_2, while B would be CO_2.

In the optically pumped system, a strongly allowed transition connects the ground state (0) of the laser ion (Cr^{3+} in ruby) to a broad electronic energy level (1) that lies at an energy above that of the upper laser level (2). Since this energy level is broad a large amount of the radiation from the pump can be absorbed, making for efficient operation. Electrons transferred to energies within this band rapidly settle to the bottom of the band where they can lose their energy either by making the radiative transition (1) → (0) or by undergoing a radiationless transition to level (2). In ruby, the radiative transition (1) → (0) occurs with less probability than the radiationless (1) → (2) transition. Thus, most of the electrons transferred into level (1) by the absorption of pump radiation rapidly relax into level (2). If level (2) is metastable, that is if it has a long radiative lifetime $\tau_{20} = A_{20}^{-1}$, then this population can build up until stimulated emission becomes important. When the pumping is continued, a population inversion may be created between levels (2) and (0). Note that as the number of ions in the system is finite, the ground state population is reduced by optical pumping, which aids the attainment of inversion between levels (2) and (0).

The system shown in Fig. 1.3b is representative of the situation in a CO_2 laser discharge. The discharge excites N_2 molecules electrically to establish a population in energy level (1). Practically, the only way in which this energy may be dissipated is by means of resonant energy transfer to a state (2) of the CO_2 molecule. This causes the colliding CO_2 molecule to be raised from its ground state (0) to the excited state (2). As a similar excitation mechanism is not possible for the lower laser level (3), a population inversion can be built up between levels (2) and (3). The decay from (2) $\rightarrow$ (3) results in the transfer of population to level (3), and for efficient operation some method must be provided for returning the molecules in this level to the ground state or the population buildup in level (3) will reduce or eliminate the inversion between levels (2) and (3). This is accomplished in high-power CO_2 laser systems by the addition of helium, which quenches the excitation on the lower laser levels through collisions, returning CO_2 molecules to their ground state.

We see that laser action in the system of Fig. 1.3b is controlled in a very specific way by collisional activation and deactivation rates and does not rely solely on radiative processes. This implies that a wide variety of parameters (gas pressure, composition, temperature, discharge current, electron temperature, etc.) will affect the behavior of such devices. In the system of Fig. 1.3a, however, excitation and deexcitation rates are controlled by radiative and nonradiative decay rates, which are intrinsic properties of the laser ion and its host matrix and are therefore less amenable to external variation.

Figures 1.4 and 1.5 show in a simplified way how both of these pumping mechanisms can be obtained in practical systems. The traces in the lower part of Fig. 1.4 illustrate the variation in $N_2 - N_0$ and the intensity of a probe beam at the laser frequency with time during optical excitation. The time scale for these traces would typically be of the order 1 msec.

The pumping methods shown in Fig. 1.5 are well suited to cw lasers. The next chapter will discuss some further ways in which CO_2 lasers may be pumped to obtain both cw and pulsed laser outputs.

1.4 THE THRESHOLD FOR LASER OSCILLATION

When a population inversion exists between two energy levels, the system can act as an amplifier for radiation whose frequency satisfies the criterion $\nu_{ab} = (E_b - E_a)/h$. To turn this system into an oscillator a feedback loop must be created. This can be accomplished by putting the amplifier inside the cavity formed by two partially reflecting mirrors in a Fabry–Perot configuration (Fig. 1.6). As the mirrors of this cavity have a reflectivity R that is less than 100%, light waves traveling along the optical axis of the system will be partially reflected back in the opposite direction when they encounter one of the reflectors. This reflection back into the amplifying medium constitutes an optical feedback loop that causes the

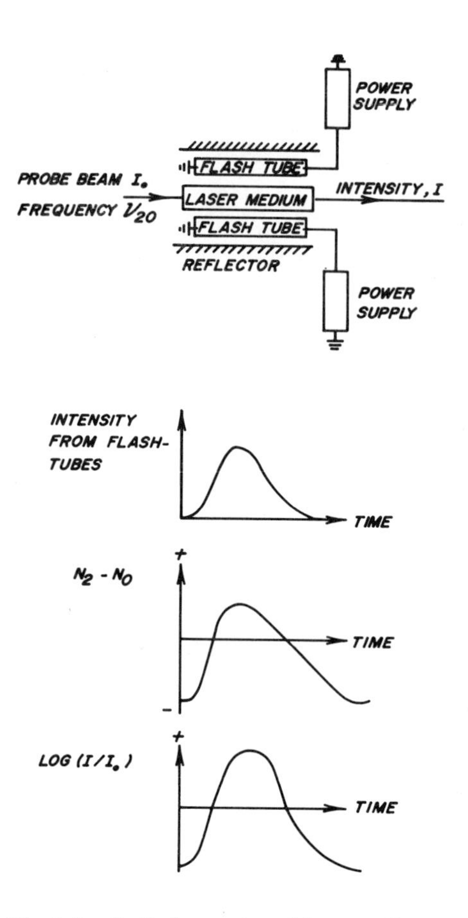

Fig. 1.4. Optical pumping of laser medium.

electromagnetic field strength to rise rapidly within the cavity. When the single pass gain due to stimulated emission exceeds the losses per pass arising from scattering or some other process within the optical amplifier and the "leakage" of $(1 - R)$ of the field through the reflectors, then oscillation can occur. This condition will first be reached for a particular value of the population inversion. The threshold population inversion can be obtained from the following simple analysis. In the absence of an amplifying medium, an electromagnetic wave propagating back and forth within the Fabry–Perot resonator would continuously decrease in amplitude. After n passes the energy in this wave would decrease to $1/e$ of its initial value, so that

$$R^n = 1/e$$

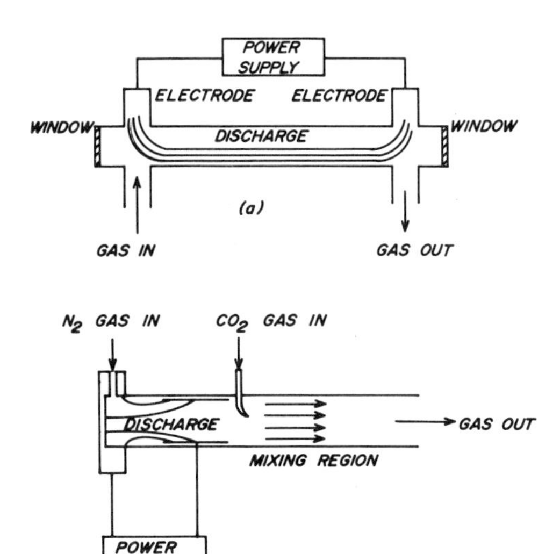

Fig. 1.5. Two methods of exciting a CO_2 gas laser. (a) Discharge applied to CO_2, N_2, He mixture directly. (b) Only N_2 excited in discharge followed by resonant energy transfer to CO_2 downstream.

We will assume that R is large; then

$$n \simeq 1/(1 - R)$$

If the separation between the reflectors of the cavity is d, then the time taken for the energy to reduce to $1/e$ of its initial value is

$$\tau = nd/c = d/c(1 - R)$$

where c is the velocity of light. The power required due to stimulated emission to balance this loss will be approximately

$$P_L = E/\tau \tag{9}$$

where E is the energy stored in the electromagnetic field propagating in the

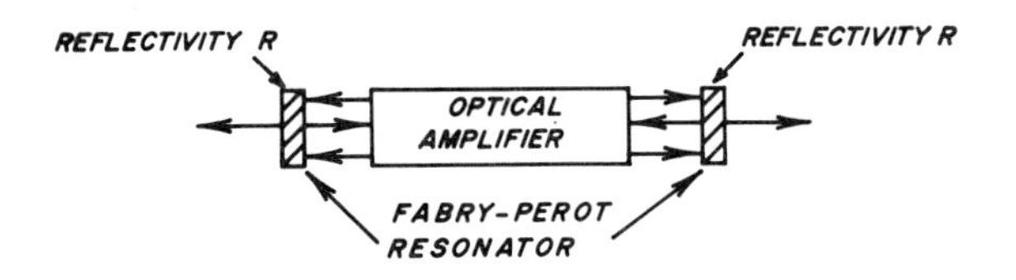

Fig. 1.6. Optical amplifier inside a Fabry–Perot resonator, which provides feedback.

cavity. The power due to stimulated emission can be obtained from the equation

$$P_s = B(N_b - N_a)h\nu_{ab}\rho(\nu_{ab})A'd \tag{10}$$

where the cross-sectional area of the mirrors and amplifying section is A'. B can be expressed in terms of D, the dipole matrix element (which measures the strength of the $b \rightarrow a$ transition), as

$$B = 2\pi^2 D^2/h^2\epsilon_0 \tag{11}$$

where ϵ_0 is the permittivity of free space [$=8.85 \times 10^{-12}$ $C^2/(N\text{-}m^2)$]. Then

$$P_s = \frac{2\pi^2 D^2}{h\epsilon_0}\nu_{ab}A'd\rho(\nu_{ab})(N_b - N_a) \tag{12}$$

To balance the losses P_L we must have

$$P_s > P_L \tag{13}$$

and hence the following condition on the population inversion:

$$N_b - N_a > \frac{hc\epsilon_0 E(1 - R)}{2\pi^2 D^2 \nu_{ab}A'd^2\rho(\nu_{ab})} \tag{14}$$

But the energy stored in the electromagnetic field within the cavity,

$$E = f\rho(\nu_{ab})\ \Delta\nu_{ab}A'd \tag{15}$$

where f is a numerical factor that depends on the exact shape of the spectral line emitted on making the $b \rightarrow a$ transition* and $\Delta\nu_{ab}$ is a characteristic width for this line (in hertz). As a result, the threshold condition becomes

$$N_b - N_a > \frac{\epsilon_0 hc(1 - R)f}{2\pi^2 dD^2\nu_{ab}}\Delta\nu_{ab} \tag{16}$$

For the very special case of a line broadened by the Doppler effect

$$f = (\pi \log 2)^{1/2}, \qquad \text{and} \qquad \Delta\nu_{ab} = \frac{\nu_{ab}}{c}\left(\frac{2kT}{m}\log 2\right)^{1/2}$$

where T is the gas temperature and m the mass of the emitter. Then

$$N_b - N_a > \frac{\epsilon_0 h(1 - R)\ln 2}{2(\pi)^{3/2}dD^2}\left(\frac{2kT}{m}\right)^{1/2} \tag{17}$$

* Spectral lines can never be thought of as infinitely narrow. There is always a range of energies that can be emitted in a transition $b \rightarrow a$, leading to a broadening of the emitted line.

It is evident that given a particular laser material, the threshold for oscillation is reduced by keeping the linewidth small and by increasing the length of the laser cavity (assuming it is completely filled with the amplifying medium). The threshold is also reduced by increasing R.

As a numerical example, $R = 0.95$, $T = 300°\text{K}$, $m = 50$ amu, $d = 1$ m, and $D = 0.6 \times 10^{-30}$ C-m, which is a typical value for an infrared laser, we obtain

$$N_b - N_a > 1.6 \times 10^{16}\ \text{cm}^{-3}$$

Since a gas at NTP contains 3×10^{19} molecules/cm^3 we see that the threshold condition requires a partial pressure of $\simeq 0.4$ Torr for molecules in the upper laser level.

1.5 OPTICAL RESONATORS

As in a microwave cavity, only certain distributions of electromagnetic field can be maintained without loss in the Fabry–Perot resonator. These field distributions are called modes of the cavity. We will postpone a full discussion on this subject to Section 3.6; however, it is evident that two main types of modes will exist. Longitudinal modes of the resonator will be defined by the number of half-wavelengths of the electromagnetic field that can be contained between the reflectors. This number is

$$q = 2d/\lambda$$

where λ is the wavelength. The frequencies of these modes will be spaced by

$$\Delta\nu = c/2d$$

For a 1-m cavity, this separation would be 150 MHz.

Simultaneously, various configurations of the electromagnetic field perpendicular to the optical axis will be found. The notation for these modes is TEM_{mn} (TEM, transverse electromagnetic) so that a complete description of a mode of the cavity would be through the label TEM_{mnq}.

The width of an emission line corresponding to a transition of the type $b \rightarrow a$ in a typical gas laser system can be many times larger than the spacing between longitudinal modes. When the system has high gain, oscillation may occur simultaneously on more than one of these longitudinal modes. Various methods can be used, however, to discriminate against all but one longitudinal mode (see Section 2.24) so that single-frequency operation is obtained. A laser operating in this regime is said to be *mode-locked.*

It is obvious that oscillation can only be obtained in a system in which the resonator provides sufficient feedback to allow the optical field intensity to build up to the point where the gain compensates for the loss per pass. High peak power output pulses can often be obtained from high-gain laser media by withholding the feedback until the population inversion maximizes. At this point the feedback loop is switched on allowing the field to rise rapidly (in times of the order d/c) to a very large value. This process, which involves spoiling the Q of the cavity until the optimum amplification conditions are established, is called *Q-switching*. It may be accomplished mechanically by rotating one of the resonator mirrors or electrically through a variety of electro-optic or acousto-optic devices. The pulsed TEA CO_2 laser exhibits a variation of this effect called *gain-switching*.

1.6 CHARACTERISTICS OF LASER LIGHT

The distinguishing properties of laser radiation are

(a) the radiation is highly monochromatic,
(b) laser radiation exhibits high spatial coherence,
(c) laser radiation exhibits high temporal coherence.

The monochromaticity of laser radiation compared to that attainable from conventional light sources can be understood by realizing that discrete spectral lines emitted from a low-pressure discharge lamp will still show the effect of Doppler broadening. Laser oscillation occurs, however, with the aid of modes of the optical cavity that have intrinsic widths many times smaller than this Doppler width. Indeed, as we have seen above, a given Doppler-broadened line profile may contain many longitudinal modes. The high Q of the laser cavity automatically ensures a narrow output linewidth.

The quantum mechanical uncertainty principle can be used to relate the linewidth $\Delta\nu$ to the coherence time Δt:

$$\Delta\nu \, \Delta t \simeq 1$$

For a laser linewidth of 1 MHz, this predicts that $\Delta t \simeq 10^{-6}$ sec. The coherence length L_c is then given by

$$L_c \simeq c/\Delta\nu$$

or $\simeq$300m in our example. A linewidth of 1 MHz is really quite conservative and coherence lengths many times this value can easily be obtained. An experiment in which the light from a laser produces fringes in a Michelson-type interferometer can in principle be used to demonstrate the concept of coherence length. When the path length between the interfering beams exceeds L_c, interference fringes will be of low contrast. Note that the linewidth of pulsed lasers is often limited by the length of the laser pulse through the uncertainty relation; for a nanosecond pulse, $\Delta\nu$ would be 1 GHz. Further discussion on coherence time and coherence length, as well as the means by which these are measured, is given by Allen and Jones (1967) and Heard (1968).

While temporal coherence can be thought of as the correlation between the values of the radiation field at the same point in space at two different times, spatial coherence is measured by the correlation between the values of the radiation field at two different points in space at the same time. Thus a source may exhibit spatial coherence without time coherence or vice versa. Laser outputs are, however, both temporally and spatially coherent. Spatial coherence can be demonstrated by a Young-type interference experiment in which light from the laser source irradiates two pinholes in an opaque screen. Since the light from the laser is spatially coherent, a screen placed behind the pinholes will show an interference pattern as illustrated in Fig. 1.7. A similar experiment performed with a spatially incoherent source requires a source pinhole as shown in Fig. 1.7b.

The spatial coherence of laser light accounts for the high brightness or radiance of laser sources. A perfectly coherent plane wave will be diffracted on encountering an aperture of diameter D through the solid angle

$$\Delta\Omega \simeq \lambda^2/D^2$$

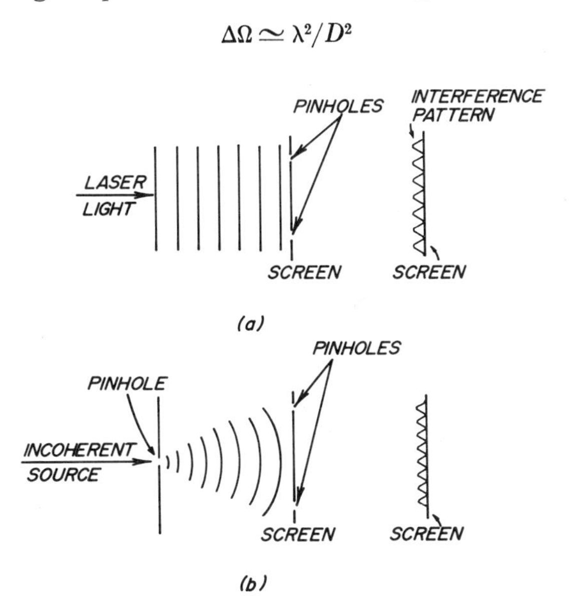

Fig. 1.7. Experiments demonstrating spatial coherence. (a) Laser source with uniphase wavefront, no source pinhole required. (b) Incoherent source, source pinhole required to obtain spatial coherence at second screen.

When D is simply the diameter of the aperture provided by the finite diameter of the laser itself (or the beam diameter) $\Delta\Omega$ will be the angular divergence of the beam. If the laser emits P W of power over a cross-sectional area $\pi D^2/4$ cm², then the brightness or radiance of the source will simply be

$$R \simeq P/(\pi D^2/4)\ \Delta\Omega\ \mathrm{W/cm^2/ster}$$

For $\Delta\Omega = \lambda^2/D^2$, this becomes

$$R \simeq 4P/\pi\lambda^2$$

At the CO_2 laser wavelength $\lambda = 10.6\ \mu\mathrm{m} = 1.06 \times 10^{-3}$ cm, a 100-W beam would then have a brightness $R \simeq 10^8$ W/cm²/ster. For comparison, an incoherent 1000-W arc lamp would typically have a brightness $\simeq 10^3$ W/cm²/ster. The difference from the spectral radiance

$$R/\Delta\nu = 4P/\pi\lambda^2\ \Delta\nu\ \mathrm{W/cm^2/ster/Hz}$$

where $\Delta\nu$ is the laser linewidth in frequency units, is even greater. A 100-W cw laser at 10.6 μm with $\Delta\nu = 10^6$ Hz has

$$R/\Delta\nu\,|_{\mathrm{laser}} \simeq 10^2\ \mathrm{W/cm^2/ster/Hz}$$

while

$$R/\Delta\nu\,|_{\mathrm{arc}} \simeq 10^{-10}\ \mathrm{W/cm^2/ster/Hz}$$

The brightness of pulsed lasers can be enormous since P is large. For example, a 100-mJ pulse of 1-nsec duration at 10.6 μm has $P = 10^8$ W and $R \simeq 10^{14}$ W/cm²/ster. However, the spectral radiance is not increased correspondingly since $\Delta\nu \simeq 1/\Delta t$, where Δt is the pulse length, and thus $\Delta\nu$ increases as the pulse length diminishes. For our example $\Delta\nu \simeq 10^9$ Hz and $R/\Delta\nu \simeq 10^5$ W/cm²/ster/Hz.

The properties of coherence, directionality, and high brightness give rise to a variety of special applications involving laser light sources. Spatial coherence and high brightness have made the laser attractive in many areas of material fabrication. The monochromaticity of laser light sources has opened up wide analytical possibilities in the area of atomic and molecular spectroscopy. Temporal coherence is of value in systems involving interferometric measurements and in nonlinear optics. These and other applications of laser light will be discussed in subsequent chapters.

)0 W/cm^2 has been obtained. Smith and McCoy (1969) and Christense
t al. (1969) concluded that this variation could be due to the finite are
of the sampling probe beam. Tyte (1970) suggests that temperature gradi
ents between the axis of the laser tube and its walls may also affect th
saturation parameter.

2.2.1.5 Discharge Current and Gas Pressure. The discharge current determines the rate at which CO_2 molecules in the laser tube ar
pumped by direct electron excitation and via collision with excited N_2 molecules. The amplifier gain and the maximum output power obtained from a
particular laser tube would therefore be expected to increase continuously
with current in the discharge. However, a point is reached on increasing
current at which the heating effect at the tube axis becomes substantial
hat the gain decreases. The output power will then saturate at a par-
lar point as the discharge current is increased and may actually de-
ise as the current is further increased. The discharge current for maxi-
n power output from a particular tube will depend on the gas pressure
the tube diameter. Tyte (1970) has shown that as the tube diameter
eases, the optimum current increases, while the maximum total gas
ssure for highest output decreases. For a 5-cm diameter tube, optimum
ent is in the range 100–125 mA and the maximum gas pressure is about
orr. For a 2.5-cm diameter tube these values are 80 mA and 10 Torr,
ectively. With a suitable ballast resistor, a current of 100–125 mA in a
n diameter, 3-m long tube at a pressure of 6–7 Torr requires a voltage
2–15 kV.

.2.1.6 Efficiency. The efficiency of conventional cw CO_2 laser
charges may approach 30% at low laser output (Rigden and Moeller,
66). Roberts *et al.* (1967) have shown that the efficiency depends strongly
n wall temperature and the flow rate. It is also usually true that maximum
efficiency of a particular system may not occur at the same discharge parameters as the point at which maximum power output is obtained. However, the efficiency of a 2.3-kW multimodule cw laser described by Roberts
et al. (1967) was found to be as high as 9.4% at full laser output power.

2.2.1.7 Cavity Parameters. Most high-power lasers of this type now
use output couplers consisting of plane disks of germanium or another semiconductor coated on one side to produce the desired reflectivity at 10.6 μm
and antireflection coated on the other side. The question of what reflectivity will give highest performance in a particular system is often answered
by trial and error, although some general rules have been given by Allen
(1968) and Tyte (1970). Tyte has shown that a plot of $\log(R)$ versus l/d,
where R is the reflectivity, l the length of the cavity, and d the diameter of
the discharge, is linear. This plot is shown in Fig. 2.2. A 10-m cavity con-

Chapter 2

The CO_2 Laser

2.1 INTRODUCTION

Improvements in the means of excitation of CO_2 lasers have resulted in a rapid increase in the power attainable from these devices in the ten years since Patel (1964) first announced cw laser oscillation in gaseous CO_2. In this chapter the development of both cw and pulsed CO_2 lasers will be discussed. We will also review some of the work that has been done on energy transfer mechanisms and excitation processes in CO_2 laser discharges.

2.2 AXIAL FLOW CO_2 LASERS

2.2.1 Conventional CO_2 Lasers

2.2.1.1 Low-Flow Devices. While it is true that low axial flow or conventional cw CO_2 lasers are no longer "state of the art" as regards high-power generation, the simplicity of these devices and the ease with which they can be fabricated make them attractive for applications that may require cw powers of up to about 500 W. Basically the conventional cw CO_2 laser is nothing more than a water-cooled tube with mirrors on both ends through which the laser mixture is flowed and excited electrically. A simple two-section laser of this type is shown schematically in Fig. 2.1a and an actual device is shown in Fig. 2.1b. Under optimized conditions one may count on obtaining output powers of about 80 W/m for short ($\lesssim$3 m) tubes to somewhat less than 50 W/m for long (50 m or more) tubes. Exceptions to this general rule exist, however. As an example Roberts *et al.*

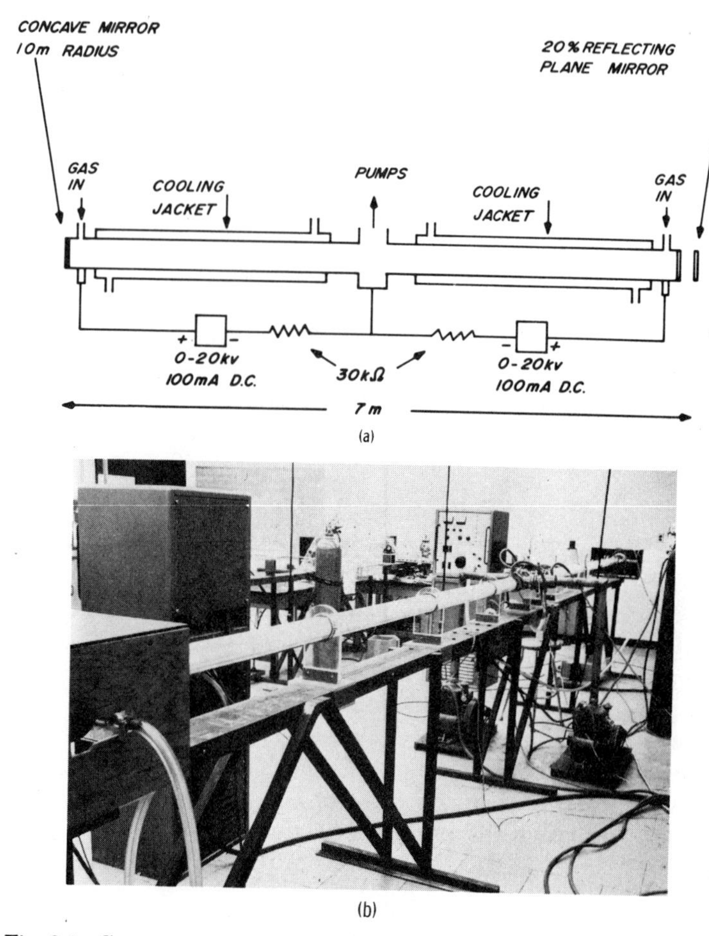

Fig. 2.1. Conventional CO_2 laser. (a) Schematic, (b) actual photograph.

(1967) obtained 100 W/m from an 8.2-m long laser of this sort. The longest and most powerful conventional cw CO_2 laser seems to have been reported by Horrigan *et al.* (1969), who developed a folded system with a total length of 750 ft, which was capable of generating 8.8 kW of cw power. However, such systems have now been replaced by new laser designs based on rapid transverse gas flows.

In this section, we will discuss some aspects of the design and construction of conventional cw CO_2 lasers. For a more comprehensive treatment the reader is referred to the excellent review on this subject by Tyte (1970).

2.2.1.2 Gas Composition. A wide variety of different three-component gas mixtures have been investigated in conventional flowing CO_2 laser systems but the highest output power is obtained from a mixture of CO_2, N_2, and He. The optimum ratio of these gases is approximately 0.8 : 1 : 7, although maximum output from a given system is usually found empirically by varying the mixture ratio during operation. In addition,

such parameters as tube diameter, flow rate, and o
will also determine the optimum mixture in a given d
output power is not too sensitive to changes in the [CO_2
but will depend quite strongly on CO_2 pressure and the [C
In practice, to determine optimum operating conditions one
[CO_2] : [N_2] ratio constant at about 0.8 : 1 and then vary
[He] until peak power was obtained. The [CO_2] : [N_2] ratio
be "fine-tuned" by varying the N_2 flow rate to find a point at
system was optimized.

2.2.1.3 Gas Flow. In an otherwise optimized system, the p
output will increase steadily with gas flow rate. This increase is most ra
in the regime where the flow rate produces less than about 100 changes
gas in the laser tube per minute (Tyte, 1970) and is thought to be due
the enhanced removal rate of dissociation products such as CO and
Above 100 gas changes per minute the enhancement of output power
be due in part to convective cooling of the discharge. De Maria (1
shows that the ratio of the power obtained from a diffusion-cooled las
one with convective cooling $P_d/P_c \propto \Lambda v_t/Dv$, where Λ is the mean
path of the CO_2 molecules in the mixture, v_t their thermal molecular sp
D the diameter of the tube, and v the flow velocity. Since Λ/D is very s
at pressures of 10 Torr and with a tube diameter of several centime
P_d/P_c will be small even for small v. As v increases, however, into the r
where $v \to v_t$, convective cooling dominates and P_c can be very m
greater than P_d. (A variety of convectively cooled laser devices wil
described in later sections.) One other advantage of fast flow is that
incident electrical power that can be dissipated in the flowing gas can of
be increased as the flow rate increases.

2.2.1.4 Tube Diameter. Rigden and Moeller (1966) have determined that both the output power and conversion efficiency of electrical power to laser output are essentially independent of tube diameter for diameters of up to 50 mm. This is only true when the gas pressure and discharge current are optimized for each tube diameter. The gain for 10.6-μm radiation has, however, been found to depend in a complex way on tube diameter (Cheo and Cooper, 1967) although the peak gain decreases with increasing tube diameter. In the limit of extremely small-diameter cw dielectric wave
guide discharge tubes, the gain can be as high as 5.3%/cm (Chester a
Abrams, 1972; Burkhart *et al.*, 1972). Such systems have generated ou
power densities of up to 15 W/cm³ of active discharge volume (see S
2.2.2).

The saturation intensity of low-pressure conventional CO_2
charges has been measured by many groups (Hotz and A
Kogelnik and Bridges, 1967; Christensen *et al.*, 1969) and a

Chapter 2

The CO_2 Laser

2.1 INTRODUCTION

Improvements in the means of excitation of CO_2 lasers have resulted in a rapid increase in the power attainable from these devices in the ten years since Patel (1964) first announced cw laser oscillation in gaseous CO_2. In this chapter the development of both cw and pulsed CO_2 lasers will be discussed. We will also review some of the work that has been done on energy transfer mechanisms and excitation processes in CO_2 laser discharges.

2.2 AXIAL FLOW CO_2 LASERS

2.2.1 Conventional CO_2 Lasers

2.2.1.1 Low-Flow Devices. While it is true that low axial flow or conventional cw CO_2 lasers are no longer "state of the art" as regards high-power generation, the simplicity of these devices and the ease with which they can be fabricated make them attractive for applications that may require cw powers of up to about 500 W. Basically the conventional cw CO_2 laser is nothing more than a water-cooled tube with mirrors on both ends through which the laser mixture is flowed and excited electrically. A simple two-section laser of this type is shown schematically in Fig. 2.1a and an actual device is shown in Fig. 2.1b. Under optimized conditions one may count on obtaining output powers of about 80 W/m for short ($\lesssim 3$ m) tubes to somewhat less than 50 W/m for long (50 m or more) tubes. Exceptions to this general rule exist, however. As an example Roberts *et al.*

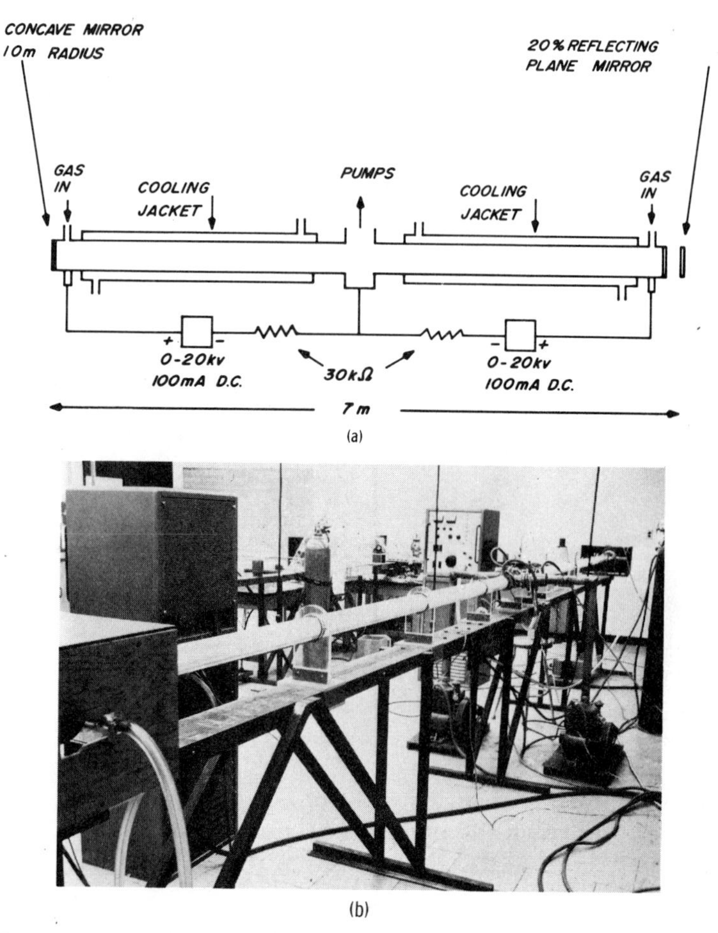

Fig. 2.1. Conventional CO_2 laser. (a) Schematic, (b) actual photograph.

(1967) obtained 100 W/m from an 8.2-m long laser of this sort. The longest and most powerful conventional cw CO_2 laser seems to have been reported by Horrigan *et al.* (1969), who developed a folded system with a total length of 750 ft, which was capable of generating 8.8 kW of cw power. However, such systems have now been replaced by new laser designs based on rapid transverse gas flows.

In this section, we will discuss some aspects of the design and construction of conventional cw CO_2 lasers. For a more comprehensive treatment the reader is referred to the excellent review on this subject by Tyte (1970).

2.2.1.2 Gas Composition. A wide variety of different three-component gas mixtures have been investigated in conventional flowing CO_2 laser systems but the highest output power is obtained from a mixture of CO_2, N_2, and He. The optimum ratio of these gases is approximately 0.8 : 1 : 7, although maximum output from a given system is usually found empirically by varying the mixture ratio during operation. In addition, such parameters as tube diameter, flow rate, and optical output coupling will also determine the optimum mixture in a given device. Generally, the output power is not too sensitive to changes in the [CO_2, N_2] : [He] ratio but will depend quite strongly on CO_2 pressure and the [CO_2] : [N_2] ratio. In practice, to determine optimum operating conditions one would set the [CO_2] : [N_2] ratio constant at about 0.8 : 1 and then vary [CO_2, N_2] : [He] until peak power was obtained. The [CO_2] : [N_2] ratio would then be "fine-tuned" by varying the N_2 flow rate to find a point at which the system was optimized.

2.2.1.3 Gas Flow. In an otherwise optimized system, the power output will increase steadily with gas flow rate. This increase is most rapid in the regime where the flow rate produces less than about 100 changes of gas in the laser tube per minute (Tyte, 1970) and is thought to be due to the enhanced removal rate of dissociation products such as CO and O_2. Above 100 gas changes per minute the enhancement of output power may be due in part to convective cooling of the discharge. De Maria (1973) shows that the ratio of the power obtained from a diffusion-cooled laser to one with convective cooling $P_d/P_c \propto \Lambda v_t/Dv$, where Λ is the mean free path of the CO_2 molecules in the mixture, v_t their thermal molecular speed, D the diameter of the tube, and v the flow velocity. Since Λ/D is very small at pressures of 10 Torr and with a tube diameter of several centimeters, P_d/P_c will be small even for small v. As v increases, however, into the range where $v \rightarrow v_t$, convective cooling dominates and P_c can be very much greater than P_d. (A variety of convectively cooled laser devices will be described in later sections.) One other advantage of fast flow is that the incident electrical power that can be dissipated in the flowing gas can often be increased as the flow rate increases.

2.2.1.4 Tube Diameter. Rigden and Moeller (1966) have determined that both the output power and conversion efficiency of electrical power to laser output are essentially independent of tube diameter for diameters of up to 50 mm. This is only true when the gas pressure and discharge current are optimized for each tube diameter. The gain for 10.6-μm radiation has, however, been found to depend in a complex way on tube diameter (Cheo and Cooper, 1967) although the peak gain decreases with increasing tube diameter. In the limit of extremely small-diameter cw dielectric waveguide discharge tubes, the gain can be as high as 5.3%/cm (Chester and Abrams, 1972; Burkhart *et al.*, 1972). Such systems have generated output power densities of up to 15 W/cm^3 of active discharge volume (see Section 2.2.2).

The saturation intensity of low-pressure conventional CO_2 laser discharges has been measured by many groups (Hotz and Austin, 1967; Kogelnik and Bridges, 1967; Christensen *et al.*, 1969) and a range of 13 to

100 W/cm^2 has been obtained. Smith and McCoy (1969) and Christensen *et al.* (1969) concluded that this variation could be due to the finite area of the sampling probe beam. Tyte (1970) suggests that temperature gradients between the axis of the laser tube and its walls may also affect the saturation parameter.

2.2.1.5 Discharge Current and Gas Pressure. The discharge current determines the rate at which CO_2 molecules in the laser tube are pumped by direct electron excitation and via collision with excited N_2 molecules. The amplifier gain and the maximum output power obtained from a particular laser tube would therefore be expected to increase continuously with current in the discharge. However, a point is reached on increasing the current at which the heating effect at the tube axis becomes substantial so that the gain decreases. The output power will then saturate at a particular point as the discharge current is increased and may actually decrease as the current is further increased. The discharge current for maximum power output from a particular tube will depend on the gas pressure and the tube diameter. Tyte (1970) has shown that as the tube diameter increases, the optimum current increases, while the maximum total gas pressure for highest output decreases. For a 5-cm diameter tube, optimum current is in the range 100–125 mA and the maximum gas pressure is about 6 Torr. For a 2.5-cm diameter tube these values are 80 mA and 10 Torr, respectively. With a suitable ballast resistor, a current of 100–125 mA in a 5-cm diameter, 3-m long tube at a pressure of 6–7 Torr requires a voltage of 12–15 kV.

2.2.1.6 Efficiency. The efficiency of conventional cw CO_2 laser discharges may approach 30% at low laser output (Rigden and Moeller, 1966). Roberts *et al.* (1967) have shown that the efficiency depends strongly on wall temperature and the flow rate. It is also usually true that maximum efficiency of a particular system may not occur at the same discharge parameters as the point at which maximum power output is obtained. However, the efficiency of a 2.3-kW multimodule cw laser described by Roberts *et al.* (1967) was found to be as high as 9.4% at full laser output power.

2.2.1.7 Cavity Parameters. Most high-power lasers of this type now use output couplers consisting of plane disks of germanium or another semiconductor coated on one side to produce the desired reflectivity at 10.6 μm and antireflection coated on the other side. The question of what reflectivity will give highest performance in a particular system is often answered by trial and error, although some general rules have been given by Allen (1968) and Tyte (1970). Tyte has shown that a plot of $\log(R)$ versus l/d, where R is the reflectivity, l the length of the cavity, and d the diameter of the discharge, is linear. This plot is shown in Fig. 2.2. A 10-m cavity con-

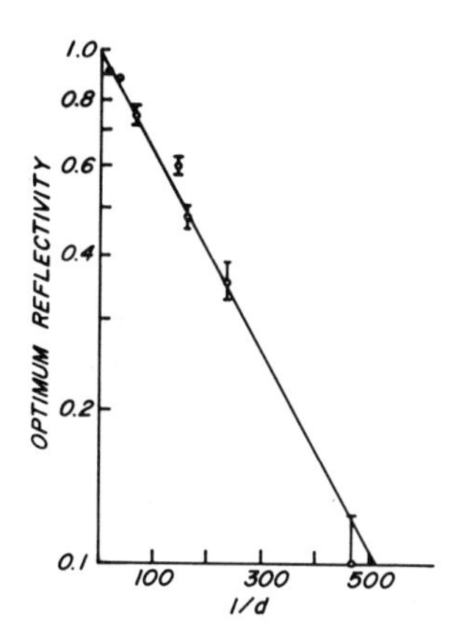

Fig. 2.2. Optimum reflectivity as a function of the ratio of laser length to diameter (Tyte, 1970).

taining a 5-cm diameter discharge would require $R \simeq 0.4$ for optimum output.

2.2.1.8 Sealed-Off CO_2 Lasers. In many industrial applications of CO_2 lasers it is an advantage to have a self-contained laser tube that does not require an input of gas during operation. Such systems do not require auxiliary gas cylinders and vacuum pumps and thus lend themselves more readily to portable operation. The main problem involved in the operation of a closed CO_2 laser is in providing a reaction path whereby the products of the dissociation of CO_2 can be regenerated to form CO_2. These dissociation products are mainly CO and O_2.

The problem of stable, long-term operation of sealed CO_2 laser tubes has been the subject of extensive investigation by Witteman (1965, 1966a,b, 1967a,b,c, 1968, 1969) and by Carbone (1967, 1968, 1969). Witteman's system relies on the admixture of a small amount of H_2O, H_2, or H_2 and O_2 to the CO_2, N_2, He laser gas. These species reduce the amount of CO present in the discharge presumably through the reaction

$$CO^* + OH \rightarrow CO_2^* + H$$

Carbone found that the dissociation products from CO_2 reacted with nickel electrodes to yield relatively weakly bound $Ni(CO)_4$ and carbonate compounds that could be dissociated by thermally heating the electrode to about 300°C. The product of this thermal dissociation (CO_2) regenerated the gas mixture. However, this process requires interrupting operation of the tube while regeneration is carried out. Witteman has used a special design of platinum electrode in his tubes, which may continuously catalyze the reverse reaction involving O atoms and CO:

$$CO + O \xrightarrow{Pt} CO_2$$

Sealed operation for many thousands of hours is now possible with output powers of about 60 W per meter discharge length.

Recently Seguin *et al.* (1972) have reported details of a sealed-off CO_2 + CO cw laser that can be operated at either 5 or 10 μm. This system has generated 4 W of cw laser power at either 5 or 10 μm from a 1.1-m long tube. They also report that lifetimes of one year have been obtained from sealed CO_2 lasers developed in their laboratory.

2.2.2 Waveguide CO_2 Lasers

The principles of a waveguide gas laser were first discussed by Marcatili and Schmeltzer (1964) and waveguide operation of He–Ne was reported by Smith (1971). Ordinarily operation of a laser in an extremely small bore ($\lesssim$1 mm) tube greatly enhances the radiation loss due to diffraction. However, when the tube is constructed in the form of a dielectric waveguide diffraction losses are minimized and advantage may be taken of the proximity of the walls of the discharge tube to reduce the gas temperature and to facilitate deexcitation of molecular species through collisions with the walls. These factors result in the possibility of operating at high pressures with an attendant increase in gain, power output per unit volume, linewidth, and saturation intensity (see, however, the discussion on similarity relations by Abrams and Bridges, 1973). CO_2 waveguide lasers have been reported by Bridges *et al.* (1972), Jensen and Tobin (1972), Chester and Abrams (1972), and Burkhardt *et al.* (1972). A schematic diagram of such a system is shown in Fig. 2.3.

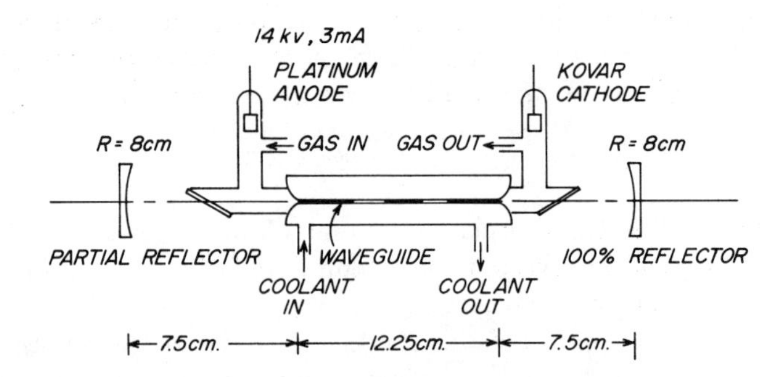

Fig. 2.3. Dielectric waveguide CO_2 laser (after Bridges *et al.*, 1972).

Since the bore diameter of these tubes is typically 1 mm, an appreciable pressure gradient exists along the length of the discharge capillary. Bridges *et al.* (1972) report inlet and outlet pressures of 100 and 20 Torr, respectively, in their system with a gas flow rate of 10 cm^3-STP/sec or 1200 gas changes/sec. Cooling the walls of the waveguide discharge channel results in an enormous increase in gain, $-70°C$ reportedly giving a gain of 8.5%/cm from about 5.3%/cm at room temperature. The saturation intensity of these devices is substantially higher than that for large bore axial flow tubes. Values of up to 22.5 kW/cm^2 have been reported (deMaria, 1973). Capillaries have been constructed from Pyrex (Jensen and Tobin, 1972; Bridges *et al.*, 1972) and from beryllia tubing (Burkhardt *et al.*, 1972; Abrams and Bridges, 1973). These systems have the advantage of stable output power and mode pattern and are mechanically rugged. The combination of high gain and high-pressure operation provides the opportunity of single-frequency operation over a wide tuning range. Bandwidth-limited pulsewidths in mode-locked operation should be less than 1 nsec at 350 Torr and trains of 3-nsec mode-locked pulses have been obtained using acoustooptic modulation (Smith *et al.*, 1972). A tuning range of several hundred megahertz has been demonstrated by Beterov *et al.* (1974), and Abrams (1974) has continuously tuned the output of a cw sealed-off waveguide CO_2 laser over a range of 1.2 GHz. Recently McMullen *et al.* (1974) have reported gain measurements on a planar waveguide laser where the gas flow and discharge current are collinear and are transverse to the optic axis.

2.2.3 *Q*-Switching

The use of *Q*-switching to obtain CO_2 laser pulses of high peak power has now been largely superseded by the rapid development of electrically pulsed or gain-switched lasers of the TEA type (see Section 2.5). However, the conventional CO_2 laser discharge can be *Q*-switched in a variety of ways and indeed, because of the long lifetime of the upper laser levels, is well suited to this mode of operation. *Q*-switching has been accomplished by means of rotating mirrors, intracavity chopping, reactively by moving one cavity mirror rapidly along the optic axis, and passively by using a variety of saturable absorbers. Detailed references to this work may be found in the review articles by Tyte (1970) and Cheo (1971).

With rotating *Q*-switches, the peak power obtainable is usually about 10 kW/m. Pulses are of $\simeq$100-nsec duration and the maximum pulse repetition frequency in tubes of a few meters length is less than 1 kHz. After a *Q*-switched pulse has drained the population inversion in the CO_2 laser gas, the discharge will start to reestablish this inversion. If the next cavity resonance is established in a time short compared to the pumping time, then the equilibrium population inversion will not have a chance to be created and this second pulse will be of diminished power. If, however, the second resonance is established just as the population inversion once again reaches its maximum value, then a pulse of the same power will be generated. In this way, both the peak Q-switched pulse power and the average output power under Q-switched conditions depend sensitively on the frequency at which the rotating mirror establishes resonances in the cavity.

Higher but more irregular pulse rates can be obtained with reactive Q-switching but here the pulsewidths may vary up to several microseconds. Passive Q-switching using hot CO_2, SF_6, BCl_3, and other saturable absorbers has been reported in the literature (Izatt *et al.*, 1974). Pulse rates can approach 100 kHz and pulsewidths are in the 0.5–2 μsec range. Selective operation on various rotational–vibrational lines in the 10-μm band can be accomplished by incorporating wavelength-dispersive elements in the cavity.

2.2.4 Mode-Locking and Frequency Stabilization

Mode-locking of a conventional CO_2 laser was first reported by Caddes *et al.* (1968) using a GaAs crystal as an intracavity acousto-optic loss modulator. The estimated pulse width was 5 nsec. A system developed by Bridges and Cheo (1969) that generated spontaneous 20-nsec pulse trains during Q-switching with a GaAs electro-optic Q-switch is shown in Fig. 2.4. Single 20-nsec pulses could be dumped from the cavity through an output

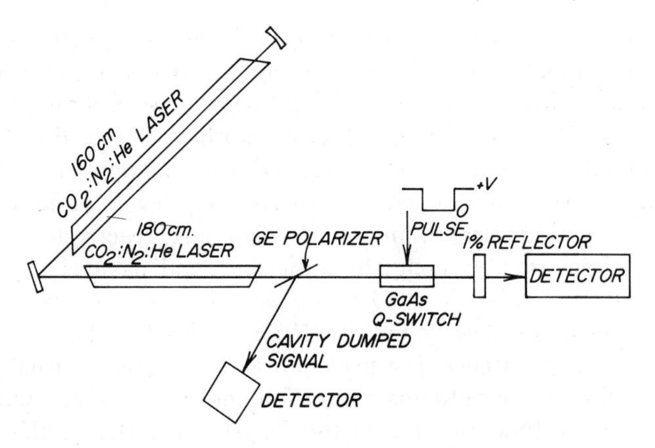

Fig. 2.4. System for self-pulsing and single-pulse generation in a CO_2 laser (after Bridges and Cheo, 1969).

coupling polarizer. These pulses had a peak power of about 10 kW. Before Q-switching, the voltage V applied to the GaAs crystal turned it into a quarter-wave plate, which together with the Ge polarizer prevented oscillation. Switching V to 0 in less than 10 nsec restored the Q of the cavity and allowed the laser signal to build up in amplitude. The peak intensity of the resulting self-generated pulses reached a maximum about 250 nsec after the GaAs was switched to its isotropic condition. These pulses could be observed through the 1% transmitting window at one end of the cavity. The interval between pulses was equal to the round trip transit time in the resonator (30–60 nsec). Switching on the voltage to the electro-optic Q-switching during a null in the output pulses resulted in a single pulse being reflected from the Ge polarizer.

Communications and "radar" applications of the CO_2 laser require high stability sources with little change in laser frequency and amplitude over long periods of time. The narrow amplification bandwidth of conventional cw CO_2 lasers (50–100 MHz under typical operating conditions) makes it a relatively simple matter to maintain a single-frequency, single-mode output even at quite high output powers. Nevertheless great care must be taken to eliminate such sources of fluctuation as thermal changes in the refractive index of the laser gas and thermal or mechanical disturbances in the resonator system. These requirements are thoroughly discussed in the review article by Polanyi and Tobias (1968). Freed (1968) has obtained frequency stabilization of the order of 10 kHz (or 0.3×10^{-9}) for periods of up to 1 sec through stabilization of the cavity structure. More recently, the Lamb-dip method employed with intracavity saturable absorbers (see Section 8.4) has been effectively used to obtain highly stabilized output frequencies from cw CO_2 lasers. Stabilization of the output from a waveguide CO_2 laser tunable over a range of 1 GHz has recently been demonstrated (Nussmeier and Abrams, 1974) using the Stark shift in an absorption line in NH_2D. A long-term frequency stability of ± 100 kHz was reported.

2.2.5 Wavelength Selection

The CO_2 laser can be made to emit on at least 400 individual vibration–rotation lines in the 8.7–11.8-μm wavelength region when one takes into account that isotopes other than $^{12}C^{16}O_2$ can also be used. Usually without any attempt to select the wavelength emitted, oscillation will occur simultaneously on several lines, the strongest of which are $P(18)$, $P(20)$, and $P(22)$ of the 00^01–$[10^00, 02^00]_I$ band. Wavelength selection may be accomplished by means of a grating or prism in the laser cavity. When a grating is used, it can be incorporated as one reflector in the cavity. Alternatively a Fabry–Perot etalon plate may be inserted to suppress oscillation on all but one frequency. A list of $^{12}C^{16}O_2$ laser wavelength has been given by Laures and Ziegler (1967). Transitions in bands other than 00^01–$[10^00, 02^00]_I$ can be observed in emission during pulsed operation.

2.2.6 Electrical Pulsing

Pulses with peak powers exceeding the average power obtainable from the same tube under cw conditions by several orders of magnitude may be produced through electrical pulsing. Tyte (1970) reports peak powers 500 times larger than the cw power from a 50-mm diameter tube at pulsing frequencies of up to 100 Hz. At higher rates the peak power drops to the cw level. The pulse shape obtained under these conditions consists of a broad peak, which may last for 300 μsec, preceded by a 1–2 μsec spike of high power. A significant increase in both peak output power and pulse energy was obtained by Hill (1968) using a megavolt pulser at higher than normal pressure ($\simeq$50 Torr) in a 7.5-cm diameter, 2.5-m long tube. 10-J pulses of 1-MW peak power at 20% efficiency were generated at a rate of 30 pps (Hill, 1970). This corresponded to 1 J/liter of discharge volume. However, it was found that both the energy per pulse and the average power obtained dropped markedly for pulse repetition rates exceeding 30–100 Hz. This was attributed to thermal effects (Hill, 1970), which populated the (01^10) level of CO_2. When the tube length was reduced to 1 m and the flow velocity was increased to 1000 ft/sec, operation at 30–150 Torr yielded 2–3 kW of average power at an efficiency of 13%. Direct scaling to higher mass flow rates to obtain higher average output powers was indicated.

2.2.7 Fast Axial Flows

The work described in the previous sections clearly points to advantages that would be obtained by the operation of axial flow lasers in the regime where gas cooling occurs via convection instead of by diffusion. Breakthroughs in this area occurred in 1969 with the work of Lavarini *et al.* (1969) and Deutsch *et al.* (1969). The system developed by Deutsch *et al.* is shown in Fig. 2.5. This system produced 1.4 kW/m at a pressure of about 70 Torr from a 1-m tube. In fact, this system is much longer than need be since laser action occurs only in a small subvolume of the flow tube. Rapid scaling to larger volumes and higher mass flow rates culminated in the announcement of 20- and 27.2-kW cw output powers by Hill (1971) and Brown and Davis (1972), respectively, from more sophisticated systems. At this point in the development of high-power cw CO_2 lasers the geo-

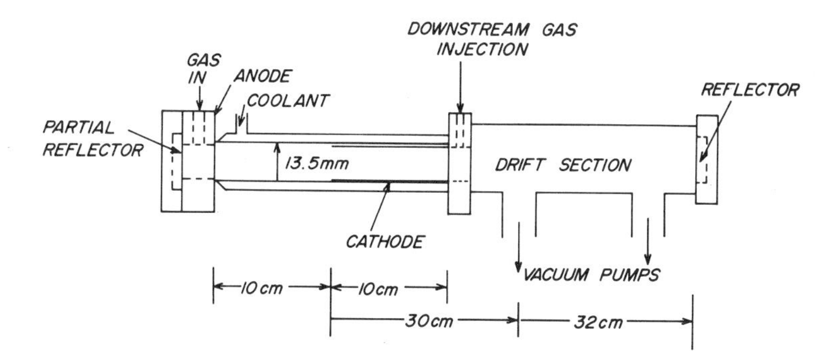

Fig. 2.5. Convectively cooled axial flow cw CO_2 laser (after Deutsch *et al.*, 1969).

metrical picture of the interrelation of the optical axis, the axis of gas flow, and the discharge direction defined by the conventional CO_2 laser system is obscured and it becomes necessary to examine a whole new family of lasers based on rapid gas flow techniques. This is the subject of the next section.

2.3 ELECTRIC DISCHARGE CONVECTION LASERS

The development of cw CO_2 lasers based on diffusion cooling effectively ended when it was realized that much higher average output powers could be obtained from lasers utilizing fast gas flow rates and convective cooling. These devices were capable of generating previously unheard of powers from quite modest discharge volumes. However, experimental problems that previously centered on ways to condense long discharge columns into physically reasonable volumes shifted to the area of high-pressure, high-flow fluid dynamics. The physics of convective flow through laser discharges pointed nevertheless to higher and higher powers as the mass flow rate increased. It is safe to say that limits on obtainable power from these devices have not yet been reached, the remaining problems centering on the provision of high mass flow rates, adequate stable electrical excitation, and the design of optical elements capable of handling cw powers in the 100-kW range.

Some of the advantages of convective cooling can be seen from the following simple analysis of a two-level laser system based on the description by De Maria (1973). If the population in the lower level is N_1 while that in the upper level is N_2, then the rates of change of these populations due to pumping, stimulated emission, collisional relaxation, and streaming through the discharge region are

$$\frac{\partial N_1}{\partial t} = R_1 - \frac{N_1}{\tau_1} + (N_2 - N_1)\frac{\sigma I}{h\nu} + \frac{(N_{10} - N_1)}{\tau_F}$$

$$\frac{\partial N_2}{\partial t} = R_2 - \frac{N_2}{\tau_2} - (N_2 - N_1)\frac{\sigma I}{h\nu} + \frac{(N_{20} - N_2)}{\tau_F}$$

where

- R_1, R_2 lower and upper level volume pumping rates
- τ_1, τ_2 lower and upper level collisional relaxation times
- N_{10}, N_{20} lower and upper level populations in the absence of stimulated emission
- σ cross section for stimulated emission
- I laser beam intensity
- $h\nu$ photon energy
- τ_F x/v_F
- x length of discharge region parallel to gas flow
- v_F gas flow rate

When the system is in equilibrium at a particular output intensity, flow rate, and pumping rate, $\partial N_1/\partial t = \partial N_2/\partial t = 0$ and the gain coefficient

$$\alpha = \sigma(N_2 - N_1) = \frac{\sigma(R_2\tau_2 - R_1\tau_1)}{1 + (I\sigma/h\nu)[\tau_2\tau_F/(\tau_2 + \tau_F) + \tau_1\tau_F/(\tau_1 + \tau_F)]}$$

In the absence of stimulated emission $I = 0$ and $\alpha = \alpha(0)$, where $\alpha(0)$ is the small signal gain coefficient. Then

$$\alpha = \frac{\alpha(0)}{1 + I/I_s}$$

where I_s is the saturation intensity,

$$I_s = \frac{h\nu}{\sigma}\,\frac{1}{[\tau_2\tau_F/(\tau_2 + \tau_F) + \tau_1\tau_F/(\tau_1 + \tau_F)]}$$

These expressions simplify in the regimes of low ($\tau_F \gg \tau_1, \tau_2$) and high flow rate ($\tau_F \ll \tau_1, \tau_2$) to give

v_F small:

$$\alpha = \frac{\alpha(0)}{1 + (\sigma I/h\nu)(\tau_2 + \tau_1)}, \qquad I_s = \frac{h\nu}{\sigma(\tau_2 + \tau_1)}$$

v_F large:

$$\alpha = \frac{\alpha(0)}{1 + 2\sigma I \tau_F / h\nu}, \qquad I_s = \frac{h\nu}{2\sigma\tau_F}$$

It is evident that the saturation intensity increases linearly with increasing flow speed at high flow rates and that the gain asymptotically approaches the small signal gain as v_F increases. As predicted from this analysis, the output power from such convectively cooled lasers should increase continuously with flow rate. This has been experimentally observed (De Maria, 1973) and a steady increase in output power with gas pressure at a particular flow rate has also been noted.

Several configurations of gas flow electrical excitation axis and optical axis have been reported in the literature, and three of these arrangements are shown schematically in Fig. 2.6a,b,c. The rapid axial flow system in Fig. 2.6a (Deutsch *et al.*, 1969) has been discussed previously and was historically one of the first devices to show the benefits to be obtained from convective gas cooling. In a modification of this system (Fig. 2.6b), the optical axis is perpendicular to the direction of gas flow, and the electrical discharge and a volume discharge is obtained by the provision of many cathode–anode pairs in the gas flow. This system has been used by Hill (1971) and Brown and Davis (1972). The third configuration (Fig. 2.6c) has the optic axis, the discharge axis, and the flow direction in mutu-

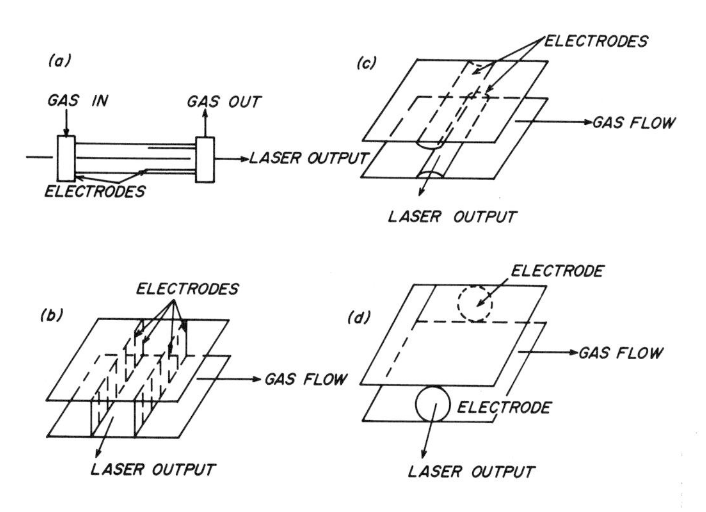

Fig. 2.6. Laser systems involving convective cooling. (a) Axial; (b) transverse (gas discharge) TGD system; (c) transverse gas, transverse discharge TG TD system; (d) transverse gas TG system.

ally orthogonal directions (Brandenberg *et al.*, 1972). A final arrangement is shown schematically in Fig. 2.6d. Here the discharge and optical axes coincide, while the flow is transverse to both. The tendency for the discharge to run downstream in the flow direction can be overcome by providing a magnetic field in a direction perpendicular to the discharge and flow vector (Buczek *et al.*, 1970). Data on the performance of some of these devices are summarized in Table 2.1. The notation used for geometrical configurations is given in the legend to Fig. 2.6.

One system that is also capable of generating high cw laser powers that is not included in Fig. 2.6 is the electrical discharge mixing laser (EDML) (Brown, 1970). Here nitrogen is vibrationally excited upstream from a source of cool CO_2 gas. Vibrational excitation of the CO_2 occurs by collisions with hot N_2 in an interaction region. The laser output is obtained transverse to the gas flow downstream from the mixing volume. High-flow axial lasers have also been operated in this mode (Deutsch *et al.*, 1969).

The tendency of high-pressure, rapid-flow laser systems to develop plasma instabilities during operation and thus to switch from a stable glow discharge regime to one in which part of the discharge constricts to an arc (Eckbreth and Davis, 1971; Nighan and Wiegand, 1974) provides limits to the amount of power that can be dissipated in the laser gas, especially at high pressure. Eckbreth and Davis (1972) and Brown and Davis (1972) have shown that augmentation of the high-power discharge by an rf discharge greatly improves discharge stability, particularly in closed-cycle operation at high input powers. Obviously this is just one method of influencing the density of charged particles in the discharge and hence the plasma stability. Direct injection of electrons and photoionization by uv or other radiation can also influence these concentrations and thus condition the discharge for higher power operation.

Recently, Hoag *et al.* (1974) have reported a cw high-flow-rate system that utilizes preionization by the direct injection of electrons from an external source. This device is capable of generating cw output powers of up to 17 kW. The electron source produces a volume ionization density of 3.4×10^{10} electrons/cm^3. Input power is tailored to yield a ratio E/N of electric field to the total number of neutral molecules per cm^3 of 1.2×10^{-16} V-cm^2. The small signal gain was reported to be $\simeq 0.7\%$/cm. An output power of 15 kW was obtained in a nearly diffraction-limited beam. McLeary *et al.* (1974) describe a method of preionization using plasma injection that allows up to 150 kW/liter of power to be dissipated in cw discharges at atmospheric pressure.

McLeary and Gibbs (1973) have described cw operation in a linear fast-flow system at atmospheric pressure using a flow-conditioning technique.

Table 2.1

Representative Performance of Several CO_2 Laser Systems Utilizing Convective Cooling

System	Output power	Gain (%/cm)	Flow	Comments	Reference
Axial	—	4.15	194 m/sec	CO_2 mixed downstream with excited N_2	Cool and Shirley (1969)
	225 W	2.4	>10 liters-STP CO_2/min		Deutsch *et al.* (1969)
TGD	1000 W	1.8	35 m/sec	Closed system	Tiffany *et al.* (1969)
TG	540 W	5	10–50 m/sec	Magnetically stabilized	Buczek *et al.* (1970)
EDML	900 W	4.3	150 m/sec	CO_2 mixed downstream with excited N_2	Brown (1970)
	1200 W	6	300–425 m/sec		Eckbreth *et al.* (1971)
TGD	1400 W	1.2	75–125 m/sec	Used as multiple-pass amplifier	Eckbreth and Davis (1971)
	20 kW	1.9	600 m/sec	—	Hill (1971)
TG TD	34 W/cm^3 (av)		Mach 3	Pulsed operation	Brandenberg *et al.* (1972)
TGD	—	0.8		Discharge augmented by rf auxiliary source; closed system	Eckbreth and Davis (1972)
	27.2 kW			Closed system; used as multiple-pass amplifier; rf augmentation	Brown and Davis (1972)

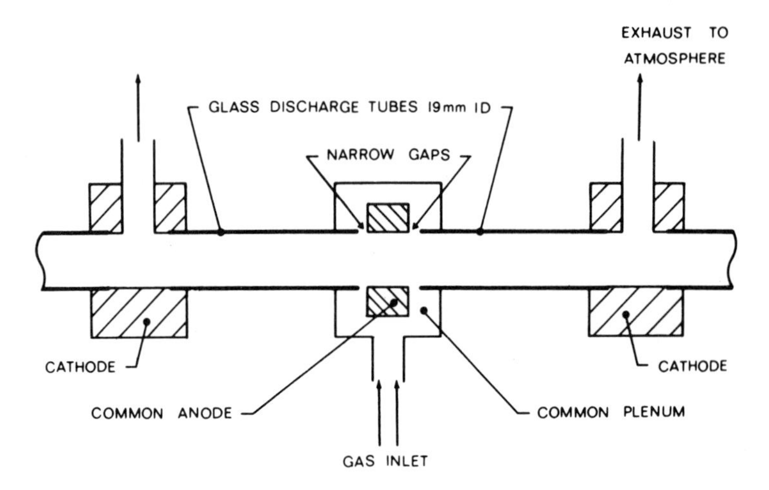

Fig. 2.7. Representation of cw atmospheric laser of McLeary and Gibbs (1973). The gas flow velocity is approximately sonic.

The gas is injected at near sonic velocities as shown in Fig. 2.7. Energy inputs of up to 500 J/gm were possible without arc formation. Under these conditions, six cascaded discharge sections each 200 cm long and 19 mm in diameter yielded cw output power of $\simeq$500 W at an efficiency of $\simeq$5%. Mixtures were 1 : 19 : 300 of CO_2 : N_2 : He.

With the enormous mass flow rates that are now being used in convectively cooled lasers, the provision of gas recirculation would seem to be necessary to avoid high operating costs and the problems involved in coping with massive amounts of exhaust gas. It appears, however, that contaminant species in the gas phase may promote plasma instabilities (De Maria, 1973) and thus some renewal of the circulating gas may be necessary for stable long-term operation. Alternatively, impurities may be removed catalytically during recycling.

2.4 GAS DYNAMIC LASERS

As early as 1963 before the properties of the N_2–CO_2 laser system had been discovered, Basov and Oraevskii (1963) suggested that population inversions could be produced thermally by rapid gas expansion. The promise of a CO_2 laser system based on the rapid expansion of a gas flowing through a supersonic nozzle was soon discussed by Konyukhov and Prokorov (1966). Similar studies by Hurle and Hertzberg (1965) indicated the feasibility of producing population inversions in the fast expansion of an arc-heated plasma. A laser based on these theoretical predictions was discussed in detail by Gerry (1970) and by Konyukhov *et al.* (1970) and a multimode output power of 60 kW cw was reported.

If a gas such as CO_2 is heated to a high temperature and allowed to equilibrate at high pressures the population of excited vibrational levels will be given by the well-known Boltzmann distribution $n_i = n_0 \exp(-\Delta E_i/kT)$, where n_i is the population in the ith level, n_0 the ground state population, ΔE_i the energy separation between the ith level and the ground state, and T the temperature, with k = Boltzmann's constant. In equilibrium the population of all nondegenerate levels of the excited state will be less than n_0. If this gas is then allowed to expand rapidly in a time that is short compared with the vibrational relaxation time of one upper vibrational level while, by the addition of a quencher for a lower vibrational level, this level is caused to relax at a higher rate, then the upper state population may be "frozen" at a value corresponding to the Boltzmann distribution at the original temperature. However, the lower level population is still characterized by the lower temperature reached on expansion. Under the correct conditions a volume downstream of the expansion nozzle will contain a highly inverted population between these two states. In the CO_2 gas dynamic laser system a mixture of typically 7.5% CO_2, 91.3% N_2, and 1.2% H_2O quencher is heated to a temperature $\simeq$1400°K at a pressure of 17 atm before being allowed to expand supersonically through a carefully designed nozzle to produce the desired population inversion (Gerry, 1970). This inversion is reached only a few centimeters downstream from the nozzle and persists for many centimeters farther. The power that can be extracted from this flow is enormous, since it is effectively given by the population of the upper laser level at the initial temperature times the energy of a 10.6-μm quantum ($\simeq$0.12 eV). This is 35 J/gm/sec of gas flow when the initial gas temperature is 1400°K. Gerry reports that, allowing for system inefficiencies, up to 0.5 of this energy may be extracted from the flowing gas. This represents the direct conversion of thermal energy to power. An interesting aspect of this direct conversion process is that, since thermal energy is involved, practical considerations concerned with the maximum attainable reservoir temperature limits efficient cw operation to wavelengths in the infrared range. For example, at 1000°K the peak of the black-body distribution lies at a wavelength of about 3 μm. Efficient operation would therefore be possible only at laser wavelengths $\lesssim$3 μm. This region does, however, correspond to the region of vibrational–rotational transitions of many polyatomic molecules so that efficient emitters are available. The overall efficiency of gas dynamic laser (GDL) systems is limited by the fact that only a small fraction of

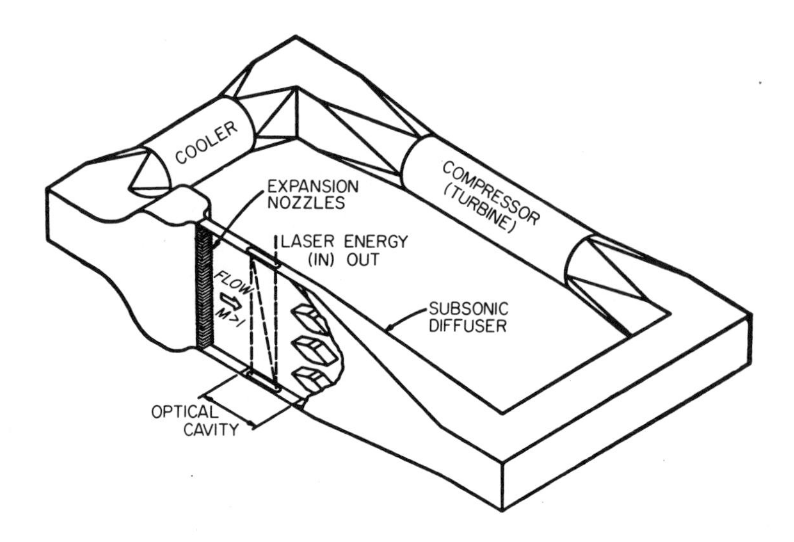

Fig. 2.8. Closed-cycle gas dynamic laser system (after Hertzberg *et al.*, 1972).

the total enthalpy of the laser mixture at high temperatures in the stagnation region is in the form of vibrational energy. For pure N_2 the ratio of the energy stored in the $v'' = 1$ level of N_2 to the total enthalpy of the gas at 2000°K is only $\simeq 6\%$ (Christiansen and Hertzberg, 1973). Although much of this vibrational energy can subsequently be extracted, the overall efficiency of the energy conversion process is limited by the necessity of disposing of most of the energy/unit volume in the stagnation volume as waste heat. Hertzberg *et al.* (1972) have discussed the possibility of recovering the major part of the gas enthalpy not used for lasing in a closed system. This system is shown schematically in Fig. 2.8. In the limit of ultimate efficiency such a system would completely convert the shaft work on the compressor to output laser power. A full discussion of technical problems associated with such a system can be found in the papers by Hertzberg *et al.* (1972) and Christiansen and Hertzberg (1973). The reverse process, in which absorbed laser radiation is converted to shaft work, is also possible and the combination of such an engine with a GDL generator would yield an effective power transmission system. Such a system might be used for the transmission of power to orbiting space stations (Hansen and Lee, 1972).

Efficient extraction of laser power requires attainment of the highest possible population inversion in the expanded laser mixture. Extensive theoretical analyses of the flow kinetics have been given by Christiansen and Hertzberg (1973) and by others (Konyukhov and Prokhorov, 1966;

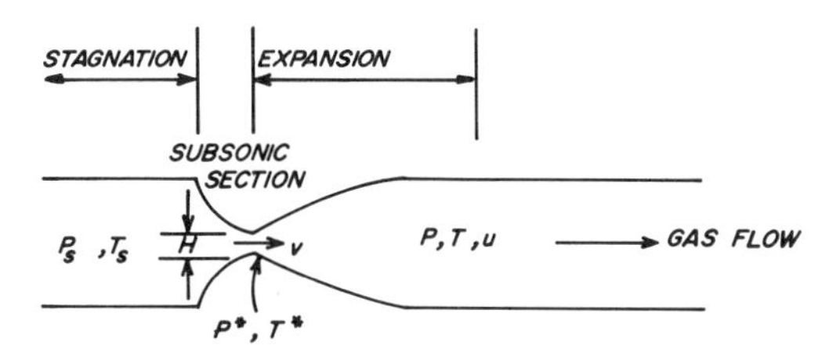

Fig. 2.9. Supersonic expansion nozzle. P, pressure; T, temperature; u, velocity; v, velocity; H, throat height. Note $P_s > P$, $T_s > T$.

Basov *et al.*, 1969). Ideally the expansion through the nozzle should occur instantaneously but this can only be approximately obtained in practice. Design parameters for nozzle shapes that promote effective freezing of vibrational populations have been investigated by Kuehn (1972). Nozzles with small throat heights contoured to give the maximum rate of expansion and expansion ratio are most effective. A fundamental requirement is that the flow time through the throat of the nozzle must be less than the time required for relaxation of the CO_2 upper level and N_2 ($v'' = 1$) in the throat. This requirement can be expressed as

$$H/v < (P\tau_{\text{eff}})_{T^*}/P^*$$

where v is the flow velocity in the throat, τ_{eff} the relaxation time, and the other parameters are as shown in Fig. 2.9. Since $P^* \simeq 0.5P_s$, the stagnation pressure, this requirement may be rewritten

$$P_sH < 2(P\tau_{\text{eff}})_{T^*}v$$

and thus it is evident that efficient freezing of the upper state population in CO_2 occurs only for a selected range of stagnation pressures and temperatures for given nozzle geometry.

Kuehn (1972) has shown that the optimum reservoir temperature T_s increases with stagnation pressure for $P_s \to 100$ atm. On the other hand an increase in T_s while keeping P_s constant shows that the highest values of T_s are not necessarily the best for obtaining high output power. At least two competing effects are responsible for this dependence. First, the vibrational energy stored in the gas increases with increasing T_s. This tends to raise the maximum power output. On the other hand, high temperature also promotes dissociation of CO_2, so that the number of emitters decreases with increasing T_s. A second effect that tends to mediate the increase of output with T_s is the increase in relaxation times (τ_{eff}), which occurs at high T_s. This makes the freezing out of the excited state population more difficult to achieve. Kuehn concludes that since the optimum T_s increases

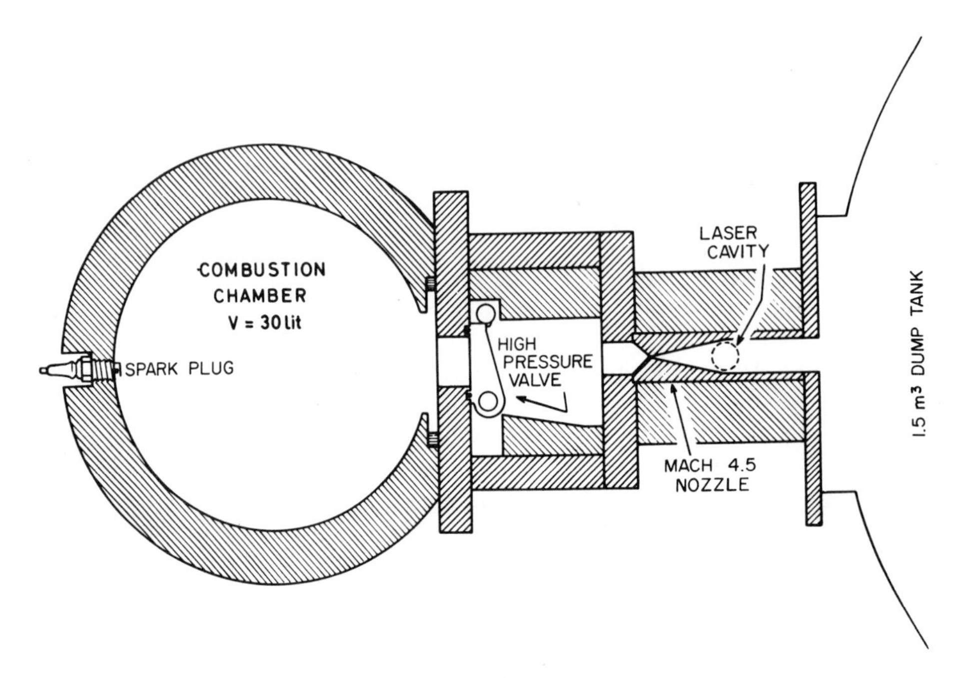

Fig. 2.10. Combustion-operated GDL (after Yatsiv *et al.*, 1971).

with P_s, the effect of relaxation is not dominant as T_s increases. Instead it appears that power is limited more by the dissociation of CO_2 produced at high T_s. With proper nozzle design and variation of T_s, the output from Kuehn's laser system increased almost linearly with P_s up to 120 atm, the maximum stagnation pressure used. Similar dependencies of gain at 10.6 μm on T_s were reported by Lee and Gowen (1971) in CO_2, N_2, He mixtures. The gain was essentially independent of P_s at high gas pressures. Required stagnation temperatures may be obtained by combustion of CO (Gerry, 1970) or by arc heating (Bronfin *et al.*, 1970). The system of Bronfin *et al.* is unusual in that arc-heated N_2 is expanded through a supersonic nozzle to mix downstream with a cold CO_2, He mixture. This expansion occurs quickly enough that the vibrational temperature of N_2 is maintained while its translational temperature is reduced. Thermal energy to optical energy conversion efficiencies of 0.6% were reported from this system.

So far only cw GDL's have been discussed. Laser oscillation is also possible under pulsed conditions using shock-tube (Kuehn and Monson, 1970; Dronhov *et al.*, 1970) or combustive (Yatsiv *et al.*, 1971; Tulip and Seguin, 1971a) excitation of a gas mixture that is subsequently expanded to supersonic velocities. There has been much interest in such systems following these initial reports and various groups have reported experimental or theoretical investigations (Dzhidzhoev *et al.*, 1971; Marchenko and Prokhorov, 1971; Yatsiv *et al.*, 1972; Christiansen and Hertzberg, 1973). The combustion operated CO_2 GDL developed by Yatsiv *et al.* (1971) is shown in detail in Fig. 2.10. A mixture of CO, O_2, H_2 and N_2 was ignited in the combustion chamber by a spark plug. The high-pressure valve shown is released after a preselected time interval following the initiation of the explosion to allow the heated gas to expand through a supersonic nozzle where the population inversion is obtained. The laser pulse generated lasts for several hundred milliseconds. Output energies of 20 J were obtained. A similar system developed by Tulip and Seguin (1971b) gave pulses of 60-W peak power and 5-J energy but ran on mixtures of acetylene, propane, or natural gas with oxygen. In contrast to shock-tube GDL's, the time required to recycle the system between pulses was short ($\simeq$30 sec).

Much higher peak power pulses have been obtained from shock-tube excited GDL's. A theoretical prediction of the performance of these devices has been made by Christiansen and Hertzberg (1973). Their theoretical plot of pulse power versus tube diameter and stagnation pressure is reproduced in Fig. 2.11. Apparently this ideal performance has been approached in practice; Christiansen and Hertzberg (1973) report a peak

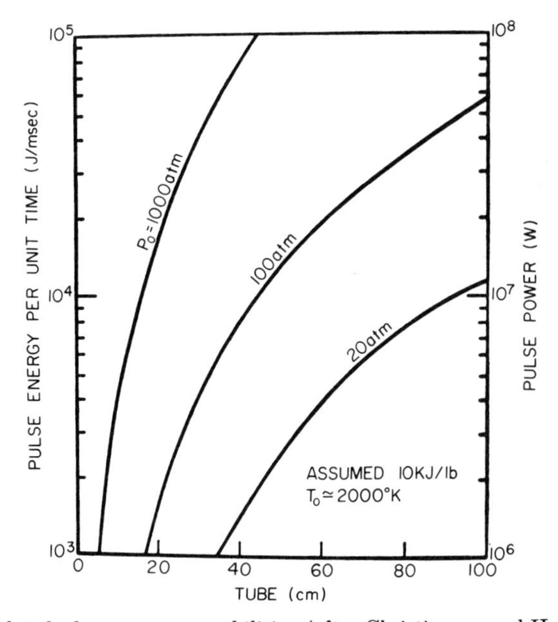

Fig. 2.11. Shock-tube laser power capabilities (after Christiansen and Hertzberg, 1973).

power of 450 kW from a 10.7-cm diameter tube under conditions where $P = 10^4$ lb/in^2 and $T = 2000°$K. The duration of this pulse was 4 msec.

The gas dynamic laser has also been used to excite CO mixtures (McKenzie, 1970; Watt, 1971; Brunet and Mabru, 1972; Kan *et al.*, 1972; Rich *et al.*, 1971) and N_2O (Bronfin *et al.*, 1970). Although CO_2 is ideally suited to excitation in this way, there would seem to be many other molecules that might be suitable candidates for GDL systems. Chemical reactions in these flow systems leading to inverted populations may also be of interest. Vallach *et al.* (1972) report laser emission from chemically excited CO formed by a discharge-initiated $CS_2 + O_2$ reaction in a supersonic flow.

2.5 PULSED TRANSVERSELY EXCITED CO_2 LASERS

2.5.1 Devices

The astoundingly rapid increase in the maximum power attainable from CO_2 lasers in all of their modifications received considerable impetus late in 1969 with the announcement that the CO_2 laser could be driven in a pulsed transverse discharge configuration at all pressures up to and slightly above one atmosphere (Beaulieu, 1970; Dumanchin and Rocca-Serra, 1969). Transverse excitation, which had previously been used by Leonard (1965, 1967) with other gases lasing at lower pressures, enabled the high voltages required for gas breakdown at high pressures (Hill, 1968) to be reduced substantially. As an example, the initial report by Beaulieu (1970) showed that a glow discharge using the transverse electrode structure shown in Fig. 2.12 could be obtained by exciting the gas with a 25,000-V pulse of about 2-μsec duration. Rapid excitation together with the incorporation of series resistors for each point electrode reduced the tendency for the discharges to develop into arcs. Normally, a glow discharge at atmospheric pressure is unstable and rapidly develops into an arc. However, the time to develop an arc is finite (Johns and Nation, 1972) and

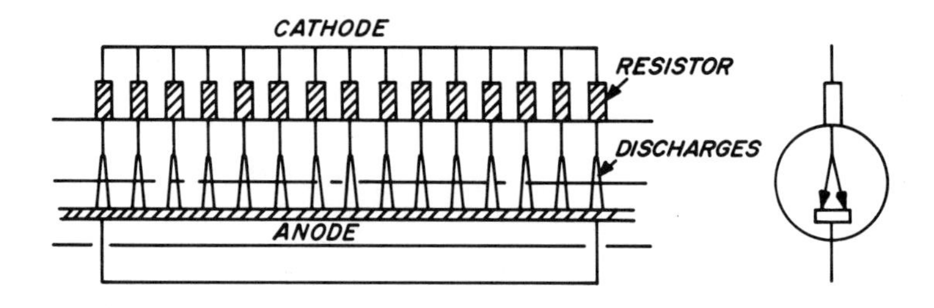

Fig. 2.12. Original TEA CO_2 laser configuration (after Beaulieu, 1970).

hence formation can be inhibited by excitation with pulses whose duration is less than the arc formation time. Series resistors tend to stabilize the discharge by preventing large currents from being drawn through any one pin electrode. The pin–rod configuration has, however, been successfully used without series resistors (Laurie and Hale, 1971) but requirements on the duration and shape of the applied current pulse are more severe if arcs are to be avoided. Elimination of resistors was, however, reported to increase efficiency. Tan *et al.* (1972) have obtained an output power of over 15 MW from a resistorless pin–curved-rod system excited with voltages of up to 288 kV from a Marx generator at atmospheric pressure. The great advantage of this system lies in the fact that high-pressure gases can be easily excited. Hidson *et al.* (1972) report obtaining laser action from mixtures at pressures as high as 6 atm using 20–50 nsec duration pulses from a 200-kV Marx generator. Volume discharges between a stainless steel grid cathode and a planar copper anode have been excited by 20-nsec, 500-kV pulses from a Marx generator (Morrison and Swail, 1972).

One problem that occurs with the use of series resistors is that repeated discharges cause the resistors to develop short or open circuits due to the transient high-current densities that are passed through them. When this happens resistors will often explode during a current pulse destroying one of the pin–rod discharge paths. This problem can be eliminated, but the stabilizing properties of series resistances can be maintained by the use of a conducting solution (NaCl in water will suffice), which acts as a distributed resistor in series with the pin electrodes. A suitable system is shown in Fig. 2.13a.

Direct control over the energy delivered to each pin in a resistorless

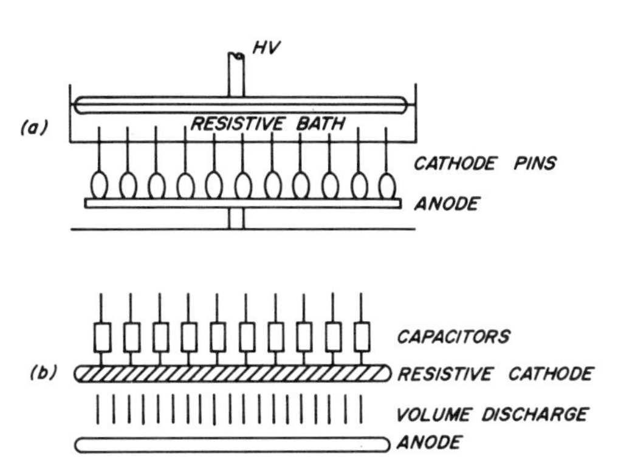

Fig. 2.13. (a) Pin–rod system using distributed cathode resistance. (b) Two-electrode system using distributed resistance and multiple capacitive excitation (after Johns and Nation, 1973).

configuration can be obtained by using small capacitors to drive each pin–rod discharge separately (Johnson, 1971). Johnson obtained 1.2-J pulses with peak powers of $\simeq$0.5 Mw from a 1.3-m long laser containing 101 pin–rod discharges, each driven by a 500-pF capacitor. Up to 300 J/liter of electrical energy has been deposited in an atmospheric pressure laser without arc formation by using a distributed resistive electrode driven by individual 570-pF capacitors approximately 1 cm apart along the resistive electrode (Johns and Nation, 1973). The resistive electrode was constructed by mixing bone carbon in an acrylic matrix until a resistivity of 12 Ω/cm was attained. No pins are needed as the discharge terminates directly on the exposed surface of this electrode (Fig. 2.13b). Belanger *et al.* (1972) describe a similar laser system, which uses semiconducting plastic electrodes.

In all of these pin–rod configurations, the active amplifying medium consists of a series of roughly conical-shaped volumes located periodically along the optic axis of the system. The effective volume is therefore much less than that of the total volume between anode and cathode. Furthermore, since only part of the gas is heated during a laser pulse, substantial refractive index variations occur along and transverse to the optic axis. Both of these effects tend to limit the output power that can be obtained from this configuration. By using multiple staggered rows of pins (Robinson, 1971) the active volume can be increased substantially, but the excitation is still nonuniform and much scattering and deflection of the laser beam occurs as it passes down the axis of the system. These effects have been studied in detail by Seguin (1972) and by O'Neil *et al.* (1972). The helical pin–pin discharge configuration described by Fortin *et al.* (1971), Nakatsuka *et al.* (1972), Rampton and Gandhi (1972), and Verreault *et al.* (1974) minimizes this effect but residual refractive index variations have been shown (Otis and Tremblay, 1971; Fortin *et al.*, 1971) to introduce the equivalent of a time-dependent long focal length diverging lens into the laser. Verreault *et al.* (1974) have found that the grouping of electrodes in a helical laser permits operation in specific transverse modes, i.e., TEM_{00} or TEM_{01}.

In the quest for higher output powers and more stable operation it was soon realized that other discharge configurations first reported by Dumanchin and Rocca-Serra (1969) and by Laflamme (1970) offered the possibility of more uniform excitation of large volumes than that feasible with pin–rod systems. Attention then shifted to the "double-discharge" method of excitation shown schematically in Fig. 2.14. In both these systems, breakdown of the spark gap applies the voltage on the storage capacitor to the cathode. As the voltage on this electrode rises, the field gradient be-

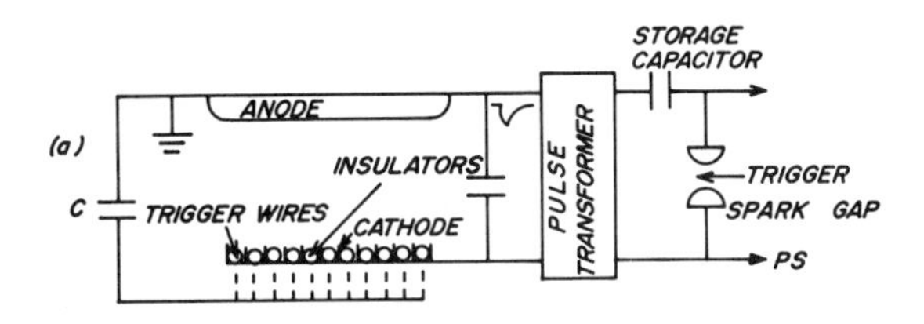

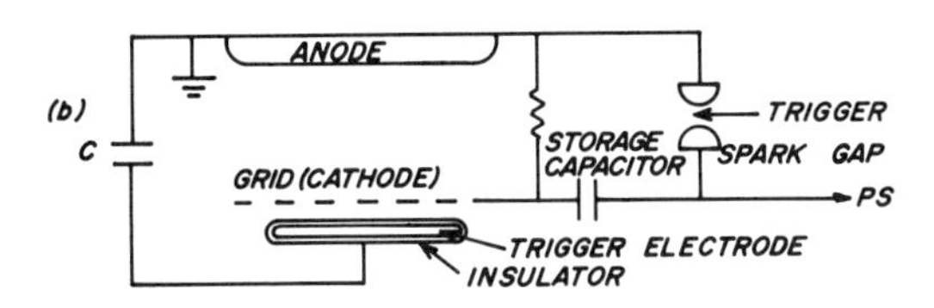

Fig. 2.14. (a) Double-discharge system of Dumanchin *et al.* (1972). (b) System of Laflamme (1970).

tween the cathode and the insulated trigger electrodes grows more rapidly than does that between the cathode and anode. This forms a corona discharge between the trigger electrodes and the cathode. The small capacitor C then charges, reducing the field between trigger and cathode and trapping electrons in the vicinity of the cathode. These electrons are subsequently released into the main discharge volume lowering the discharge impedance and initiating the main discharge. When the main current pulse is shaped to preclude arc formation, the preionization electron pulse will permit the formation of a uniform glow discharge between anode and cathode. Pan *et al.* (1972) have determined that best performance of these devices occurs when the initial voltage pulse applied to the cathode rises slowly (typically over a period of $\simeq 2$ μsec). To inhibit arc formation, the voltage applied across the gap between anode and cathode must be reduced immediately after the current pulse peaks. Pan *et al.* discuss some circuits that can be used to accomplish this shaping.

The importance of pulse shaping in optimizing the output and efficiency of these double-discharge devices as well as the high efficiency that is possible with lasers of this type are shown in Table 2.2, which compares results obtained by different groups. It should be noted that the maximum attainable energy density that can be stored in one liter of pure CO_2 gas at NTP is about 500 J (Beaulieu, 1971) while the absolute limiting efficiency based on the energy levels in the CO_2 molecule is $\simeq 40\%$.

Table 2.2

Output Energy (J/liter of Excited Mixture) and Efficiency (Output Pulse Energy/Input Energy) of Some Double-Discharge Lasers

Energy output (J/liter)	Efficiency (%)	Reference
3	—	Dumanchin and Rocca-Serra (1969)
6	6.3	Pearson and Lamberton (1972)
5.49	7.14	Laflamme (1970)
10	10	Dyer *et al.* (1972)
18	17.4	Dumanchin *et. al.* (1972)
17	24	Pan *et. al.* (1972)

In contrast to the spatial distribution of the laser output with pin–rod lasers, which is often quite irregular, the output from double-discharge devices is usually much more uniform. Laflamme (1970) reported an output beam with a cross section of 2.5 × 2.5 cm from an electrode structure that was 3.2 cm wide and separated by 3.8 cm. The distribution of intensity across the output beam can be further improved by stacking individual laser sections along the optic axis with a rotation of 90° between adjacent sections (Dumanchin *et al.*, 1972).

Modifications to the basic double-discharge system have been described by Merchant and Irwin (1971) and by Otis (1972). Merchant and Irwin obtained a volume discharge between two brass electrodes of square cross section mounted with sharp edges facing one another across the gap and with flat dielectric coated trigger strips placed parallel to these electrodes halfway between them but far removed from the optic axis. Otis describes a double-discharge system in which the trigger electrode has a distributed resistance obtained by mixing graphite with an acrylic matrix. The variable resistivity of the trigger electrode is reported to facilitate pulse shaping in the trigger circuit.

An important modification of the double-discharge system shown in Fig. 2.15 has been described by Lamberton and Pearson (1971) and by Pearson and Lamberton (1972). Trigger wires are placed parallel to the optic axis in a plane offset toward the cathode. These wires are connected via small capacitors to the cathode. When the storage capacitor is connected across the cathode and anode by breaking down the spark gap, a short discharge is initiated between these trigger wires and the anode. The energy of this discharge is limited by the size of the trigger capacitors (typically 300 pF).

Charges liberated by this small discharge due to direct ionization and to photoemission from the cathode excited by the uv radiation from the discharge condition the mixture so that a glow discharge can be formed between anode and cathode. The streak photographs of Pearson and Lamberton (1972) show that the small initial discharge lasts for only $\simeq$20 nsec. After a delay of some 10 nsec, the main discharge is initiated and sustained for a few hundred nsec.

The solid electrodes used in this and other devices to be described below are designed to have profiles that provide a nearly uniform field throughout the anode–cathode volume. Such electrodes were first discussed by Rogowski (1923) and later by Bruce (1947), Felici (1950), Harrison (1967), and Chang (1973). Seguin *et al.* (1972) give details of a profile milling cutter that is suitable for the machining of electrodes having a Rogowski profile.

Figure 2.16 shows some results of a parametric study on the device described by Pearson and Lamberton (1972). The total pulse energy is seen to increase with charging voltage, although the range of stable operation (i.e., operation without arc formation) decreases drastically as the charging voltage is increased. Highest peak powers and pulse energy are obtained using the parameters given in Table 2.3.

Extensive constructional details for a larger double Rogowski TEA laser of this type have been given by Seguin *et al.* (1972). Three 60-cm long electrode sections were driven from the same power supply and triggered spark gap. The system could be repetitively pulsed at rates of up to 10 pps. Pulse energies in excess of 15 J and peak powers of 100 MW in a 100-nsec pulse were obtained. Other similar laser systems have been described by Denes and Farish (1971), Grigoriu and Brinkschulte (1973), and Balochin *et al.* (1972). Denes and Farish obtained an output energy density of up to 17 J/liter and an overall efficiency of 10.4%. By incorporating a small amount of xylene in the laser gas mixture Grigoriu and Brinkschulte found it possible to uniformly excite a 4 : 1 : 1 He : CO_2 : N_2 mixture at pressures up to 1 atm in a system with plane-parallel electrodes. The output energy density was 21 J/liter. In this device it would seem that the addi-

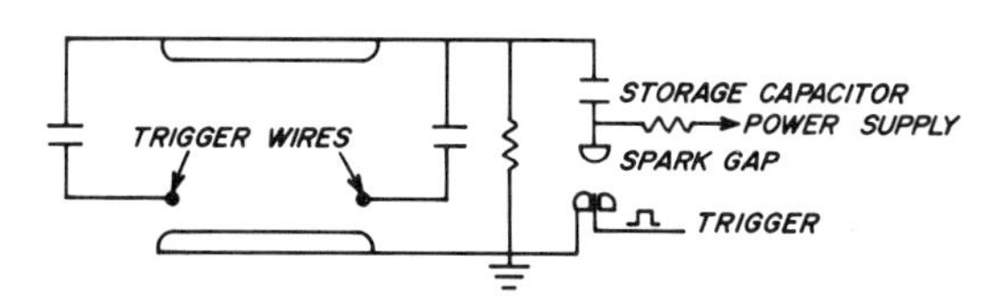

Fig. 2.15. TEA laser system developed by Lamberton and Pearson (1971) and Pearson and Lamberton (1972). The trigger wires excite photoelectron emission from the cathode to provide preionization.

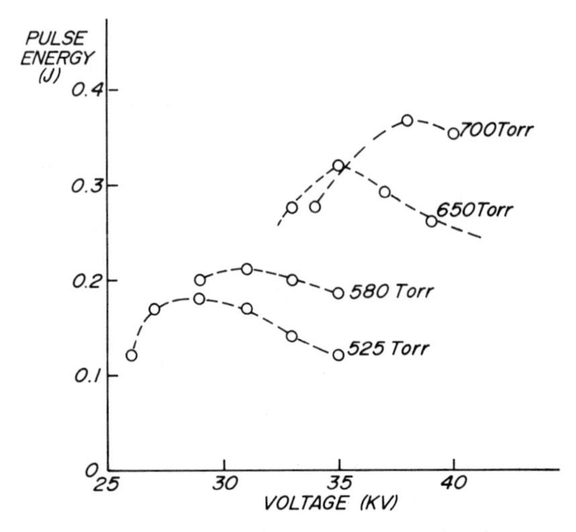

Fig. 2.16. Pulse energy vs. voltage at various gas pressures. Gas mixture 75% He, 12.5% N_2, 12.5% CO_2. Open circles indicate experimental curves.

tion of an impurity with a relatively low ionization potential such as xylene acts to increase the density of precursor electrons through photoionization by light from the trigger discharge (Javan and Levine, 1972; Levine and Javan, 1972). Chang and Wood (1972b) describe a modification of the Lamberton–Pearson laser that when driven by a voltage doubler at 2 × 30

Table 2.3

Optimum Operating Parameters for the Double Rogowski Laser of Pearson and Lamberton (1972)

Discharge length	28 cm
Discharge height	2.6 cm
Discharge width	1.5 cm
Discharge volume	110 cm^3
Cavity length	68 cm
Mirror radius of curvature	8 m
Reflectivity of plane mirror	70%
Total circuit inductance	100 nH
Storage capacitance	0.026 μF
Trigger capacitance	330 pF
Charging voltage	60 kV
Input energy	47 J
Output energy	2 J
Efficiency	4.3%
Mixture by volume CO_2:N_2:He	1.5:1.2:2
Output energy density	18 J/liter

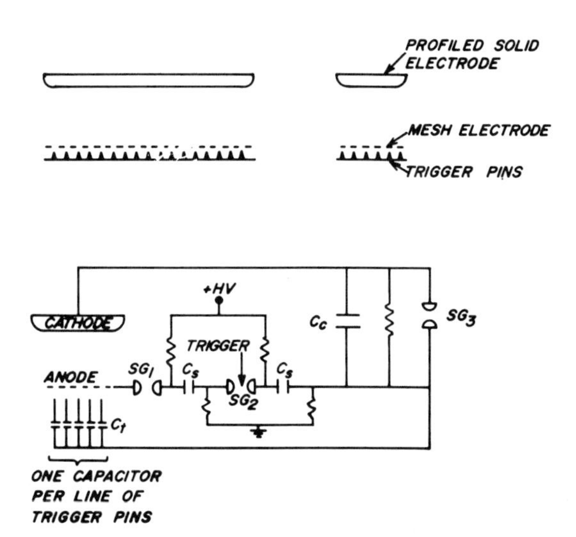

Fig. 2.17. Double-discharge system of Richardson *et al.* (1973a). $C_s = 0.1\ \mu F$; $C_t \simeq$ 100–160 pF; SG_1, SG_2, SG_3, pressurized nitrogen spark gaps.

kV yields a 22 J/liter multimode output energy or self-mode-locked pulses with peak powers greater than 40 MW.

A significant improvement in double-discharge lasers was obtained by Richardson *et al.* (1973a) using the electrode structure and triggering scheme shown in Fig. 2.17. A seven-module system was capable of generating 300-J pulses with peak powers exceeding 3 GW at an efficiency of $\simeq$10%. In the circuit shown in Fig. 2.17, SG_2 is triggered and SG_1 breaks down applying the Marx bank voltage between the point electrodes and the grid. This causes a corona discharge to form in the volume between the grid and the point electrodes. The corona discharge rapidly develops into a series of arcs spreading from the tips of the point electrodes. The light emitted from these arcs, which is rich in uv radiation, causes preionization in the cathode–anode volume. When this preionization has reached an optimum value, SG_3 fires, dumping the bulk of the energy stored in the two C_s capacitors into the preionized gas. It was found that up to 300 J/liter of electrical energy could be passed into the laser medium without deterioration in the character of the discharge through arc formation. The time delay between the preionization discharge and the main discharge can be varied up to 400 nsec by changing the breakdown voltage requirements of spark gap SG_3. This enables optimization of preionization conditions within the anode–cathode volume before the main discharge is initiated.

The role of volumetric photoionization and photoemission excited by a precursor arc or spark discharge has been studied by Seguin and Tulip (1972), Cohn and Ault (1973), Judd (1973), Seguin *et al.* (1973a,b), and Figueira (1974). Seguin and Tulip passed the main discharge current through a series spark gap within the laser cavity. The light from this discharge was shown to initiate and sustain the main discharge through bulk ionization formed by photoemission from the cathode and a volume ionization produced by short-wavelength radiation from the auxiliary spark. A significant development was the observation that the maximum energy density that could be dumped into the laser mixture increased almost linearly with electrode separation. This suggests that photoionization and photoemission may be useful methods of preionizing the gas in large aperture lasers.

Richardson *et al.* (1973b) have shown that volumetric preionization with uv radiation may be extended to large-aperture high-pressure laser systems simply by optimizing the uv source–laser electrode configuration. Using an array of spark discharges generated from a series of closely spaced electrodes on an insulating substrate, it was found possible to initiate volumetric discharges with cross-sectional areas of $\simeq 600\ cm^2$ in a system with 30-cm separation between anode and cathode. It was found that a simple relationship exists between

$$P = (P_{CO_2} + P_{N_2})/(P_{CO_2} + P_{N_2} + P_{He})$$

the partial pressure of CO_2 and N_2 in the laser mixture, and the electric field E required in the main discharge volume for stable uniform discharges. This relationship is

$$E = 27.8\, P^{2/3}\ \mathrm{kV/cm}$$

It was suggested that the limiting cross-sectional area for such devices may be greater than $10^3\ cm^2$ and that output pulse energies of 10^4 J may be possible.

Measurement of the electron density in an experimental system without a cathode (Seguin *et al.*, 1973a) showed that electron densities as high as $10^{12}/cm^3$ could be produced 12 cm away from a single uv spark source in typical low-pressure laser mixtures. Surprisingly, the photoelectron density was highest in pure He gas even at pressures approaching 1 atm and was lowest in CO_2 and O_2. Since the photoelectron density is highest in the gases with the lowest uv absorption (i.e., He), Seguin *et al.* (1973a) suggested that residual impurities with low ionization potentials may be responsible for the observed photoelectron densities. At STP a gas phase impurity with a partial pressure of only 10^{-8}–10^{-9} Torr would be sufficient to generate electron densities of 10^{10}–$10^{11}/cm^3$ when exposed to a high flux of near vuv radiation. In fact, Javan and Levine (1972), Levine and Javan (1972), and Schriever (1972) have suggested that volumetric ionization of a laser gas could be accomplished by seeding the gas with a small quantity of impurities having low ionization potentials and a quantum efficiency for photoionization of nearly unity. Seguin *et al.* (1973b) examined the role of impurities such as triethylamine and tripropylamine in a controlled experiment and found that trace amounts of these molecules were sufficient to raise the volumetric photoelectron density by up to four orders of magnitude in typical laser mixtures. This effect was most noticeable at high ($\rightarrow$100 Torr) pressures. Incorporation of these impurities was found to increase the maximum obtainable energy output density to 60 J/liter in a photosustained TEA laser.

The observation of volume ionization at distances of up to 10 cm away from a spark source at several hundred Torr pressure in gas mixtures that strongly absorb vuv radiation raises a number of pertinent questions concerning the mechanism of propagation of ionizing radiation over long distances in absorbing gases. It is almost certain that in the absence of direct seeding with low ionization impurities, only wavelengths $\lesssim$1200 Å are effective in producing photoionization (Seguin *et al.*, 1973a; Judd, 1973). Absorption spectra of N_2 and CO_2 (Inn *et al.*, 1953) show that while only sharp discrete spectral features are present in N_2 gas in the wavelength region $\lambda > 1000$ Å, CO_2 has a complex spectrum shortward of about 1750 Å. This spectrum consists of at least three continua on which are superimposed a complicated system of diffuse absorption bands. There is, however, a minimum in absorption from about 1190 to 1200 Å where the absorption coefficient drops to <1 cm^{-1} at STP. Thus an optical depth of unity at 1190–1200 Å would correspond to a path length of $\simeq$3–4 cm in CO_2 at a partial pressure of 300 Torr. This path length is compatible with the distances over which volumetric photoionization can be produced in typical laser mixtures at atmospheric pressure. Below 1000 Å both CO_2 and N_2 have rich absorption spectra with values of absorption coefficient in the 10^2–10^3 cm^{-1} range at STP. There would seem to be few, if any, gaps in this absorption at wavelengths down to 100 Å. Thus, in the absence of two photon effects it seems likely that direct photoionization of impurity molecules occurs through a "window" at 1190–1200 Å to yield the observed volume ionization. However, recent results of Judd and Wada (1974), Seguin *et al.* (1974), and Lind *et al.* (1974) indicate that the energy transfer mechanism is far from this simple. Seguin *et al.* note that the radial dependence of photoionization density $n(r)$ should follow the relation

$$n(r) = (A/r^2) \exp(-r/L_p)$$

where r is the radial distance from a point source, A a constant, and L_p the absorption length. This relation should describe the dependence of photoionization density on distance from a radiation source if the physics of radiative transfer is simple. Measurements of this dependence by Seguin *et al.* (1974) show that the above equation describes $n(r)$ in doped mixtures only when $r \lesssim 15$ cm at 200 Torr total pressure. $n(r)$ is larger than predicted for r greater than this amount. In pure helium, the decrease with distance is less than $1/r^2$. Thus, there is no simple explanation for the dependence of the charge density on distance at the present time. An obvious experiment to resolve this equation would involve a high-resolution spectroscopic analysis of the light from one of these spark sources transmitted through the laser mixture.

Clark and Lind (1974) have studied the spatial and temporal dependence of the gain in a uv-sustained TEA discharge containing tripropylamine. Tripropylamine is ionized by a single-step process involving radiation wavelengths between 1200 and 1700 Å (Lind *et al.*, 1974). Optimum energy input to the laser gas is a sensitive function of the partial pressure of tripropylamine and the CO_2 pressure. At low CO_2 pressures the effective mean free path for photons is determined by the seed gas concentration. As the seed gas concentration is increased, the photogenerated charge density is initially too low for optimum performance but then becomes too large and limits the photon mean free path. An optimum seed gas concentration results in good volume excitation together with a high charge density. When the CO_2 gas concentration is raised the photon mean free path diminishes due to CO_2 absorption, so that full use cannot be made of the seed gas to generate charges. Lind *et al.* (1974) show that an optimized gas mixture produces output energy densities and pulse durations that are competitive with electron-beam-sustained devices.

It is evident that the creation of a high density of electronic charge within the laser medium before and during the application of the main voltage pulse facilitates the deposition of larger quantities of electrical energy into the laser gas. Fenstermacher *et al.* (1971) were the first to show that this process could be enhanced and the range of operation of high-pressure CO_2 lasers extended by direct deposition of electrons from an external source into the laser mixture. When the preionization electron density is sufficiently large, the main discharge may be operated at a field strength that would be less than that required to operate a self-sustained discharge. The electron beam then controls the main discharge and the device is known as an electron-beam-controlled laser. A schematic diagram of such an electron-beam-controlled CO_2 laser is shown in Fig. 2.18. Electrons emitted from a series of hot cathode sources are accelerated by a 200-keV pulse toward a thin metal film that forms part of one wall of the laser

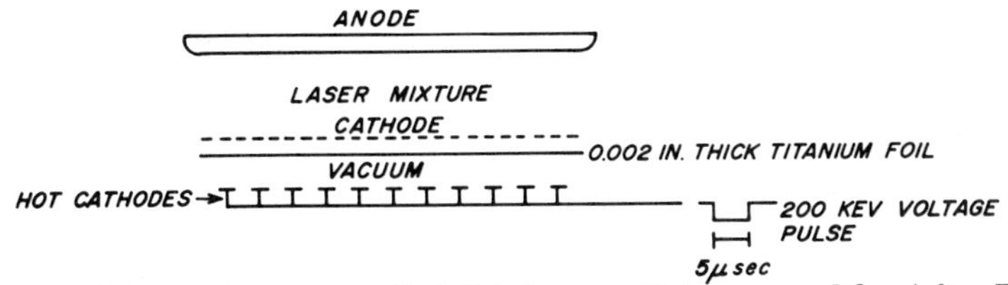

Fig. 2.18. Electron-beam-controlled CO_2 laser oscillator or amplifier (after Fenstermacher *et al.*, 1972).

container. The energy of these electrons is chosen so that their range (in mg/cm^2) is substantially larger than the metal window area density. Most of the electrons then pass through the metal film and excite the laser gas mixture. This excitation involves the creation of electron–ion pairs with individual primary electrons producing about 100 such pairs per centimeter of gas traversed (Fenstermacher *et al.*, 1972) and losing about 25–35 eV of their energy per pair created (Smith, 1972). The primary current density during this process may be as large as 1 A/cm^2. Advantages of this method of ionizing the laser medium prior to and during the main discharge have been summarized by Fenstermacher *et al.* (1972). The main advantage involves the separation of the source of ionization from the electric field that produces pumping of the laser medium. Thus, the electric field E may be independently tailored to yield the optimum value for the ratio E/N, where N is the total number of neutral molecules/cm^3 in the gas. Furthermore, as ionization can be sustained over relatively long periods of time by the external electron source, the duration of the electric field can be matched to the relaxation time of the gain (several microseconds) to maximize energy deposition. Daugherty *et al.* (1972) have reported excitation of a 40-liter volume of a 1 : 2 : 3 mixture of $CO_2 : N_2 : He$ over a 4000-cm^2 area using 130-keV electron beam ionization and have obtained 2000-J pulses for an output energy density of 50 J/liter. This result points out quite clearly another advantage of the electron-beam-controlled configuration: the fact that it lends itself to scaling to large volumes and to high pressures. [Basov *et al.* (1971c,d) reported laser action in a $CO_2 : N_2 : H_2O : He$ mixture at a pressure of about 15 atm using an electron-beam-controlled device. See also the article by Wood (1974) for a review of other Soviet work in this area.] Furthermore, long ($\simeq$50 μsec) pulses can be obtained from devices of this sort, which may make electron-beam-controlled systems attractive for certain cutting, welding, or machining operations.

Ahlstrom *et al.* (1972) describe a cold-cathode emission source that was used to control a CO_2 laser amplifier. They point out that cold-cathode sources are capable of generating larger electron currents than thermionic sources, although for shorter periods of time. Marcus (1972) used a 3-nsec pulse of 600-keV electrons incident along the optical axis of the laser and contained by a pulsed magnetic field. The maximum laser pulse length was 120 μsec and an output energy of 17 J/liter was obtained. In this case the electron beam does not control the discharge but acts only to provide a copious preionization density. A similar method of preionization using an external source of high-energy electrons has been described by Garnsworthy *et al.* (1971). Their system consisted of a central anode running down the optic axis surrounded by a titanium foil tube mounted coaxially. External to this tube another cylindrical electrode acted as an electron beam cathode. The region between the outermost cylindrical electrode and the foil tube contained low-pressure helium in which a discharge was initiated by 120-keV pulses from a Marx generator. Electrons from this discharge passed through the foil into the main discharge volume to act as sources of preionization. About 180 J/liter could be delivered to this preionized gas without the formation of arcs.

A possible limitation on the maximum energy that can be extracted from high-pressure laser mixtures due to gas breakdown within the laser cavity has been pointed out by Berger and Smith (1972). Since the breakdown threshold will decrease with increasing gas pressure while the saturation energy flux will increase with increasing pressure, Berger and Smith conclude that an optimum operating pressure of 2–4 atm with an output flux of 3–1.8 J/cm^2 will be the limit at which breakdown-free operation is possible. Thus, large aperture devices are favored for the generation of high-energy pulses. A discussion of volumetric heating effects and the effect of acoustic waves on the optical quality of the output from *E*-beam lasers has recently been presented by Pugh *et al.* (1974).

2.5.2 High-Repetition-Rate Pulsed TEA Lasers

Most of the lasers described in the previous section can easily be pulsed at rates of up to 10 pps. The gas must be flowed through the system to avoid the buildup of degradation products and heating of the gas, but pulse rates in this range do not put stringent requirements on the gas flow system. At higher pulse repetition frequencies (prf) these problems become severe and a rapid transverse flow of gas is required to maintain high output. One of the first high-prf TEA lasers was reported by Beaulieu (1971) but this device was able to operate at its rated output of 1200 pps for only a few seconds before serious degradation of the discharge occurred. A similar pin–rod system, which had a transverse flow that provided a gas change in the laser cavity between pulses, was operated successfully at 1000 pps for up to 20 min (Turgeon, 1971). However, the average power was found to drop steadily during operation. This drop in power was most severe for low gas flow rates, but even at the highest rate attainable (40 liter/min) significant degradation in the output power was observed.

Brandenberg *et al.* (1972) have operated a transversely excited high prf laser in a supersonic (Mach 3) flow for times of the order of 0.3 sec. The maximum pulse rate was 17 kHz and 34 W/cm^3 of average power was extracted at a static pressure of 160 Torr. Scaling to atmospheric pressure predicts that average output powers of 150 W/cm^3 should be attainable. A modification to this system to permit preionization by means of a radio frequency discharge was later described by Nichols and Brandenberg (1972).

The double-discharge laser developed by Dumanchin *et al.* (1972) has been operated in a closed-loop recirculation system at rates of up to 100 pps and pulse energies of 20 J at atmospheric pressure. One problem with such a system involves the design of a heat exchanger capable of accepting the large residual heat left in the laser mixture after excitation. Typically this may be 200 J/pulse at high output energy. For a prf of 1 kHz, this would correspond to an average power of 200 kW to be dissipated. However, there would seem to be no major problems involved in operating transversely excited lasers of this sort at rates of up to and including 1 kHz. An extensive study by Brown (1973) on repetition rate effects in a fast flow system with an electrode structure similar to that of Dumanchin *et al.* (1972) showed that the limitation on pulse rate was occasioned by the occurrence of arcing rather than gas heating. The average output power scaled linearly with prf up to the point where arcs occurred in the laser cavity. This point occurred at a constant value of the ratio of prf to gas flow rate.

2.5.3 Mode-Locking

Shortly after the TEA laser was announced, Wood *et al.* (1970) reported the mode-locking of a TEA device using an intracavity acoustic loss modulator. The width of the output pulses was estimated to be less than 1 nsec. Subsequently, passive (Nurmikko *et al.*, 1971; Gilbert and LaChambre, 1971; Gibson *et al.*, 1971, 1974; Fortin *et al.*, 1973; Alcock and Walker, 1974; Feldman and Figueira, 1974) and active (Rheault *et al.*, 1972; LaChambre *et al.*, 1972; Davis *et al.*, 1972; Sakane, 1974; Alcock and Walker, 1974) mode-locking have generated considerable interest. Self-mode-locking has also been noted (Lyon *et al.*, 1970; Smith and Berger, 1971; Crocker and Lamberton, 1971; Gilbert and LaChambre, 1971; Nakatsuka *et al.*, 1972; Chang and Wood, 1972b).

Gilbert and LaChambre (1971) found that spontaneous self-locking of axial modes occurred in a pin–pin helical high-pressure laser. This self-locking occurred without wavelength selection and the width of the mode-locked pulses was typically 5 nsec. In general, the occurrence of mode-locking was insensitive to electrical excitation parameters, gas pressure, and the $CO_2 : N_2$ ratio. Multipulsing at beat frequencies of the cavity round-trip frequency $c/2L$ was observed most strongly with longer cavities. Insertion of a SF_6 saturable absorber in the laser cavity greatly reduced the tendency for multipulsing. Lyon *et al.* (1970) incorporated a grating in the cavity and found that spontaneous mode-locking occurred on 11 lines centered about $P(20)$. The pulse duration was 4 nsec FWHM. [Volume-excited lasers similar to those developed by Dumanchin and Rocca-Serra (1969) and by Lamberton and Pearson (1971) were shown to exhibit spontaneous mode-locking at atmospheric pressure (Crocker and Lamberton, 1971). The FWHM of the pulses obtained was about 3 nsec.]

Nurmikko *et al.* (1971) found that a cell containing SF_6 in the laser cavity yielded operation on only one longitudinal mode of the system with output power equal to 80% of the multimode output. Heated CO_2 (Gibson *et al.*, 1971) produced operation on two simultaneously oscillating modes in a similar configuration. Until recently, the shortest pulses reported from a CO_2 laser using passive mode-locking had a duration of 2 nsec (FWHM) (Fortin *et al.*, 1973). Active mode-locking was shown (Abrams and Wood, 1971) to yield pulses with a FWHM of 0.7 nsec. Since the pressure-broadened linewidth of individual rotational lines is $\Delta\nu \simeq 3 \times 10^9$ Hz at 1 atm (5% CO_2, 95% He) one would expect that bandwidth-limited pulsewidths $\tau \simeq 1/\pi\ \Delta\nu \simeq 0.1$ nsec should be possible. However, it has been shown (Siegman and Kuizenga, 1969; Kuizenga and Siegman, 1970; Abrams and Wood, 1971; Kuizenga *et al.*, 1973) that the minimum pulsewidth obtainable in mode-locked operation with an intracavity amplitude or phase modulator is instead

$$\tau = 0.445 (g_0/\delta) (f_c\ \Delta\nu)^{-1/2}$$

where g_0 is the saturated single-pass excess gain of the laser, δ the modulation depth of the modulator, f_c the mode-locking frequency, and $\Delta\nu$ the laser linewidth. At 1 atm this pulsewidth is typically 1 nsec. Some methods of reducing this limit have been discussed by Abrams and Wood (1971).

Attention has recently shifted to systems passively mode-locked by means of p-type germanium absorbers (Gibson *et al.*, 1974; Alcock and Walker, 1974; Feldman and Figueira, 1974). Gibson *et al.* (1972) have shown that the absorption of this material saturates at an intensity of about 10 MW/cm². Use of p-type germanium as a saturable absorber has resulted in the mode-locking of a 12-atm CO_2 laser and the observation of output pulses with durations $\lesssim$150 psec (Alcock and Walker, 1974).

Feldman and Figueira (1974) found that later pulses in a mode-locked train are sharpened by about an order of magnitude due to the fact that they make a larger number of passes through the saturable absorber.

Two other approaches to obtaining subnanosecond pulses from 10.6 μm lasers have been reported by Richardson (1974) and by Yablonovitch and Goldhar (1974). Richardson used a GaAs electro-optical gate to sharpen 20-nsec pulses from a TEA uv-preionized laser to $\simeq$600 psec. The rise time of transmitted 10.6-μm pulses was $\lesssim$300 psec. Yablonovitch and Goldhar produced pulses of 100–500 psec duration by switching with a laser breakdown spark followed by optical free induction decay in a sample of heated CO_2 gas exposed to the laser output pulse passing through the breakdown region. When breakdown occurs, direct excitation of the heated CO_2 gas ceases and the gas radiates a pulse of the same power as the incident laser beam but of opposite phase and with a duration of the order of the molecular collision time.

Single 1-nsec pulses have been generated from a TEA laser oscillator actively mode-locked with an acousto-optic loss modulator in conjunction with a pulse selector similar to that shown in Fig. 2.4 (Davis *et al.*, 1972). Pan *et al.* (1974) report the selection of single 10-J, 1-nsec pulses using a similar technique to select the pulse and subsequent amplification in a two-stage amplifier to increase its peak power into the multigigawatt range. Amplification of nanosecond pulses in electron-beam-pumped amplifiers has also been reported (Figueira *et al.*, 1973). Single 1-nsec pulses containing multiple frequencies in the 10.4 and 9.4 μm bands of CO_2 have been generated by Figueira and Sutphin (1974). 2-nsec pulses containing several lines in the 10.4-μm band have been obtained by Sakane (1974).

2.5.4 The Spin–Flip Raman Laser

In 1967, Slusher *et al.* (1967) demonstrated that the Raman scattering of 10.6-μm CO_2 laser radiation from electrons in a sample of n-type InSb in a magnetic field exhibited spectral peaks at $w_0 - \mu_B g_{eff} B$, $w_0 - 2w_c$, and $w_0 - w_c$, where w_0 is the laser frequency, $w_c = eB/m^*c$ the cyclotron frequency for electrons of effective mass m^*, μ_B the Bohr magneton, B the magnetic field strength, and g_{eff} the effective gyromagnetic ratio for the electrons. This was followed soon after (Patel and Shaw, 1970) by the observation of tunable stimulated Raman scattering in the same material pumped by 2-kW pulses from a *Q*-switched CO_2 laser. The Raman output was tunable over the range $\simeq$11.7–13.0 μm by varying the magnetic field from 48 to 100 kG. Cw operation of a spin–flip Raman laser pumped by the output from a cw CO laser at 5.32 μm was then reported by Mooradian *et al.* (1970) and Brueck and Mooradian (1971). Extension of the operating range to include anti-Stokes (short wavelength) components (Shaw and Patel, 1971) provided a tunable pulsed output from 10.6 to 9.4 μm with a 10.6-μm pumping wavelength. The need for a high magnetic field was overcome by the use of low electron-density InSb by Patel (1971b), and cw operation on the first and second Stokes as well as the anti-Stokes components was reported using a CO laser pump. This paper also reported tunable cw operation on anti-Stokes frequencies short of 1888 cm^{-1}. High-intensity operation using a transversely excited CO_2 laser pump was subsequently reported by Aggarwal *et al.* (1971).

The considerable interest generated by the availability of these devices has been prompted by possible applications in the areas of high-resolution infrared spectroscopy (Patel *et al.*, 1970; Wood *et al.*, 1972; Patel, 1972, 1974) and the detection of pollutants in the atmosphere (Kreuzer and Patel, 1971). Further discussions on these applications will be found in Sections 8.4 and 10.5.1, respectively.

The frequencies given above for the inelastic scattering of 10.6-μm radiation from conduction band electrons in n-type InSb by Slusher *et al.* (1967), $w_0 - \mu_B g_{eff} B$, $w_0 - 2w_c$, and $w_0 - w_c$, correspond to a spin–flip transition, an excitation at twice the cyclotron frequency, and an excitation at the cyclotron frequency, respectively. The spin–flip transition, which is the one observed in stimulated emission, occurs at the electron spin resonance frequency of the conduction electrons in the applied magnetic field. The frequency of this transition and hence the frequency of the output can be varied by changing B. In the absence of stimulated emission, the linewidth of the spin–flip transition is typically $\simeq 2$ cm^{-1} and the intensity of the spin–flip satellite line increases more or less linearly with the pump power. As the threshold for stimulated Raman scattering is exceeded, the output power rises rapidly, while the linewidth of the spin–flip satellite narrows by several orders of magnitude (Patel and Shaw, 1970). The conversion efficiency of these devices can be quite high: Brueck and Mooradian (1971) report an efficiency of $<50\%$, while DeSilets and Patel (1973) obtained a conversion efficiency of 80% and were able to observe Stokes satellites at up to four times the spin–flip frequency. These high efficiencies were obtained in n-type InSb samples excited with 5-μm CO laser radiation with collinearity between the incident and Raman scattered beams. It should be noted that the 5-μm output of the CO laser enhances the spin–flip scattering cross section since this frequency corresponds quite closely to the InSb band gap. At the same time as the cross section for scattering increases, the threshold power decreases and threshold powers as low as 50 mW have been reported (Brueck and Mooradian, 1971) using a CO laser as the pump. Interest in these devices as sources for infrared spectroscopy can be understood when one realizes that the narrow linewidth of the spin–flip output can be combined with high output powers [1 kW pulsed (Aggarwal *et al.*, 1971) and >1 W cw (Brueck and Mooradian, 1971)].

2.5.5 Optically Pumped High Pressure Lasers

An alternative method of pumping the CO_2 laser using direct excitation of the CO_2 (00^01) level by absorption of 4.23-μm HBr laser radiation has been reported by Chang and Wood (1972a, 1973). Recently, operation of a CO_2 laser at 33 atm has been accomplished using this pumping technique (Chang and Wood, 1973). Laser oscillation occurs on the $P(16)$–$P(20)$ and $R(10)$–$R(20)$ transitions of the 10.4-μm band and the $P(16)$ transition of the 9.4-μm band for CO_2 pressures <10 atm. Above 10 atm the laser output occurs mainly on the $R(10)$–$R(20)$ transitions of the 10.4-μm band. The energy levels involved and the optical pumping transition are shown in Fig. 2.19. Very strong absorption occurs in room temperature CO_2 gas at the HBr laser output wavelength and the transitions involved in this absorption are not known with certainty. It appears that many (00^0n) levels may be simultaneously populated due to multiple absorption of incident 4.2-μm photons. Chang and Wood (1973) show that total absorption of the incident laser radiation occurs in a path length of <1 mm at CO_2 pressures >4 atm. In fact, the resonator used at 33 atm was only 1 mm long.

Pumping of this device was with 0.4-μsec pulses. The energy threshold for oscillation at 10 μm increased steadily with pressure, but even at 33 atm was still only 30 mJ. Output pulses were observed to have a width of about 2 nsec at 20 atm. The tuning range of such a high-pressure laser is expected

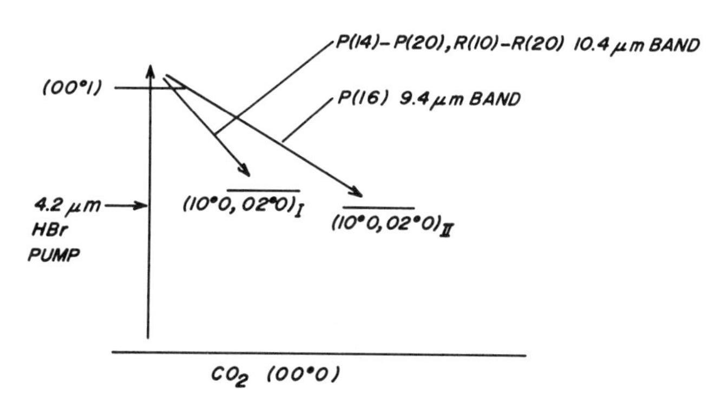

Fig. 2.19. Energy level diagram and laser transitions observed with optical pumping of high-pressure CO_2 laser using 4.2-μm HBr laser output.

to be $\simeq 5\ cm^{-1}$, although Chang and Wood (1973) report that continuous tunability is compromised by the tendency for oscillation to occur on a large number of transverse modes.

Optical pumping has been used effectively in other infrared laser systems. A pulsed CO_2 laser was used to obtain laser emission from methyl fluoride (Brown *et al.*, 1972; DeTemple *et al.*, 1973; Chang and Bridges, 1970) and methanol (Brown *et al.*, 1972). HF has been optically pumped with the output from a HF laser (Skribanowitz *et al.*, 1972a,b). Laser emission from N_2O at pressures of up to 42 atm has been reported on optically pumping CO_2 with a HBr laser (Chang and Wood, 1974) in N_2O–CO_2 mixtures. It is likely that other systems will be discovered in which optical pumping is effective. One advantage of this method of excitation is that it is selective and involves transfer of energy only to the desired energy levels. This makes optical pumping attractive for high-pressure and perhaps even liquid or solid state infrared laser systems, where collisional excitation can no longer occur.

2.6 CHEMICAL TRANSFER LASERS

The term "chemical laser" has been conceived as a description of devices in which chemical energy is converted directly into electromagnetic radiation. In such systems the energy of a chemical reaction may be converted in part to vibrational or electronic excitation of the reaction products. Under appropriate conditions, population inversions may be established within one or more components of these reaction products and laser action can result. This situation occurs in the HF (Deutsch, 1967) and CO (Pollack, 1966) chemical lasers. The exciting reactions are

$$F + H_2 \rightarrow HF^* + H + 32\ \text{kcal/mole}$$

$$O + CS_2 \rightarrow SO + CS + 30\ \text{kcal/mole}$$

and

$$O + CS \rightarrow CO^* + S + 85\ \text{kcal/mole}$$

Another type of chemical laser, which will be described here in more detail, involves the creation of a population of highly excited chemical species, which then transfer vibrational energy selectively to a "cool" component in the gas, yielding a population inversion in this component. These devices are called chemical transfer lasers. Chemical energy is used to produce the initial vibrational excitation, which is then transferred to the lasing molecule.

Laser emission from CO_2 excited by the transfer of chemical energy from HCl was first reported by Chen *et al.* (1968). Subsequently it was found that transfer could be obtained from other molecules, including DF (Gross, 1969; Cool *et al.*, 1969, 1970; Brunet and Mabru, 1971; Basov *et al.*, 1971a,b, 1972), HF (Cool *et al.*, 1969), and HBr (Cool and Stephens, 1970b). Laser action from chemically excited CO_2 was first observed in pulsed systems (Chen *et al.*, 1968; Gross, 1969). Subsequent development of cw chemical transfer lasers based on HCl–CO_2, HBr–CO_2, HF–CO_2, and DF–CO_2 was rapid (Cool *et al.*, 1969; Cool and Stephens, 1970). Supersonic chemical transfer CO_2 lasers have been discussed by Cool (1973). A high-pressure DF–CO_2 chemical transfer laser initiated by a transverse discharge has been reported by Poehler and Walker (1973). The subject of chemical transfer lasers has recently been reviewed by Cool (1973).

In the DF–CO_2 chemical transfer laser, the reaction mechanism is typically

$$F + D_2 \rightarrow DF^* + D + 97.4 \text{ kcal/mole}$$

$$D + F_2 \rightarrow DF^* + F + 31.0 \text{ kcal/mole}$$

followed by

$$DF^* + CO_2\,(00^00) \rightarrow CO_2\,(00^01) + DF + 558 \text{ cm}^{-1}$$

Fluorine atoms can be obtained from the reaction

$$F_2 + NO \rightarrow ONF + F - 18 \text{ kcal/mole}$$

The enormous energy defect in the transfer $DF^* \equiv DF\ (v'' = 1)$ to CO_2 (00^00) would seem to imply that this process would be very inefficient indeed, since kT at 300°K is only $\simeq$200 cm^{-1}. In fact, measured rate constants for this process show that it occurs readily despite the energy defect and with a rate constant that can exceed that for the $N_2^* \rightarrow CO_2\ (00^00)$ energy transfer (Stephens and Cool, 1972; Stephenson *et al.*, 1972; Airey and Smith, 1972). It appears that large amounts of excess energy may be transferred directly to rotation (Stephens and Cool, 1972; Stephenson *et al.*, 1972). This may be due to the existence of a strong attractive potential interaction between species such as HF and DF, and CO_2.

A schematic diagram of a cw CO_2 chemical transfer laser based on DF is shown in Fig. 2.20. It is interesting that such a device can be operated on a variety of wavelengths (not simultaneously, however) simply by changing the gas mixture composition. This system was capable of generating cw laser powers of 160 W at 10.6 μm at a chemical efficiency of 4.6% (Cool *et al.*, 1970b). The flow speed was 200 m/sec and the static pressure was 15.4 Torr. Optimum partial flow rates were He, 112 mmole/sec; CO_2,

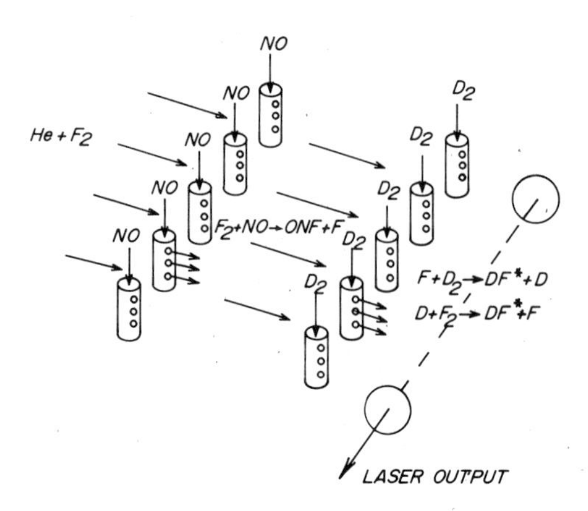

Fig. 2.20. Chemical transfer laser based on DF–CO_2. Laser output: DF, 3.8 μm; HF, 2.7 μm; DF–CO_2, HF–CO_2, 10.6 μm (after Cool, 1973).

57 mmole/sec; F_2, 7.3 mmole/sec; D_2, 6.5 mmole/sec; and NO, 1.2 mmole/sec. Higher powers have subsequently been reported (Cool, 1973).

The chemical transfer laser involving transfer from hydrogen or deuterium halides to CO_2 may be initiated by flash photolysis of a quiescent mixture of H_2 (or D_2) + F_2 + CO_2 + He. An extensive study of such a laser has been described by Poehler *et al.* (1973). Light from a xenon flash-lamp dissociates F_2 in the process

$$F_2 + h\nu \rightarrow 2F \; - \; 37.7 \text{ kcal/mole}$$

and the resulting F atoms undergo the reactions with D_2 listed above. A parametric study of laser output shows that for constant flash-lamp energy the output laser pulse energy increases linearly with increasing pressure, while the pulse duration decreases. A peak power of 200 kW was obtained in a pulse of 25-μsec duration. The small signal gain coefficient was found to increase with an increase in flash-lamp energy. The maximum value obtained was about 2.5%/cm. Efficiencies of these devices are small; Poehler *et al.* report that the ratio of the output pulse energy to the energy released in the flash-initiated exothermic reactions is only 3.2%. When one looks at the ratio of output energy to that of the initiating flash, the efficiency is even smaller. However, when the mode volume of the cavity is taken into account, the efficiency increases to 15%. Cool (1973) suggests that chemically pumped lasers of this sort may eventually yield specific energy outputs comparable to those of transversely excited, electrically pulsed N_2–CO_2 lasers. Detailed numerical simulation of pulsed DF–CO_2 devices have been reported by Kerber *et al.* (1973).

2.7 LASER MECHANISMS

2.7.1 Energy Levels in CO_2 and Laser Transitions

Since CO_2 is an unreactive, relatively simple polyatomic molecule its spectrum is quite well known (Herzberg, 1967) particularly in the infrared (Courtoy, 1957). Vibrational levels in the infrared derive from the three fundamental modes shown in Fig. 2.21. In the symmetric stretching mode of frequency ν_1, the two oxygen atoms move in opposite directions while the carbon atom is stationary. The asymmetric stretching mode shown in Fig. 2.21 has the two O atoms moving together while the C atom moves in the opposite direction. The bending mode with frequency ν_2 consists of two degenerate vibrations perpendicular to and within the plane of the page.

Spectroscopists have developed a concise notation that permits a simple description of the vibrational state of excitation of such a molecule. The vibrational state is defined by the notation (n_1, n_2^l, n_3) where $n_{1,2,3}$ are the number of quanta of frequency $\nu_{1,2,3}$, respectively, possessed by the molecule. The superscript l on the quantum number of the degenerate vibration takes the value $l = n_2, n_2 - 2, \ldots, 1, 0$, with each l giving rise to a sublevel. When $n_2 = 1$ the only value that l can take is $l = 1$. When $n_2 = 2$, $l = 2, 0$, and two sublevels result. If no other vibrations of the molecule are excited at the same time, these states would be written (01^10) and (02^20), (02^00), respectively.

The notation Σ_g^+, Σ_u^+, etc., that accompanies the vibrational states of CO_2 is the label for the irreducible representation of the point group $(D_{\infty h})$ of CO_2 to which the eigenfunction of the vibration belongs. The eigen-

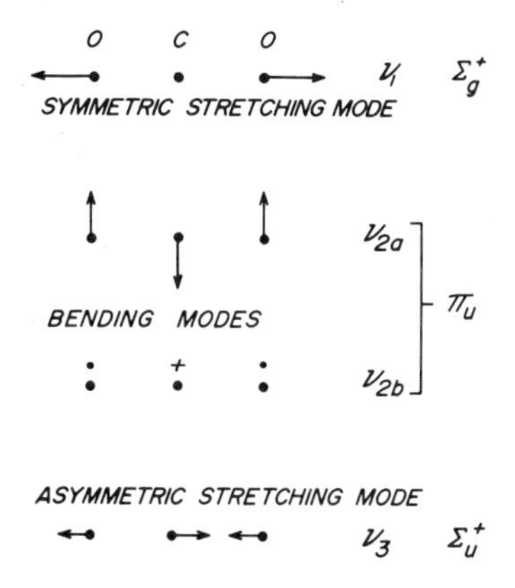

Fig. 2.21. Normal vibrations of CO_2.

function of a particular vibrational state of the molecule will transform in a particular way under the symmetry operations of the point group. However, only certain transformations are possible consistent with the symmetry of the molecule and these are known as irreducible representations of the point group. A given eigenfunction will then transform in the way prescribed by one of these irreducible representations and the symmetry of the wavefunction is given by the symmetry of its corresponding irreducible representation.

It happens that a near resonance occurs between the energies of the (10^00) and (02^00) vibrational states. This leads to a perturbation of both these levels of the type first discussed by Fermi (1931), and a mixing of the eigenfunctions of the two levels results. Thus, the designations (10^00) and (02^00) for these states are no longer valid, since the wavefunction for each is actually an admixture of the wavefunctions of both the (10^00) and (02^00) states. As a result the correct designation of these levels is (Amat and Pimbert, 1965) $(10^00, 02^00)_{\mathrm{I}}$ and $(10^00, 02^00)_{\mathrm{II}}$, with the $(10^00, 02^00)_{\mathrm{II}}$ state lying lowest. Fermi resonance is not restricted to the (10^00) and (02^00) levels, it produces mixing of many other vibrational levels of CO_2 and accounts for the occurrence of what would appear to be forbidden transitions on the basis of the inexact notation.

Since the vibrations ν_2 and ν_3 are antisymmetric and involve a change in dipole moment of the molecule, these vibrations can be excited by direct absorption of an infrared photon. They are consequently known as infrared-active fundamentals. The symmetric mode ν_1 involves no change in dipole moment and hence is infrared inactive or Raman active. Figure 2.22 shows some vibrational levels of CO_2 with energies less than about 0.25 eV.

A series of rotational levels are superimposed on each of these vibrational states. The quantum number of these levels is given the label J. Because of the symmetry of the CO_2 molecule, odd rotational levels of $\Sigma_g{}^+$ states and even rotational levels of $\Sigma_g{}^+$ states are missing. This structure shows up in a simplification of certain vibration–rotation transitions as observed spectroscopically. The selection rules for transitions between various vibrational and rotational states are as follows:

vibrational transitions: $\Delta n = 1, \quad \Delta l = 0, \pm 1, \quad \mathrm{g} \rightarrow \mathrm{u}, \quad \mathrm{u} \rightarrow \mathrm{g}$

rotational transitions: $\Delta J = 0, \pm 1, \quad + \leftrightarrow -, \quad \mathrm{s} \leftrightarrow \mathrm{a}$

where s and a refer to symmetric and antisymmetric, respectively. This designation refers to the symmetry of the rotational wavefunction. + and − denote the change in sign of the total eigenfunction of the molecule under inversion. For symmetric vibrational levels of species Σ^+ even rotational levels are positive while odd levels are negative. In antisymmetric

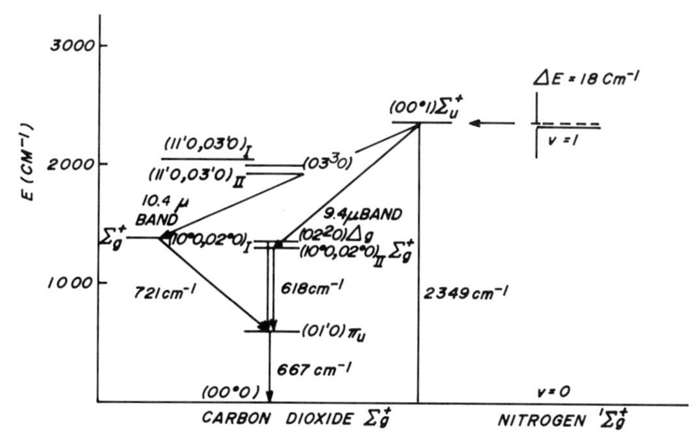

Fig. 2.22. Energy level diagram for low-lying states of CO_2 and N_2.

levels (Σ^-) even rotational levels are negative while odd levels are positive. States denoted as Π, Δ, etc., have two sublevels for each value of J at slightly different energies whose signs alternate $+-$, $-+$, $+-$, . . . , or $-+$, $+-$, $-+$, ... Branches of a vibration–rotation transition are designated by the change in J as follows:

$$P \equiv \Delta J = -1, \qquad Q \equiv \Delta J = 0, \qquad R \equiv \Delta J = +1$$

Individual lines are denoted $P(J)$, $Q(J)$, $R(J)$. The common emission lines generated by a CO_2 laser occur in the $(00^01) \rightarrow (10^00,\ 02^00)_{\rm I}$ and $(00^01) \rightarrow (10^00,\ 02^00)_{\rm II}$ bands at wavelengths of about 10.4 and 9.4 μm, respectively. In the 10.4-μm band, oscillation occurs primarily on the $P(18)$, $P(20)$, and $P(22)$ lines near 10.6 μm. Hence the wavelength of operation of the CO_2 laser can usually be taken as 10.6 μm. Tables 2.4–2.7 list vacuum wavelengths and energies for laser lines observed in the 10.4 and 9.4 μm bands as reported by Patel (1964), Frapard *et al.* (1966), Howe (1965), Barchewitz *et al.* (1965), and Legay-Sommaire *et al.* (1965). Other transitions in different bands have also been observed in the 11–18 μm wavelength range (Frapard *et al.*, 1966; Howe and McFarlane, 1966; Hartman and Kleman, 1966) but these are usually weak and some are seen only in pulsed operation. When one considers that several isotopes of CO_2 are available, the number of lines that can be obtained from CO_2 lasers increases to several hundred.

2.7.2 Excitation of the CO_2 Molecule

CO_2 is excited primarily by two mechanisms in CO_2–N_2 laser mixtures: inelastic collisions with low-energy electrons, and resonant energy transfer

Table 2.4

Measured CO_2 Laser Wavelength of the P Branch of the 00^01–$(10^00, 02^00)_I$ Vibration–Rotation Transitions

Measured laser wavelength in vacuo (μm)	Frequency (cm^{-1})	Transition
10.4410	957.76	$P(4)$
10.4585	956.16	$P(6)$
10.4765	954.52	$P(8)$
10.4945	952.88	$P(10)$
10.5135	951.16	$P(12)$
10.5326	949.43	$P(14)$
10.5518	947.70	$P(16)$
10.5713	945.96	$P(18)$
10.5912	944.18	$P(20)$
10.6118	942.35	$P(22)$
10.6324	940.52	$P(24)$
10.6534	938.67	$P(26)$
10.6748	936.78	$P(28)$
10.6965	934.88	$P(30)$
10.7194	932.89	$P(32)$
10.7415	930.96	$P(34)$
10.7648	928.95	$P(36)$
10.7880	926.95	$P(38)$
10.8120	924.90	$P(40)$
10.8360	922.85	$P(42)$
10.8605	920.77	$P(44)$
10.8855	918.65	$P(46)$
10.9110	916.51	$P(48)$
10.9360	914.41	$P(50)$
10.9630	912.16	$P(52)$
10.9900	909.92	$P(54)$
11.0165	907.73	$P(56)$

from vibrationally excited N_2 molecules. Since N_2 is a homonuclear diatomic molecule with no permanent dipole moment, transitions between vibrational levels of the same electronic state are strongly forbidden by the parity selection rule. Thus populations will tend to build up in excited vibrational levels of the ground state of N_2 when N_2 is excited in a discharge or by some other means. The first excited vibrational level of this state ($v'' = 1$) lies at an energy nearly coincident with that of the CO_2 (00^01) level. Thus energy can be transferred between N_2 ($v'' = 1$) and CO_2 (00^01) with high efficiency when N_2 collides with CO_2. The transfer

Table 2.5

Measured CO_2 Laser Wavelengths of the R Branch of the 00^01–$(10^00, 02^00)_I$ Vibration–Rotation Transitions

Measured laser wavelength in vacuo	Wavenumber (cm^{-1})	Transition
10.3655	964.74	$R(4)$
10.3500	966.18	$R(6)$
10.3335	967.73	$R(8)$
10.3190	969.09	$R(10)$
10.3040	970.50	$R(12)$
10.2860	971.91	$R(14)$
10.2855	972.24	$R(16)$
10.2605	974.61	$R(18)$
10.2470	975.90	$R(20)$
10.2335	977.18	$R(22)$
10.2200	978.47	$R(24)$
10.2075	979.67	$R(26)$
10.1950	980.87	$R(28)$
10.1825	982.08	$R(30)$
10.1710	983.19	$R(32)$
10.1590	984.35	$R(34)$
10.1480	985.42	$R(36)$
10.1370	986.49	$R(38)$
10.1260	987.56	$R(40)$
10.1150	988.63	$R(42)$
10.1050	989.61	$R(44)$
10.0955	990.54	$R(46)$
10.0860	991.47	$R(48)$
10.0760	992.46	$R(50)$
10.0670	993.34	$R(52)$
10.0585	994.18	$R(54)$

is given by the equation

$$N_2\ (v'' = 1) + CO_2\ (00^00) \leftrightarrow N_2\ (v'' = 0) + CO_2\ (00^01) - 18\ \text{cm}^{-1}$$

and the rate of energy exchange is $k_l = 1.9 \times 10^4$/Torr/sec at 300°K (Taylor and Bitterman, 1969). The energy discrepancy (18 cm^{-1}) is much less than the thermal energy of molecules in the discharge ($\simeq$200 cm^{-1} at 300°K) and thus presents no barrier to efficient energy transfer. In fact, a quenching of CO_2 (00^01) by CO ($v'' = 0$) has been shown to occur with a rate $k^{(CO)} = 0.8 \times 10^4$/Torr/sec with an energy discrepancy of 206 cm^{-1} (Moore *et al.*, 1967):

$$CO_2\ (00^01) + CO\ (v'' = 0) \leftrightarrow CO_2\ (00^00) + CO\ (v'' = 1) + 206\ \text{cm}^{-1}$$

Such a process may be important in sealed-off CO_2 lasers.

Table 2.6

Measured CO_2 Laser Wavelengths of the P Branch of the (00^01)–$(10^00, 02^00)_{II}$ Vibration–Rotation Transitions

Measured laser wavelength in vacuo (μm)	Wavenumber (cm^{-1})	Transition
9.4285	1060.61	$P(4)$
9.4425	1059.04	$P(6)$
9.4581	1057.30	$P(8)$
9.4735	1055.58	$P(10)$
9.4885	1053.91	$P(12)$
9.5045	1052.13	$P(14)$
9.5195	1050.47	$P(16)$
9.5360	1048.66	$P(18)$
9.5525	1046.85	$P(20)$
9.5690	1045.04	$P(22)$
9.5860	1043.19	$P(24)$
9.6035	1041.29	$P(26)$
9.5210	1039.34	$P(28)$
9.6391	1037.44	$P(30)$
9.6575	1035.46	$P(32)$
9.6760	1033.48	$P(34)$
9.6941	1031.56	$P(36)$
9.7140	1029.44	$P(38)$
9.7335	1027.38	$P(40)$
9.7535	1025.27	$P(42)$
9.7735	1023.17	$P(44)$
9.7940	1021.03	$P(46)$
9.8150	1018.85	$P(48)$
9.8360	1016.67	$P(50)$
9.8575	1014.46	$P(52)$
9.8790	1012.25	$P(54)$
9.9010	1010.00	$P(56)$
9.9230	1007.76	$P(58)$
9.9465	1005.38	$P(60)$

The resonant interaction of N_2 ($v'' = 1$) with CO_2 is the dominant pumping mechanism in CO_2 laser discharges even at high pressures. Only when the interaction process with the CO_2 molecules in a discharge involves a time scale <1 μsec is collisional activation by excited N_2 unimportant (Wood, 1974). This can occur, for example, when amplifying mode-locked pulses.

Both low-lying vibrational levels of CO_2 and N_2 can be excited directly by inelastic collision with low-energy ($\lesssim 5$ eV) electrons (Hake and

Table 2.7

Measured CO_2 Laser Wavelengths of the R Branch of the $(00^01)-(10^00, 02^00)_{II}$ Vibration–Rotation Transitions

Measured laser wavelength in vacuo (μm)	Wavenumber (cm^{-1})	Transition
9.3677	1067.50	$R(4)$
9.3555	1068.89	$R(6)$
9.3420	1070.43	$R(8)$
9.3295	1071.87	$R(10)$
9.3172	1073.28	$R(12)$
9.3055	1074.63	$R(14)$
9.2937	1076.00	$R(16)$
9.2825	1077.30	$R(18)$
9.2715	1078.57	$R(20)$
9.2605	1079.85	$R(22)$
9.2500	1081.08	$R(24)$
9.2397	1082.29	$R(26)$
9.2295	1083.48	$R(28)$
9.2197	1084.63	$R(30)$
9.2103	1085.74	$R(32)$
9.2010	1086.84	$R(34)$
9.1920	1087.90	$R(36)$
9.1830	1088.97	$R(38)$
9.1740	1090.04	$R(40)$
9.1660	1090.99	$R(42)$
9.1575	1092.00	$R(44)$
9.1490	1093.01	$R(46)$
9.1420	1093.85	$R(48)$
9.1340	1094.81	$R(50)$
9.1265	1095.71	$R(52)$

Phelps, 1967; Schulz, 1964). Electrons with energies in the range 1.5–4.0 eV are most effective in exciting $v'' = 1$ of N_2 with the cross section for this process exceeding 10^{-16} cm^2. $v'' = 2, 3$, etc., can also be excited via low-energy electron impact but the cross sections for these higher states are less than those for excitation of $v'' = 1$. In CO_2 the probability of excitation of the upper laser level is considerably greater than that for excitation of the lower lying laser levels. A cross section of 1.5×10^{-16} cm^2 near threshold has been reported by Nighan (1970) for direct excitation of the CO_2 (00^01) level by electron impact.

An important parameter in the electron-induced population of both CO_2 and N_2 levels in a discharge is the ratio of the electric field E to the total density of neutrals N. Nighan (1970) has performed some calculations of average electron energy in CO_2, N_2 mixtures and the fraction of discharge power transferred to vibrational levels of N_2 and CO_2 in pure N_2 or pure CO_2 as a function of E/N. The average electron energy increases steadily as E/N increases from 10^{-16} V-cm^2, reaching $\simeq$3 eV at $E/N \simeq 6 \times 10^{-15}$ V-cm^2 in a typical CO_2, N_2, He laser mixture. This value of E/N is that at which part of the incident discharge power first starts to be used in producing electronic excitation of N_2 in pure N_2. Optimum pumping of the CO_2 (00^01) level in pure CO_2 occurs when $E/N \simeq 2.5 \times 10^{-16}$ V-cm^2. It should be noted that E/N in typical high-pressure pulsed discharges is usually in the range 2×10^{-16}–8×10^{-16} V-cm^2. In electron-beam-controlled lasers E/N may be 1×10^{-16}–2×10^{-16} V-cm^2. The possibility of controlling E/N to tailor this ratio to the value most effective for pumping the upper laser level is attractive, since with optimized E/N, as much as possible is being done to adjust the discharge to yield direct electron impact excitation of CO_2 (00^01). Thus lasers in which E/N can be controlled (the EB laser is a good example) will be inherently more efficient that those in which the values of E/N tend to be relatively uncontrollable and high.

2.7.3 Relaxation Processes

Early in the development of CO_2 lasers, it was realized that adding He in quantity to the laser gas resulted in substantially increased output powers. It is now established that the primary effect of He is to relax the lower laser level while essentially unaffecting the population in the 00^01 state. Furthermore, He is also effective in depopulating the (01^10) level and may also lower the gas kinetic temperature. All of these effects are beneficial to high-power laser operation, since radiative relaxation rates are orders of magnitude smaller than those due to collisions with He atoms and other gaseous components. As examples, the Einstein A coefficient for the radiative relaxation (00^01) $\rightarrow$ (00^00) is $\simeq$10/sec, while most other rotational lines in the $J = 20$ region of the 10.4-μm band have A in the range 0.2–2/sec (Statz *et al.*, 1966; McCubbin and Mooney, 1968). For transitions between the lower laser level and the (01^10) state, $A \simeq 0.2$–2/sec (Statz *et al.*, 1966). For the (01^10) $\rightarrow$ (00^00) transition, $A \simeq 0.4$–1/sec.

Quenching processes involving the (01^10) level include the vibrational–translational (V $\rightarrow$ T) energy transfer

$$CO_2\ (01^10) + M \rightarrow CO_2\ (00^00) + M + 667\ \text{cm}^{-1}$$

Populations can be transferred between the two lower laser levels $(10^00, 02^00)_{I}$ and $(10^00, 02^00)_{II}$ through the exchange

$$CO_2\ (10^00, 02^00)_{I} + M \rightarrow CO_2\ (10^00, 02^00)_{II} + M + 103\ \text{cm}^{-1}$$

where M can be CO_2. The relaxation of these states may occur via

$$CO_2\ (10^00, 02^00)_{I} + CO_2\ (00^00) \leftrightarrow 2CO_2\ (01^10) + 64\ \text{cm}^{-1}$$

$$CO_2\ (10^00, 02^00)_{II} + CO_2\ (00^00) \leftrightarrow 2CO_2\ (01^10) - 40\ \text{cm}^{-1}$$

or $(10^00, 02^00)_{I}$ may relax through the process (Tyte, 1970)

$$CO_2\ (10^00, 02^00)_{I} + CO_2\ (00^00) \rightarrow CO_2\ (02^20) + CO_2\ (00^00) + 52.7\ \text{cm}^{-1}$$

$$CO_2\ (02^20) + CO_2\ (00^00) \rightarrow CO_2\ (01^10) + CO_2\ (01^10) + 1\ \text{cm}^{-1}$$

Rate constants associated with these processes depend on temperature, pressure, and the type of quencher. Lifetimes associated with the states involved in excitation and relaxation in actual laser mixtures are shown in Figs. 2.23 and 2.24 for two types of discharge: a low-pressure conventional cw discharge at 15 Torr (Fig. 2.24) and a 1-atm pulsed discharge (Fig. 2.23). The effect of collisional relaxation can be clearly seen in the decreasing of the lifetime of the relevant levels participating in the laser process.

Experiments to determine rotational relaxation rates have been discussed by Cheo (1971). The rate constant for relaxation due to collisions should be about 10^7/Torr/sec.

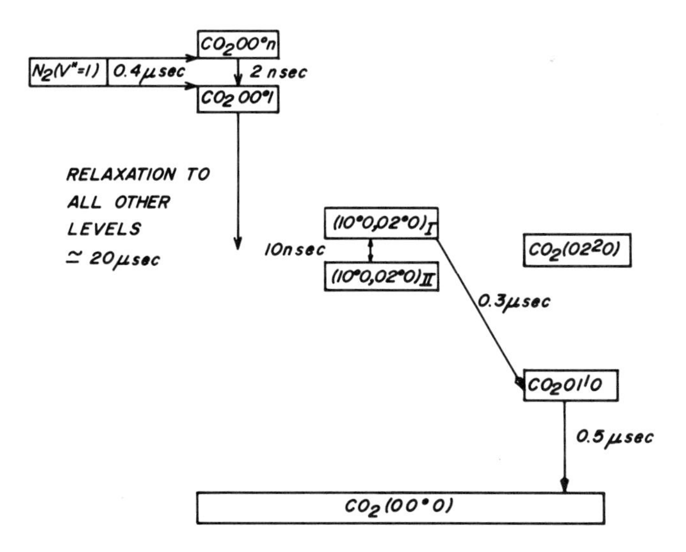

Fig. 2.23. Relaxation times in a pulsed 1-atm laser with 1:1:4 of CO_2:N_2:He (after Wood, 1974).

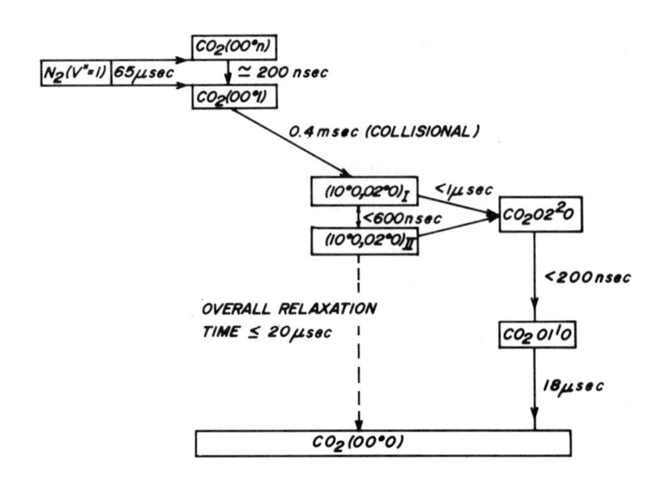

Fig. 2.24. Relaxation times in a cw discharge with 1:1:8 of CO_2:N_2:He at 15 Torr at 420°K (after Tyte, 1970).

2.7.4 Theoretical Descriptions of the Kinetics of CO_2 Lasers

In recent years there has been great interest in modeling the behavior of CO_2 laser discharges under cw (Witteman, 1966a,b; Moore *et al.*, 1967; Tyte and Wills, 1969), conventional pulsed or *Q*-switched (Meyerhofer, 1968b; Tyte and Wills, 1969; Crafer *et al.*, 1969a,b), and TEA conditions (Manes and Seguin, 1972; Lyon, 1973; Vlases and Moeny, 1972). The accuracy of these calculations is now at the stage where output power pulse shapes from TEA lasers can be predicted with little deviation from measured pulse shapes (Manes and Seguin, 1972). The model that we will discuss here is that of Witteman (1966b) as extended by Manes and Seguin (1972) to describe the conditions in a pulsed TEA laser. The original calculations of Witteman were made with a view to predicting the gain in low-pressure cw laser systems. Modifications made by Manes and Seguin were the inclusion of a cavity intensity equation and the insertion of pumping terms consistent with TEA operation.

The time development of energy densities stored in vibrational modes of CO_2 and in the vibration of N_2 are given by the following expression. E_1, E_2, E_3, and E_4 are energy densities (J/cm³) stored in the CO_2 symmetrical stretching mode, the two degenerate bending modes, the antisymmetric stretching mode, and the stretching mode of N_2, respectively. Temperatures T_1, T_2, T_3, and T_4 are associated with each of these modes.

Then

$$\frac{dE_1}{dt} = N_e(t)N_{CO_2}h\nu_1X_1 - \left(\frac{E_1 - E_1^e(T)}{\tau_{10}(T)}\right) - \left(\frac{E_1 - E_1^e(T_2)}{\tau_{12}(T_2)}\right)$$

$$+ \left(\frac{h\nu_1}{h\nu_3}\right)\left(\frac{E_3 - E_3^e(T, T_1, T_2)}{\tau_3(T, T_1, T_2)}\right) + h\nu_1\,\Delta N\,WI_\nu \tag{1}$$

$$\frac{dE_2}{dt} = N_e(t)N_{CO_2}h\nu_2X_2 + \left(\frac{E_1 - E_1^e(T_2)}{\tau_{12}(T_2)}\right) - \left(\frac{E_2 - E_2^e(T)}{\tau_{20}(T)}\right)$$

$$+ \left(\frac{h\nu_2}{h\nu_3}\right)\left(\frac{E_3 - E_3^e(T, T_1, T_2)}{\tau_3(T, T_1, T_2)}\right) \tag{2}$$

$$\frac{dE_3}{dt} = N_e(t)N_{CO_2}h\nu_3X_3 - \left(\frac{E_3 - E_3^e(T, T_1, T_2)}{\tau_3(T, T_1, T_2)}\right)$$

$$+ \left(\frac{E_4 - E_4^e(T_3)}{\tau_{43}(T)}\right) - h\nu_3\,\Delta N\,WI_\nu \tag{3}$$

$$\frac{dE_4}{dt} = N_e(t)N_{N_2}h\nu_4X_4 - \left(\frac{E_4 - E_4^e(T_4)}{\tau_{43}(T)}\right) \tag{4}$$

The cavity field intensity is given by

$$dI_\nu/dt = -(I\nu/\tau_c) + ch\nu_l\,\Delta N\,(WFI_\nu + S) \tag{5}$$

The terms used in these equations are as follows:

- $N_e(t)$ density of electrons at time t
- N_{CO_2} density of CO_2 molecules
- $h\nu_i$ energy of ith vibrational mode
- X_i effective electron vibrational excitation rate for ith mode ($X_4 \equiv N_2$)
- $E_i^e(T_i)$ equilibrium values of E_i at temperature T_i
- τ_{ij} relaxation time associated with transfer of energy between modes i and j
- τ_3 relaxation time of the antisymmetric mode
- W stimulated emission rate at the line center, $=c^2AF/(4\pi^2h\nu_l^3 \times \Delta\nu_H)$
- ν_l laser frequency
- A Einstein A coefficient
- $\Delta\nu_H$ homogeneous linewidth for laser transition

I_ν laser intensity
F ratio of mode volume filled with gain medium to total mode volume; = laser gain–medium length/optical cavity length$_{2^00)\mathrm{I}}$
ΔN population difference, $=N_{00^01}P(J) \quad - \quad (\theta_J/\theta_{J+1})N_{(10^00,0} \times P(J+1)$
θ_J $=2J+1$
J rotational quantum number
$P(J)$ $=(2hcB/kT)\theta_J \exp[-hcBJ(J+1)/kT]$
B rotational constant
N_{00^01} $=N_{CO_2}\exp(-h\nu_3/kT_3)[1-\exp(-h\nu_1/kT_1)] \times [1-\exp(-h\nu_2/kT_2)]^2[1-\exp(-h\nu_3/kT_3)]$
$N_{(10^00,02^00)_\mathrm{I}}$ $=N_{CO_2}\exp(-h\nu_1/kT_1)[1-\exp(-h\nu_1/kT_1)] \times [1-\exp(-h\nu_2/kT_2)]^2[1-\exp(-h\nu_3/kT_3)]$
T translation temperature
τ_c laser cavity lifetime, $=-2L/c \ln \mathrm{R}$
L cavity length
R output mirror reflectivity
S $ch\nu_\mathrm{L}W$

The first term in each of Eqs. (1)–(4) describes the pumping of the particular level by direct electron excitation. Terms with τ_{10}^{-1} are a measure of the rate of vibration–translation (V–T) relaxation and those with τ_{ij}^{-1} measure rates of vibration–vibration (V–V) exchange. The expressions with τ_3^{-1} show the extent of V–V exchange involving the asymmetric stretching mode. The last term in Eqs. (1) and (3), which depends on I_ν, is the rate of stimulated emission from the upper to the lower laser levels.

Manes and Seguin (1972) have solved these equations numerically for typical laser mixtures and different excitation conditions. Their calculations predict the time dependence of the population inversion and the gain. The delay of the laser output pulse and the phenomenon of gain-switching (Beaulieu, 1971) can also be accounted for. Figure 2.25 shows the results of some of their calculations. The laser pulse shown in Fig. 2.25a was obtained from a double Rogowski-type laser developed by Seguin *et al.* (1972); that in Fig. 2.25b from a pin TEA laser with a water bath as a distributed resistance. The theoretical predictions of pulse shape given in Fig. 2.25c–e are seen to be in excellent agreement with the shapes of the experimentally observed pulses. These curves show clearly the phenomenon known as "gain-switching," which occurs with high-pressure electrically pulsed lasers and is responsible for a sharp peak in the laser power output (analogous to a giant pulse from solid state lasers) after some time delay following initiation of the discharge. Gain-switching occurs because the population inversion builds up faster than the cavity intensity. The gain can then

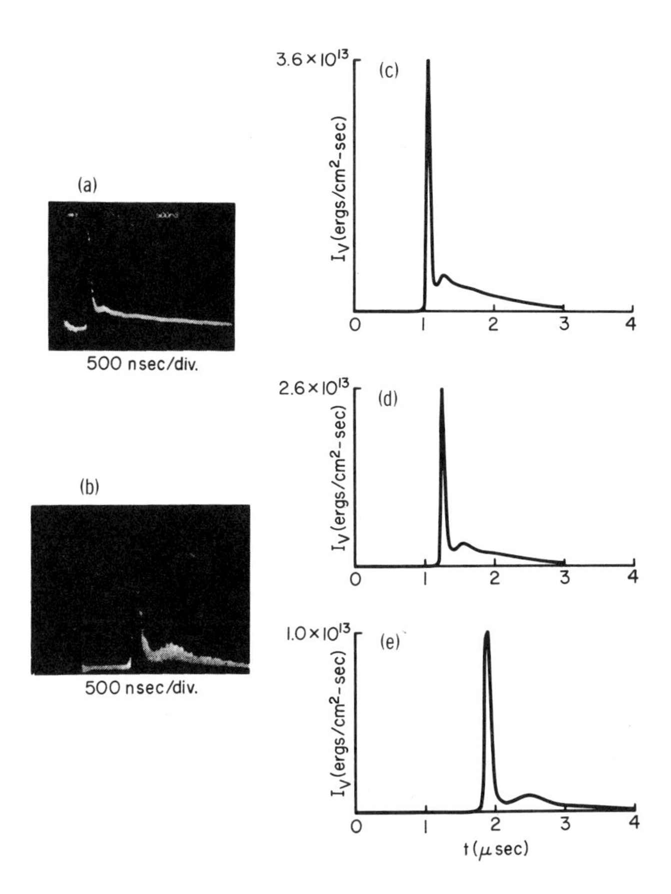

Fig. 2.25. Observed (a, b) and theoretical (c, d, e) pulse shapes for a TEA laser. Parameters for the theoretical fit were $R = 0.74$, $L = 0.48$ m, $F = 0.45$, CO_2:N_2:He = 1:1:8 (from Manes and Seguin, 1972).

be very high when the laser intensity finally builds up within the cavity to the point where the laser output intensity starts to grow and depopulation of the upper laser level due to stimulated emission begins. This is the same process that occurs in Q-switching, except that in this case the Q of the laser cavity is always high. The establishment of high gain just as the intensity of laser radiation within the cavity is growing rapidly results in the emission of a "giant" pulse. The width of this pulse is typically $\lesssim 100$–500 nsec.

Another feature of the laser pulses shown in Fig. 2.25 is the occurrence of a broad "tail" after the initial giant pulse. This follows from the fact that the initial pulse only equalizes the populations in the upper and lower laser levels. Since the lower level relaxes more rapidly than the upper level while pumping due to inelastic collisions with electrons and excited N_2 molecules continues, a population inversion can be reestablished after the termination of the gain-switched pulse. A longer low-peak-power pulse then follows the gain-switched pulse. The energy contained in this pulse depends on the $N_2 : CO_2$ ratio in the laser mixture and in some cases may exceed that in the gain-switched pulse. Girard and Beaulieu (1974) show that the length of this secondary pulse may be extended to 50 μsec by changing the $N_2 : CO_2$ ratio and optimizing the cavity resonator characteristics.

2.7.5 Gain Measurements

There have been an enormous number of experimental measurements of gain in both static (cw) and pulsed systems. Extensive references to the data on gain measurements on cw conventional systems can be found in the reviews by Tyte (1970) and Cheo (1971). Measured values of gain in convectively cooled discharges are listed in Table 2.1. The reviews by Wood (1974) and DeMaria (1973) contain concise discussions of gain in high-pressure pulsed laser discharges and high-power cw discharges, respectively. In this section representative gain measurements made on the different types of CO_2 lasers will be discussed, but because of the availability of the excellent review articles referred to above no attempt will be made to give a complete account of published work in this field.

The dependence of the small signal gain in flowing conventional cw CO_2 lasers on such factors as tube diameter, pressure, discharge current, and gas mixture has been reported in some detail by Cheo (1971). On increasing the discharge current a point will be reached at which the gain maximizes. This maximum value is, as expected, significantly higher in $CO_2 : N_2 : He$ mixtures than in mixtures with one of the N_2 or He constituents missing. Under optimum conditions, gain is highest in narrow bore tubes and decreases steadily with an increase in tube diameter. The gain is found to be relatively independent of position as the sampling beam is moved off the tube axis but decreases drastically as the wall of the tube is approached. Typically, the gain in this type of discharge is about 1%/cm or $\simeq$4 dB/m in a discharge tube with a 2.54-cm bore. In fast-flowing axial systems this value may increase to 4–5%/cm in tubes of the same diameter (Cool and Shirley, 1969).

Gain measurements on an electric discharge convectively cooled laser (Eckbreth and Davis, 1971) TGD system show that the gain increases as the probe beam is moved downstream away from the cathode. At high discharge input powers, the gain coefficient may peak in a particular region between cathode and anode; otherwise it increases steadily toward the anode. The gain also increases almost linearly with electrical power per unit volume into the discharge at low powers. At higher input powers ($\simeq$5 W/cm^3) the gain tends to level out. The maximum value obtained by Eckbreth and Davis (1971) was 1.2%/cm.

In the electric discharge mixing laser of Eckbreth *et al.* (1971), N_2 and He are excited in a discharge and then mixed with cold CO_2 downstream. The gain transverse to the gas flow in this system showed a definite peak several centimeters downstream from the CO_2 injector. Maximum values of the gain were $\simeq$6%/cm, decreasing to $\simeq$2%/cm 20 cm downstream from the injector. Brown (1970) has pointed out that the gain characteristics of an EDML should be independent of flow conditions if the ratio v/p is kept constant, where v is flow speed and p pressure, and the initial mole fractions of the excited state species are also constant. Thus the EDML lends itself well to scaling to larger volumes.

Lee and Gowen (1971) and Lee *et al.* (1972) have measured the gain in a gas dynamic laser as a function of He mole fraction, CO_2 mole fraction, stagnation temperature, and stagnation pressure. Helium was shown to be necessary for the production of positive gain (amplification); at 0% He, the gain was actually $\simeq -0.4$%/cm. Variation of the CO_2 mole fraction showed that the gain increased rapidly up to a mole fraction of 0.2. Experimental data were not available above a mole fraction of 0.2, but theoretical predictions showed that the gain should subsequently decrease. Other observations showed that gain was independent of pressure over a wide range and that maximum gain was obtained at a stagnation temperature of $\simeq$1600°K. The reasons for this behavior have been discussed previously (Section 2.4). The maximum gain was $\simeq$0.6%/cm.

The time-dependent gain in a laser similar to that of Lamberton and Pearson (1971) has been investigated by Deutsch and Rudko (1972). They found that a region of uniform gain occupies most of the volume between the two main electrodes. Near the cathode the gain rapidly increases to very high values ($\simeq$5%/cm) in a localized region and then decreases abruptly closer to the cathode. The gain in the large region of uniform gain was essentially independent of time for times in the range 5–15 μsec after the current pulse. Typically this gain was $\simeq$2–2.5%/cm. Monitoring the time-dependent gain along particular axes displaced toward the electrodes along a perpendicular to the electrodes showed that more than one gain peak was obtained. It was suggested that this effect was related to the propagation of acoustic waves at speeds of 600–1200 m/sec away from the cathode. Density variations associated with these waves may account for the gain peaks observed.

Brandenberg *et al.* (1972) have measured spatial and temporal gain profiles in a transverse pin–plane discharge excited in a supersonic gas flow. The gain was found to decrease steadily with static pressure in a Mach 3 shock for pressures from 60 to 200 Torr. This was attributed to a decrease in N_2 ($v'' = 1$) and CO_2 (00^01) vibrational temperature at high pressure. The gain was as high as 2.5%/cm at 60 Torr and decreased to $\simeq$1.2% at 180 Torr.

Gain in an electron beam pumped amplifier has been measured by Fenstermacher *et al.* (1972). The gain rises during the initial pulse of preionization before the main discharge is initiated. Subsequently the gain rises and at low-energy inputs is found to peak at the termination of the main discharge. When the energy input in the main discharge is increased the peak value of the gain is reached at earlier times. Fenstermacher *et al.* attribute this to increased heating of the gas at high-energy inputs, which tends to populate the lower laser level toward the end of the discharge pulse resulting in a decrease in gain. It was found, however, that the maximum gain achieved increased continuously with increasing field strength in the main discharge. The maximum small signal gain reported was $\simeq$4.6%/cm in a 1 : 1 : 3 CO_2 : N_2 : He mixture with a field of 3.5 kV/cm. Carmichael *et al.* (1974) show that gains of up to 10%/cm can be obtained from *E*-beam discharges containing small amounts of H_2 when the electron beam pulse and discharge are maintained for times of the order of 100 nsec. The gain in a 15-atm *E*-beam-controlled CO_2 laser has been found to scale linearly with input energy to the gas (Harris *et al.*, 1974). A small signal gain of 5.2%/cm was obtained when 115 J/liter-atm was dissipated in the laser mixture. This device when operated as a laser generated 1.2 J at an efficiency of 2.5%.

Chapter 3

Detectors, Resonators, and Optical Components

3.1 INTRODUCTION

Problems that beset experimentalists interested in CO_2 lasers during the early development of these devices were on many occasions related to the lack of suitable detectors for 10.6-μm radiation and the difficulty of obtaining high-quality optical components that could handle large cw or high-peak laser powers at 10.6 μm. Fast-sensitive infrared detectors were available but often these detectors required cooling with liquid helium. Furthermore, such devices were not capable of handling the high intensities produced by cw or pulsed CO_2 lasers. As a result, many groups investigated other devices that could be used for the measurement of the power and energy in 10.6-μm laser outputs. This resulted in the development of the pyroelectric detector which, while less sensitive than cooled photoconductive or photovoltaic detectors, was capable of operation at room temperature and of handling relatively large amounts of laser power without damage. Another type of detector developed to meet the needs of experimentalists measuring high powers from pulsed CO_2 lasers was based on the photon-drag effect in semiconductors such as germanium. These and a variety of other devices for measuring laser energy and power will be described in this chapter.

The rapid development of interest in CO_2 lasers and a mounting number of possible applications has spurred considerable effort in the perfection of optical components for use at 10.6 μm. Single-crystal specimens of Ge, CdTe, and ZnSe are now routinely available from a variety of suppliers, and coatings to produce any desired reflectivity can be obtained on demand. The properties of some of these materials will be discussed in Section 3.5.

Some fundamental principles of optical resonators used with CO_2 and other lasers will be examined in Section 3.6 and the advantages of the unstable resonator configuration for high-gain, high-aperture systems will be pointed out.

The properties of electro-optic, acousto-optic, and other types of modulator operating at 10.6 μm will be investigated in Section 3.7.

Finally, devices that have been developed to attenuate the output from CO_2 lasers and to isolate one part of a high-power laser system from other parts (optical isolators) will be discussed in Section 3.8.

3.2 PARAMETERS DESCRIBING DETECTOR OPERATION

In this section a few commonly cited parameters that are used to characterize the performance of infrared detectors will be defined. Although the quantities given here are now generally accepted by infrared physicists and engineers, this was not always the case, and care must be taken in comparing "figures of merit" given for particular detectors in some of the earlier literature on this subject.

3.2.1 Noise Equivalent Power

The noise equivalent power (NEP) is defined as the incident power that can be detected to give a signal to noise ratio, S/N, of 1 in a bandwidth of 1 Hz. Analytically one has

$$NEP = FAV_{\mathrm{N}}/V_{\mathrm{S}}(\Delta f)^{1/2}\ \mathrm{W/Hz^{1/2}} \tag{1}$$

where F is the radiant power per cm² incident on detector surface (W/cm²), A the area of detector (cm²), V_{N} the rms noise voltage ($\mathrm{V}^{1/2}$), V_{S} the rms signal voltage ($\mathrm{V}^{1/2}$) measured with the entire detector area A exposed to F, and Δf the noise bandwidth (Hz).

It is evident that a "good" detector has a *small NEP*. Standardized measurements of NEP are usually made with a blackbody radiation source kept at 500°K chopped at a frequency between 100 Hz and 1 kHz. The notation NEP(500°K, 400, 1) would mean that the NEP is specified for detection of 500°K blackbody radiation, modulated at 400 Hz with a 1-Hz bandwidth. The NEP is a function of wavelength and can vary over many orders of magnitude when measured with monochromatic light at different infrared wavelengths incident on the same detector.

3.2.2 Detectivity D and Detectors D^* and D_λ^*

Since one would like to have for a detector a figure of merit that increases with an increase in the performance of the detector the reciprocal of the NEP is occasionally used and is given the name detectivity:

$$D = 1/NEP \ (\mathrm{Hz})^{1/2}/\mathrm{W} \tag{2}$$

However, for many common types of detector (Smith *et al.*, 1968) a much more useful figure of merit is obtained by taking the product of D and $A^{1/2}$. This is called† detector D^*, or in the case of a value of a particular wavelength, D_λ^*. Then

$$D^* = A^{1/2}/NEP \ \mathrm{cm}(\mathrm{Hz})^{1/2}/\mathrm{W} \tag{3}$$

and a high value of D^* denotes a sensitive detector. As for the NEP, the conditions of measurement of D^* must be specified. Thus (500°K, 400, 1) has the same meaning as previously, while D_λ^*(10 μm, 400, 1) would mean that the value of D^* refers to that obtained with a narrow-band source at $\lambda = 10\ \mu$m, chopped at 400 Hz in a bandwidth of 1 Hz. It should be noted that not all detectors have the A dependence on NEP implied by the definition of D^*. A more meaningful figure of merit for such detectors [the thermocouple detector limited by Johnson noise is an example (Smith *et al.*, 1968)] would be the NEP.

Low-noise infrared detectors may have the ultimate value of their D^* or D_λ^* set by the detection of radiation noise from the background environment surrounding the emitter. Simply stated this means that one cannot hope to detect emission from a blackbody source at temperature T superimposed on a background blackbody source also at temperature T. A detector whose performance is limited by the background operates in the BLIP mode. D^* in this mode will depend on the solid angle Ω from which the detector can accept background radiation. A detector D^{**} normalized

† Quite often the distinction between D and D^* is neglected and D^* is simply called the detectivity.

to this solid angle is defined as

$$D^{**} = D^*(\Omega/2\pi)$$

where Ω is measured in steradians.

3.2.3 Responsivity

The responsivity R is defined as the ratio of the rms signal voltage V_S to the rms power incident on the detector, i.e.,

$$R = V_S/FA$$

This quantity can be rewritten in terms of D^* as

$$R_{BB} = D^* V_N/(A\ \Delta f)^{1/2} \tag{4}$$

where

$$R_{BB} = \int_0^\infty R_\lambda\, d\lambda$$

with

$$R_\lambda = V_S/F_\lambda A$$

where F_λ is the radiant power per cm^2 from a blackbody source at wavelength λ. In general, the responsivity will be a function of the chopping frequency in a test situation and the length of the radiation pulse to be measured in the detection of pulsed laser outputs. A full discussion of the dependence of R on chopping frequency can be found in the book by Heard (1968).

3.3 SOURCES OF NOISE IN DETECTORS

Even ideal detectors, that is, detectors that ideally approximate the ultimate performance of a particular detector type, cannot hope to circumvent some basic laws of physics and so have zero noise. In this section we will examine some fundamental sources of noise in detector systems.

3.3.1 Thermal Fluctuations

Consider a small detector element that exchanges energy with its environment to maintain a temperature T. If the heat capacity of the element is C, then a small change in thermal energy stored in the element will be accompanied by a temperature change ΔT:

$$\Delta E = C\ \Delta T$$

A fundamental theorem in statistical mechanics states that the mean square fluctuation in E due to the random nature of energy exchange between the element and its surroundings also at temperature T will be

$$\overline{\Delta E^2} = kT^2C$$

Then the mean squared temperature fluctuation due to this uncertainty in ΔE is given by

$$\overline{\Delta T^2} = kT^2/C$$

and thus the temperature is known only to within the uncertainty $[(\overline{\Delta T^2})]^{1/2}$. Any parameter of the detector that depends on temperature will be subject to fluctuations induced by this varying temperature. For example, the radiative flux emitted by the element will fluctuate, while fluxes emitted from sources to be detected will also fluctuate. For a detector at temperature T_1 exposed to a source at temperature T_2 the fluctuation in the total power absorbed and emitted by the detector element will be (Smith *et al.*, 1968)

$$\overline{\Delta W_{\mathrm{T}}^2} = 8k\epsilon\sigma A(T_1^5 + T_2^5)\ \Delta\nu$$

where ϵ is the emissivity of the detector, σ the Stefan–Boltzmann constant, and $\Delta\nu$ the bandwidth. The ultimate sensivity of detectors is then fundamentally limited by this uncertainty in incident/radiated power. For photodetectors this fluctuation is manifested as a fluctuation in the arrival rate of photons, and for thermal detectors as a variation in the flux at the surface of the detector.

3.3.2 Johnson or Nyquist Noise

The random motion of charges within a conductor does not assure a perfectly uniform distribution of charge within the conductor at all instants of time. If the voltage is measured across a conductor with a sensitive low-noise voltmeter, it will be found that, although the average voltage is zero, time-dependent voltages will be measured. The mean square value of this induced emf is

$$\overline{v^2} = 4kTR\ \Delta\nu$$

where R is resistance. It can be seen that this voltage is independent of frequency (measuring it, of course, introduces a bandwidth $\Delta\nu$) and vanishes only at $T = 0°\mathrm{K}$. Detailed considerations show that the Johnson noise voltage should start to depend on frequency only for frequencies $\nu > kT/h$. Thus, in most systems of interest the Johnson noise voltage can be considered independent of frequency. At room temperature (300°K)

$$(\overline{v^2})^{1/2} \simeq 1.3 \times 10^{-10}(R\ \Delta\nu)^{1/2} \tag{5}$$

3.3.3 Noise in Semiconductors

A variety of processes that lead to noise in semiconductor detectors have been found. Generation–recombination (GR) noise involves a fluctuation in the density of electrons and holes. It arises because electron–hole pairs are being continuously generated thermally and later recombine. There is no fundamental reason why the total number of current carriers should be absolutely constant with time because of the random nature of the generation and recombination processes. GR noise is apparent only when the semiconductor is carrying a current. GR noise (expressed as an rms voltage) is approximately independent of frequency for frequencies $<1/(2\pi\tau)$, where τ is the recombination lifetime for electron–hole pairs. Above this frequency GR noise decreases.

Current noise, which is similar to flicker or $1/f$ noise in vacuum tubes, dominates the noise spectrum of semiconductors at low frequencies. Smith *et al.* (1968) report that the rms current noise voltage is given by the approximate expression

$$(\overline{v_c^2})^{1/2} \simeq \text{const} \times [i^x/f^y] (\Delta f)^{1/2} \tag{6}$$

where x is usually $\simeq 2$, while $y \simeq 1$, and i is current.

Contact noise arises in the connections made to the semiconductor. It is dependent on current and is important at low frequencies.

Modulation noise occurs in semiconductors because current carriers can be momentarily trapped before recombining. While trapped these carriers no longer contribute to the observed current. Carriers disappearing into traps and subsequently reappearing give rise to a fluctuation in the carrier density and hence to the current carried by the semiconductor. Modulation noise is important at low frequencies and increases with the current.

In addition to these sources of noise, semiconductors are also subject to Johnson noise (which dominates the high-frequency noise spectrum) and, of course, to radiative fluctuations.

These and other sources of noise in detecting elements have been fully discussed in the work of Oliver (1965), Fleck (1966), Heard (1968), and Smith *et al.* (1968).

3.4 TYPES OF INFRARED DETECTORS

Detectors in general can be subdivided into two types: (i) thermal detectors, and (ii) quantum detectors. Thermal detectors respond only to the intensity of the incident radiation. Incident radiation is absorbed and converted into heat, which in turn produces some change in the properties of the detecting element. This change is measured to give an output proportional to the absorbed radiative intensity. It is important to note that no information can be obtained from this output concerning the discrete quantized nature of the radiation field.

Photon or quantum detectors respond to the rate at which photons arrive at the detector surface. A threshold photon energy must be exceeded before such a detector will respond to a given radiative flux. The quantum detector can count the number of photons received. The thermal detector only measures the energy deposited by these photons in a given period of time.

The result of this fundamental difference in detection mechanism can be immediately seen in the wavelength response of the two types of detector. Quantum detectors respond to only a limited range of wavelengths; thermal detectors (in principle) respond equally well to all wavelengths.

3.4.1 Thermocouple and Thermopile Devices

Historically, thermocouples were used to detect radiation as early as 1833. In its most elementary form, the thermocouple detector is simply a junction directly exposed to the flux from a radiation source. A more reliable and rugged configuration has the radiation incident on a thin foil whose temperature rise is monitored by the thermocouple. Design criteria for this sort of device are given by Smith *et al.* (1968). The conventional form of radiation thermocouple or thermopile detector is rarely used in laser studies because of its low power handling capabilities (mW/cm^2) and relatively long response time (msec). Thin film devices have, however, been reported (Day *et al.*, 1968) and the response time of these can be small. Day *et al.* formed a 1000-Å thick bismuth–silver thermocouple by vacuum deposition on a beryllium oxide substrate. The response time of this device was found to be $\simeq 10^{-7}$ sec, the *NEP* was 1.5×10^{-7} $W/Hz^{1/2}$ at 10 μm, and the responsivity (also at 10 μm) was $\simeq 4$ $\mu V/W$. Very fast response times are possible since the penetration of radiation into thin films bypasses the need for heat transfer via conduction that is dominant in conventional thermocouple detectors.

Jacobs (1971) has described a simple power meter that is suitable for measuring cw CO_2 laser powers in the 0.05–2.0 W range. A conventional carbon resistor is filed down flat on each side of its long dimension. One side is coated with an infrared blackening material, while a thermocouple is attached to the other side. The temperature rise produced by cw laser radiation incident on the blackened side yields a thermocouple voltage that can be duplicated by passing a known current through the resistor. In this way a direct comparison can be obtained between the absorbed laser power and electrical power dissipated in the resistor. Obviously such a detector is suitable only for measuring low cw laser powers.

Radiation trapping and the damage threshold can be increased by directing incident radiation into the entrance of a cone. If the cone is coated with absorbing material then multiple reflection of the incident beam will cause almost complete absorption of the incident radiation. The temperature of the walls of the cone can then be monitored with a thermocouple to obtain an estimate of the total energy absorbed. Such a device will integrate the energy in a short pulse and is called a ballistic thermopile or a cone calorimeter. Practical limitations involved in the measurement of high-power CO_2 laser pulses include a tendency for the surface of the cone to be damaged by incident radiation and the possibility that a breakdown plasma may be formed at the tip of the cone. This means that the incident beam must usually be attenuated to prevent damage to the cone and therefore that the measurement of laser energy is subjected to another possible source of error. Even in the absence of damage the effective reflectivity of cone calorimeters is often much larger at 10 μm than in the visible region of the spectrum (Preston, 1972).

Various methods have been developed to promote more effective radiation trapping and to minimize surface damage. Some devices that have been reported in the literature are shown schematically in Fig. 3.1. In the system of Stearn (1967) heat is conducted away from the absorbing cone, producing a temperature rise in the thermopile located toward the heat sink. The system is calibrated by dissipating a known power in the attached heater. Output voltage versus input power is found to be linear in the range 1–10 W.

Wilson (1969) focuses the laser output through a small hole in a spherical shell of low thermal capacity. The shell then acts as a blackbody absorber. To ensure that the incident beam is well spread out over the internal surface of the sphere, a short-focal-length lens must be used. This produces very high optical fields at the entrance hole and gas breakdown can occur unless the system pressure is reduced to several Torr.

Kellock (1969) has used a calorimeter similar to that shown in Fig. 3.1b to measure cw CO_2 laser powers in the range 1 W–1 kW. In this system a hollow sphere is cooled by a coil wound around the outside and the laser power is obtained from a measurement of the difference in inlet and outlet water temperatures. A heating element provides calibration. The system operates at atmospheric pressure.

The third calorimeter shown in Fig. 3.1c was developed by Gunn (1972) to measure the energy contained in high peak power CO_2 laser pulses. A hollow copper tube was coated with a thin layer of nickel and then polished o give a reflectivity $\simeq$0.9 at the CO_2 laser wavelength. The length of the tube was adjusted to be several times greater than the attenuation length for 10.6-μm radiation within the tube, so that effective total absorption of the incident radiation occurred. Calibration was by means of a heater wound around the outside of the tube and a precision of 0.1% in the energy measurement at large energy was reported. No damage to the surface of the absorber was evident with 0.5-J/cm^2 pulses of 100-nsec duration.

A cone calorimeter in which the rear surface of the cone is in direct contact with cooling water forms the basis for a reliable commercial cw power meter capable of handling cw CO_2 laser powers of up to 1 kW (Coherent Radiation Laboratories Model 213). In this system, thermocouples measure the temperature difference between the input and output water flows. The response time can be $<$1 sec. An elementary power meter of this sort was escribed by Rigden and Moeller (1966).

A calorimeter designed to measure the power in a laser beam of large oss section has been reported by Jennings and West (1970). A flat metallic sk coated with an absorbing layer is connected to a convectively cooled at sink by means of a thin-walled conducting tube. The temperature of is tube is measured at the end close to the disk by a series of thermouples whose reference junctions are connected to the heat sink. An elecical heater permits simulation of the laser flux and calibration of the stem. The device described by Jennings and West was capable of measurg cw laser powers in the range 1–30 W with an accuracy of 2.5%. Scaling higher cw powers and measurement of the average power of repetitively ilsed lasers was indicated. Beams up to 5.5 cm in diameter could be acmmodated. Absorption of 10.6-μm radiation in gaseous SF_6 forms the asis for another large aperture calorimeter (Reichelt *et al.*, 1974) used to easure the energy in nsec pulses having energies in the 100-J range.

An even simpler version of the disk calorimeter has been reported by Boulanger *et al.* (1973) to be useful for the measurement of the energy in pulses from a TEA CO_2 laser. This device is shown in Fig. 3.1d. 10-μm radiation is absorbed on one of the plexiglass sheets and the energy transferred to the underlying copper plate produces a temperature rise that is compared to the temperature of the reference plate. Pulse energies of 0.1–15 J could be measured at intensities of up to 20 mW/cm^2 without damage. Operation at intensities of up to 80 mW/cm^2 was possible using Makrolon instead of plexiglass. Accuracy of the energy measurement was reported to be 5%.

Jacob *et al.* (1973) have developed a similar system in which incident radiation is absorbed on the anodized surface of an aluminum plate. The thickness of the anodized layer (of Al_2O_3) was $\simeq 2.5 \times 10^{-4}$ cm. Heat

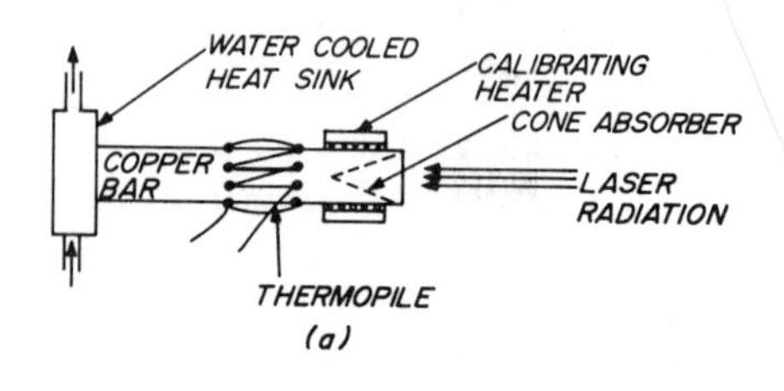

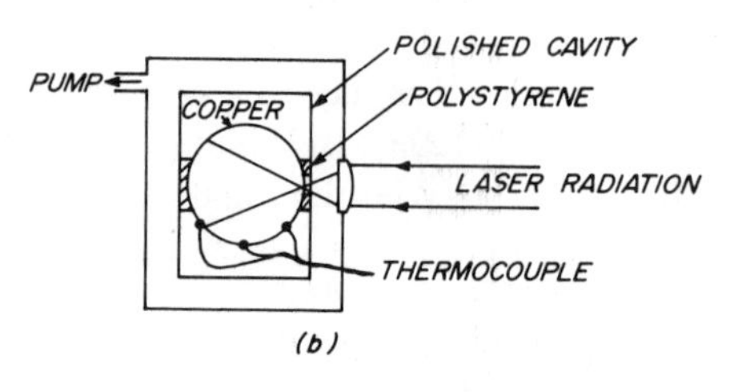

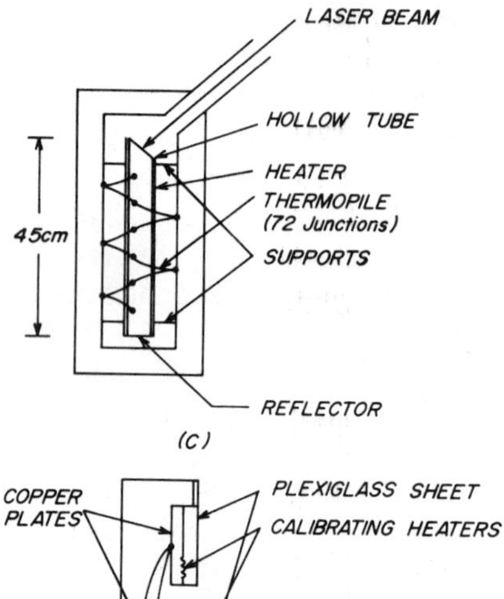

Fig. 3.1. (a) Calorimeter for measuring cw CO_2 laser power (Stearn, 19
Calorimeter for measuring the integrated energy in a laser pulse (Wilson, 1969).
lar calorimeter for high-power laser pulses (Gunn, 1972). (d) Calorimeter for
CO_2 laser pulses (Boulanger *et al.*, 1973).

transfer in this device can be defined in terms of two time constants

$$\tau_1 \simeq l_1^2\rho_1C_1/4K_1, \qquad \text{and} \qquad \tau_2 \simeq l_2^2\rho_2C_2/4K_2 \tag{7}$$

where τ_1 and τ_2 are the times for heat diffusion through the aluminum plate and the anodized layer, respectively, l is the thickness, ρ the density, C the specific heat, and K the thermal conductivity. With $l_1 = 0.32$ cm and $l_2 = 2.5 \times 10^{-4}$ cm, $\tau_1 \simeq 0.03$ sec and $\tau_2 \simeq 10^{-7}$ sec. τ_2 may be even smaller because of radiation penetration into the thin Al_2O_3 layer. When the laser pulse length $\tau_p > \tau_2$ (i.e., $\tau_p \gtrsim 10^{-6}$ sec) the maximum allowable energy flux (J/cm^2) is limited by the melting point of the aluminum plate (T_m = 660°C). Then

$$E_{max} \simeq 600(\pi\rho_1C_1K_1\tau_p)^{1/2} \tag{8}$$

or about 2.5 J/cm^2 for a 1-μsec pulse length. Convective and radiative energy losses are important only for times $>10^{-5}$ sec.

When the pulse length $\tau_p < 10^{-7}$ sec, heat is not transferred away from the Al_2O_3 surface and the limiting energy is determined by that which produces melting of Al_2O_3 ($T_m \simeq$ 2300°C). In this case,

$$E_{max} \simeq 2300(\pi\rho_2C_2K_2\tau_p)^{1/2} \tag{9}$$

and the surface should be affected when $E = 88$ mJ/cm^2 in a 1-nsec pulse.

It was found that the maximum energy flux predicted from Eq. (8) was somewhat optimistic; ablation was noted when $E \simeq 3$ J/cm^2 in a pulse with $\tau_p = 20$ μsec. A useful feature of this calorimeter is that the temperature distribution can be calculated fairly accurately. Since the Al_2O_3 surface was found to absorb more than 95% of the incident radiation, the measured temperature can be related to the absolute laser energy without the need for additional calibration.

A calorimeter designed to measure total laser energies of 3×10^4–10^7 J has been reported by Smith *et al.* (1972). The cw CO_2 laser powers that could be dissipated in this device ranged up to 10^5 W. The calibration factor was 2.267×10^6 J/V and the maximum average temperature rise produced for a 1-V output would be ≃12°C.

Some discussion of the design criteria for laser calorimeters is given by West and Churney (1970). Further instruments are described by Preston (1971), Neill (1971), Zakurenko *et al.* (1971), Buchl and Pfeiffer (1972), and West *et al.* (1972).

3.4.2 The Bolometer

The heating effect of infrared radiation can also be used to effect a change in the resistance of a metal or semiconductor. In the infrared bolometer type of detector, this change in resistance is measured and can be related to the absorbed incident radiation. Usually the resistive element to be exposed to the incident radiation is placed in a bridge circuit with an identical element that is not exposed to radiation. This helps to compensate for ambient temperature variations and local noise sources. Conventional infrared bolometers are not usually suitable as detectors for infrared radiation because of their low damage threshold powers and long response times. A number of specialized bolometers suitable for measuring laser outputs in the infrared have therefore been developed.

The thin-film bolometers described by Contreras and Gaddy (1970) and shown schematically in Fig. 3.2 were found to have a response time of less than 15 nsec and an *NEP* of $\simeq 10^{-6}$ W/(Hz)$^{1/2}$ for 10.6-μm radiation. Optimum film thickness was $\simeq$1000 Å and the maximum responsivity could be as high as 5×10^{-4} V/W. One advantage, of course, is that these devices operate at room temperature. A thin-film bolometer using V_2O_5 as the resistive element has been reported by Koren *et al.* (1973). Later studies by Contreras and Gaddy (1971) showed that thin-film bolometers can be used in heterodyne detection at 10.6 μm. The minimum detectable power in this case was 4×10^{-11} W/Hz.

Stricker and Rom (1972) have reported measurements of pulsed laser outputs at 10.6 μm using the thin-film bolometer shown in Fig. 3.2b. Radiation is absorbed in a glass light trap, which has a thin-film electrode of platinum wound in a spiral inside the trap. This electrode is in a bridge circuit whose output is monitored with a differential amplifier. In the

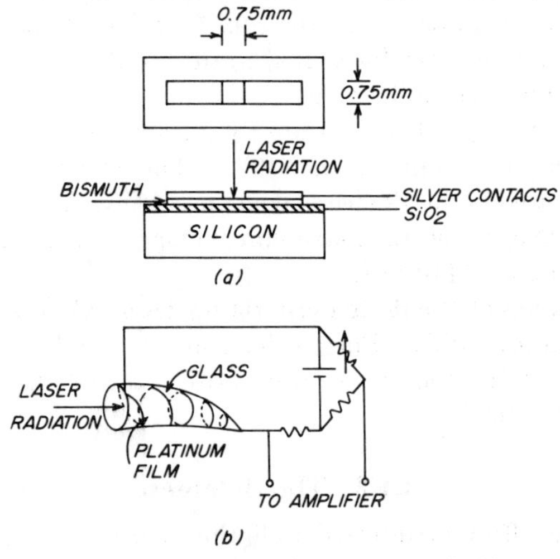

Fig. 3.2. (a) Thin-film bolometer (after Contreras and Gaddy, 1970). (b) Light trap bolometer of Stricker and Rom (1972).

range where the resistance $R(t)$ is linearly related to $T(t)$ and $V(t)$ is proportional to $R(t)$, where $V(t)$ is the output voltage, the time-dependent power delivered to the device is

$$P(t) = \Gamma\left[\frac{V(t)}{2t^{1/2}} + \frac{1}{2\pi t^{1/2}} \int_0^t \frac{\tau^{1/2}V(t) - t^{1/2}V(\tau)}{(t-\tau)^{3/2}}\, d\tau\right] \tag{10}$$

where Γ is a calibration constant that can be obtained by exposing the detector to a known CO_2 laser flux for a specific time, and $P(t)$ is in watts. Stricker and Rom found that this gauge was linear for exposure times up to $\simeq$20 msec and input energies $\simeq$100 J. The response time of the gauge was <1 μsec.

Effective absorption of incident laser power can also be obtained by passing the incident beam into an enclosure containing a tangle of insulated wire. Devices of this sort are known as "rat's-nest" calorimeters. The change in resistance of the wire is monitored in an external circuit and can be related to incident laser power. Calibration is obtained by passing a known current pulse through the tangled conductor. Rat's nest calorimeters have been developed by Baker (1963) and Schmidt and Greenhow (1969) and in modified form by Schmidt and Greenhow (1969) and Farmer (1971). Damage to the insulation on the wires usually limits operation to the measurement of energy fluxes of less than several J/cm^2.

A simple method of measuring cw CO_2 laser powers using an elementary bolometer has been described by Siekman and Morijn (1968b). A thin wire is oriented perpendicular to the output beam passing through the center of the beam. This wire absorbs a small fraction of the incident power and changes its resistance. The change in resistance can be related to the cw laser power.

3.4.3 Pyroelectric Detectors

Some materials have a permanent electrical polarization that is a strong function of temperature. If a material of this sort is cleaved in a plane perpendicular to the direction of polarization, then this plane will contain a charge. Normally this charge will not be observable under static conditions because the surface charge becomes neutralized due to the presence of stray charges of opposite sign. If, however, the temperature of the crystal is changed rapidly, the polarization will change because of an alteration in the lattice constant. The neutralizing surface charges are not able to follow this change and a net temperature-dependent surface charge will be detected. Crystals that exhibit this effect are said to be pyroelectric. Some examples are barium titanate, tourmaline, triglycine sulfate (TGS),

Rochelle salt, lithium sulfate, and $Sr_{1-x}Ba_xNb_2O_6$ (SBN). Many other pyroelectric crystals are known (Cady, 1946; Mason, 1966). The use of pyroelectric crystals to detect infrared radiation was suggested as early as 1938 by Yeou Ta (1938). Subsequent work by Cooper (1962a,b) and by Hadni *et al.* (1965) demonstrated the feasibility of pyroelectric detection. The first use of pyroelectric detectors to monitor the output of CO_2 lasers was reported by Shimazu *et al.* (1967) and by Duley (1967). Pyroelectric detectors offer the advantages of room temperature operation, fast response times, small size, and ruggedness.

Figure 3.3a shows one mode of operation of the pyroelectric detector. Electrodes each of area A are coated on planes perpendicular to the polarization vector $\bar{P}$ and radiation is absorbed by the crystal in the plane shown, which contains $\bar{P}$. If a resistance $R < R'$ (the leakage resistance of the crystal) is placed across the two electrodes, then a voltage

$$V(t) = AR\, dP/dt = AR\, (dP/dT)\, dT/dt \tag{11}$$

will be measured across this resistance. This output voltage is seen to depend on the rate of change of polarization with temperature γ $(= dP/dT)$ and the rate of change of temperature. γ is called the pyroelectric coefficient and it is evident that a large γ is desirable. Figures of merit for this type of detector are, however, difficult to define [see Putley (1971) for a discussion], since different noise mechanisms are important in different modes of operation. One useful figure is the ratio $\gamma/\rho c$, where ρc is the specific heat of the crystal in J/cm^3. Table 3.1 lists some pyroelectric detector materials and compares values of this ratio.

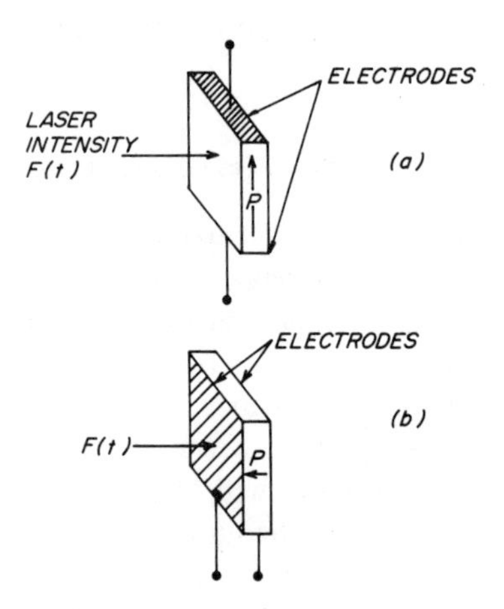

Fig. 3.3. (a) Edge electrode structure. (b) Face electrode structure for pyroelectric detectors.

Table 3.1

Some Pyroelectric Materials and Values of the Ratio $\gamma/\rho c$, Which Gives a Rough Measure of Expected Performance in Infrared Detector Applications[a]

Material	Curie temperature (°K)	$\gamma/\rho c$ (μC-cm/J)
$BaTiO_2$	399	1.7×10^{-2}
TGS	322	1.2–1.5×10^{-2}
TGS/TGSe	320	1.6–2.0×10^{-2}
SBN	333	5.3×10^{-2}
$Li_2SO_4H_2O$		0.36×10^{-2}
$LiNbO_3$	1573	0.14×10^{-2}
$NaNO_2$	437	0.2×10^{-2}
PVF[b]		0.4×10^{-3}
LZT[c]	543	0.8×10^{-2}
$PbTiO_2$	743	0.8×10^{-2}

[a] After Glass (1969), Putley (1971), Phelan *et al.* (1971), Cooper (1962a), and Yamaka *et al.* (1971).
[b] Polyvinyl fluoride (Phelan *et al.*, 1971).
[c] Lead zirconate titanate.

Glass (1968) found that the ferroelectric crystals $Sr_{1-x}Ba_xNb_2O_6$ with $x \simeq 0.25$–0.52 could be fabricated into detectors with response times <30 nsec. The responsivity at low frequencies was 2.5×10^4 V/W when the electrode configuration shown in Fig. 3.3a was used and 50 V/W when the electrode configuration was as shown in Fig. 3.3b. Sarjeant *et al.* (1971) fabricated detectors from 5-mm cubes of TGS with an electrode structure as in Fig. 3.3a that had an *NEP* of $<2 \times 10^{-8}$ W/(Hz)$^{1/2}$ and a low-frequency responsivity of 120 V/W when shunted with a 10^{10}-Ω resistor. The responsivity was virtually independent of wavelength in the range 1–4000 μm. A cross-sectional view of such a detector and its associated circuit is shown in Fig. 3.4. This type of detector is capable of handling high average laser powers. TGS crystals suitable for detector applications can easily be grown in the laboratory (Duley and Finnigan, 1973). Lock (1971) has demonstrated that doping with α-alanine lowers the Johnson noise due to the resistivity of a given element and ensures that maximum polarization is obtained. An *NEP* of 2.5×10^{-11} W/(Hz)$^{1/2}$ was possible with a detector using doped TGS.

The TGS detectors developed by Schwarz and Poole (1970) at the Barnes Engineering Co. have a $D^*(2$–$100\ \mu\text{m}, 1\ \text{kHz}, 1) \simeq 1.5 \times 10^8$ cm-

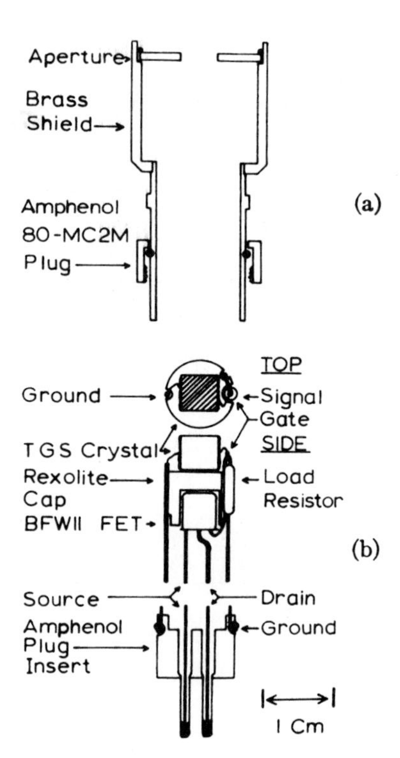

Fig. 3.4. Compact pyroelectric detector and associated circuit (Sarjeant *et al.*, 1971). (a) Case, (b) detector element with electrical connections.

$Hz^{1/2}/W$. The low-frequency detectivity $D^* \simeq 10^9$ cm-$(Hz)^{1/2}/W$ is only a little more than a factor of 10 below the photon noise limit for an ideal thermal detector viewing a 300°K background. The responsivity of these detectors was $\simeq 10^5$ V/W at 1 Hz, decreasing to $\simeq 10^2$ V/W at 1 kHz.

An enhancement of the responsivity of TGS pyroelectric detectors due to the excitation of mechanical resonances of the detector element has been reported by Ozeki and Saito (1972). Bartoli *et al.* (1973) have studied the damage produced in TGS crystals by intense laser radiation.

The fastest rise time that appears to have been reported to date was measured by Roundy and Byer (1972). Using a $LiTaO_3$ detector to detect pulses from a *Q*-switched mode-locked Nd : YAG laser at 1.06 μm a 10–90% rise time of 500 psec was observed.

Phelan *et al.* (1971) have investigated the properties of polyvinyl fluoride (PVF) plastic films as infrared detector materials. The D^* for a detector configuration as shown in Fig. 3.3b is

$$D^* = (\epsilon\gamma/\rho CL)(A/G)^{1/2}(1/4kT)^{1/2} \tag{12}$$

where ϵ is the fraction of incident power absorbed, L the distance between the electrodes, G the ac shunt conductivity, and T the temperature in °K. D^*'s as high as 3×10^8 cm-(Hz)$^{1/2}$/W for a 500°K blackbody source, modulated at 1 Hz, and a 1-Hz bandwidth were obtained. The D^* decreased with modulation frequency to $\simeq 5 \times 10^6$ cm-(Hz)$^{1/2}$/W at 1 kHz. This sort of detector lends itself quite well to scaling to large aperture devices. Further work on PVF and polyvinylidiene fluoride (PVF_2) films as detector elements has been reported by Bergman *et al.* (1971), Glass *et al.* (1971), and Phelan and Cook (1973). Day *et al.* (1974) in a study of PVF_2 detectors conclude that plastic pyroelectric detectors may be capable of having low-frequency D^*'s that are higher than those of crystalline materials. High values of D^* may be possible even in large-area detectors if particular care is paid to fabrication and poling.

Optical heterodyne detection with pyroelectric detectors was first reported by Leiba (1969) and later by Abrams and Glass (1969). With an SBN detector, the minimum detectable power at 10.6 μm was observed to be 1.5×10^{-11} W/Hz under conditions where the intermediate frequency was 1 MHz and the local oscillator power was 1 W. The question of the advantages of heterodyne detection will be discussed more fully in a later section of this chapter.

The pyroelectric effect is the basis for a very versatile calorimeter that measures the total energy of single high-power CO_2 laser pulses (Astheimer and Buckley, 1967; LaChambre, 1971). Devices of this sort are shown schematically in Fig. 3.5. When the duration of the incident light pulse is much less than the thermal and electrical time constants of the detecting element, the output voltage is predicted to be (LaChambre, 1971)

$$V(t) = \frac{\gamma}{\rho c \epsilon} \left(\frac{e^{-t/\tau} - (\tau/RC) e^{-t/RC}}{1 - \tau/RC} \right) \int_0^t F(t)\, dt \tag{13}$$

where ϵ is the dielectric constant of the pyroelectric detector, C its capacitance, R the shunt resistance, and τ the thermal time constant

$$\tau = \rho c l^2 / 2K$$

where K is the thermal conductivity of the detector material, and l its thickness. The detector element in LaChambre's calorimeter was lead zirconate titanate ceramic. It was found that this device gave a linear response to incident pulse energy up to an energy of 2 J. However, detectors of this sort must be calibrated using known radiation standards, since the calculated response is often not achieved in practice. Nowicki (1971) has reported a calorimeter utilizing barium titanate, which can be calibrated electrically.

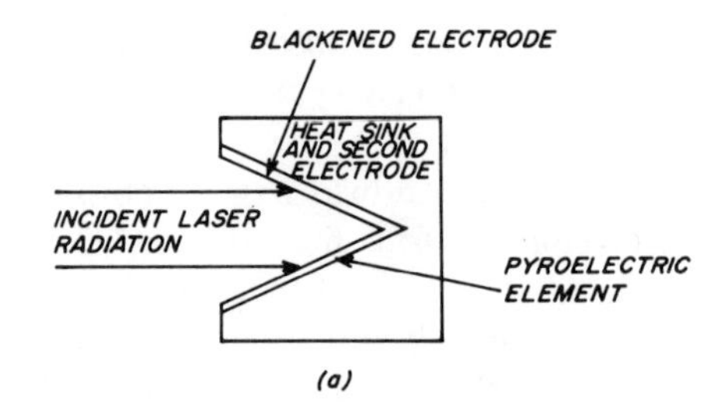

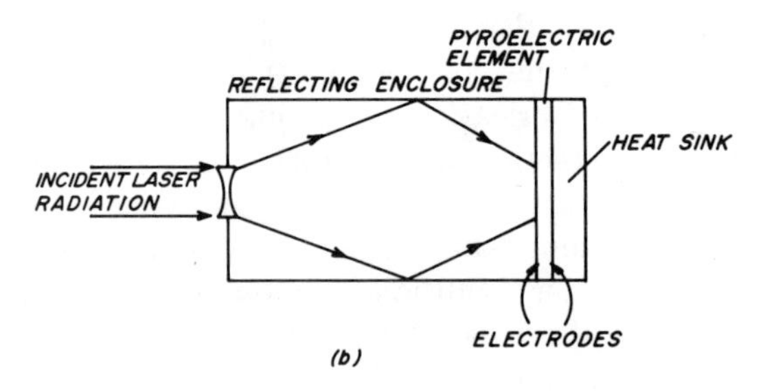

Fig. 3.5. Pyroelectric energy meters, (a) after Astheimer and Buckley (1967), (b) after LaChambre (1971).

Because of the importance of pyroelectric detectors in monitoring the output of CO_2 lasers, it is worthwhile investigating the response of a pyroelectric element to a time-dependent radiative flux in a little more detail. Suppose that the pyroelectric element is exposed to a radiative flux $F(t) = F_\omega e^{j\omega t}$; then the change in temperature of the device will be modulated at the frequency ω. The expression for $\Delta T(\omega)$ is (Cooper, 1962a)

$$\Delta T(\omega) = F_\omega / G(1 + j\omega\tau_\mathrm{T}) \tag{14}$$

where $\tau_\mathrm{T} = c'/G$ and c' is the thermal capacitance of the detector, while G is the thermal conductance connecting the detector to a heat sink and τ_T the thermal time constant of the detector. The voltage output from the detector will be

$$V = V_\mathrm{S}/(1 + 1/j\omega\tau_\mathrm{e}) \tag{15}$$

where $\tau_\mathrm{e} = R''C$ is the electrical time constant, with R'' the total shunt resistance and C the capacitance of the detector. $V_\mathrm{S} = \gamma A \, \Delta T(\omega)/C$. The equivalent circuit is shown in Fig. 3.6. V_S will therefore decrease with increasing frequency as $1/f$ ($f = \omega/2\pi$) for $\omega > \tau_\mathrm{T}^{-1}$. At the same time, the term $(1 + 1/j\omega\tau_\mathrm{e})$ will increase for frequencies up to $\omega \simeq \tau_\mathrm{e}^{-1}$ and then

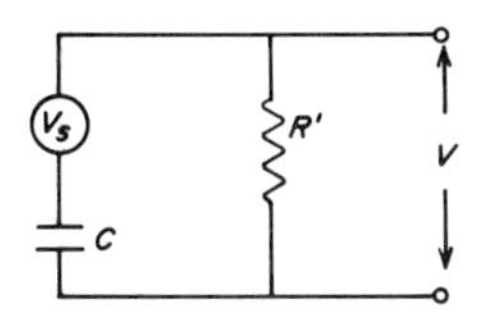

Fig. 3.6. Equivalent circuit of pyroelectric detector. C is the capacitance of detector, and R' its internal resistance.

will be independent of frequency for $\omega > \tau_e^{-1}$. At low frequencies $(1 + 1/j\omega\tau_e)^{-1} \propto f$, and hence the frequency dependence of this term will cancel that of V_S for frequencies between τ_T^{-1} and τ_e^{-1}. Since τ_T can be made very large ($\gtrsim 1$ sec) while τ_e depends only on R'' and C and thus can be made small, the voltage output from the detector can be made independent of frequency over many decades. A theoretical response curve is shown in Fig. 3.7. This figure shows that a linear response may be obtained over a wide frequency range simply by lowering the shunt resistance across the detector. On the other hand, if a high response is needed the resistance can be increased. This enhanced response will be accompanied by a decrease in the dynamic range over which the detector responds linearly.

The two electrode configurations shown previously are seen to have different capacities and different effective areas and hence will have different responsivities. The edge electrode structure will, in general, have higher responsivity than that of the face electrode structure, provided the ca-

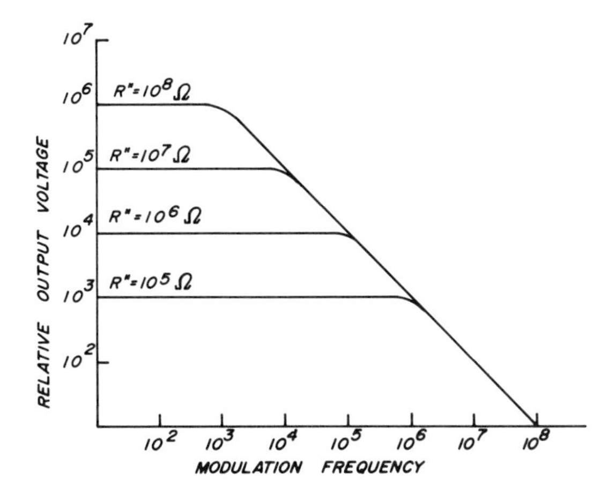

Fig. 3.7. Output voltage vs. frequency for a hypothetical pyroelectric detector with $C = 10$ pf and $\tau_T > 0.1$ sec.

pacity of the edge electrode capacitor is large enough to exceed stray circuit capacitances. This prediction was verified by Glass (1968).

The dominant source of noise in pyroelectric detectors at frequencies up to the electrical cut-off frequency is due to the Johnson noise associated with the internal resistance of the detector. In the region between τ_T^{-1} and τ_e^{-1} the *NEP* will be independent of frequency when Johnson noise dominates. For frequencies exceeding τ_e^{-1}, the *NEP* will continue to be constant since both V and the Johnson noise decrease together as $1/f$. A frequency will be reached, however, at which the noise associated with the amplifier exceeds the Johnson noise in the detector. For frequencies above this, the *NEP* will increase with f.

Further theoretical descriptions of the mechanisms involved in pyroelectric detection can be found in Cooper (1962a,b), Doyle (1970), Blackburn and Wright (1970), and Putley (1970, 1971). The response of a pyroelectric detector to repetitive pulses from a CO_2 laser has been discussed by Shaulov and Simhony (1972).

A novel application of pyroelectric crystals to optical gating has recently been reported by Glass and Negran (1974).

3.4.4 Some Other Thermal Detectors

Liquid crystals are a group of cholesteric compounds that undergo a change in structure over a very narrow temperature range. Structural changes are accompanied by a change in the wavelength of light reflected from the surface of the crystal. Thus, under appropriate conditions, the absorption of a small heat flux in a thin liquid-crystal layer will yield a significant change in optical properties. Monitoring this change either as a function of time at a particular point on the surface of the crystal or as a function of position across the crystal provides detailed information on the spatial and temporal evolution of an applied heat source. Application of the liquid-crystal effect in the monitoring of infrared laser radiation has been reported by Keilmann (1970) and by Tolmachev and Kuz'michev (1971). The system used by Keilmann is shown in Fig. 3.8. A liquid-crystal layer applied to the surface of a thin plexiglass sheet is biased at the optimum temperature for structural changes, i.e., the temperature at which the highest sensitivity with respect to small changes in incident intensity is observed. The variation in color across the liquid-crystal surface denotes the temperature distribution and hence, for absorption in a thin layer, the spatial distribution of incident laser intensity. In the experiment described by Keilmann the liquid crystal was used to display infrared interferograms of an arc jet plasma. The time constant for the approach to a steady state display pattern was 2 sec for an incident intensity of 50 mW/cm^2 at 10.6

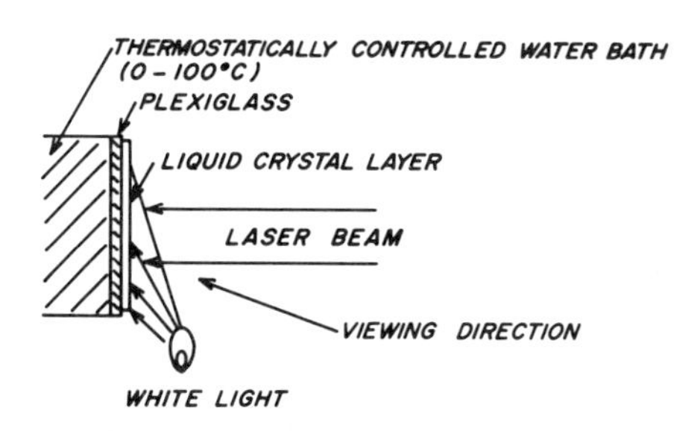

Fig. 3.8. Liquid-crystal beam monitor (after Keilmann, 1970).

μm, and in the limit <5 mW/cm^2 could be detected. There would seem to be no reason why the liquid-crystal display method could not be used for the visualization of spatial and temporal variations in the output of pulsed CO_2 lasers, with the ultimate time resolution perhaps extending to times as short as 1 μsec.

A wide variety of other materials have been used as heat detectors in the determination of the spatial distribution of radiation from pulsed and cw CO_2 lasers. In fact, almost any material that shows a controllable heating effect when exposed to 10.6-μm radiation can be used. As an example, one of the simplest ways of finding the distribution of intensity in high-power cw CO_2 laser beams is to melt a material such as foamed polystyrene using a range of beam energies (Meyerhofer, 1968a). The energy can be changed by varying the exposure time at constant laser output power. Since a certain threshold intensity is required for the production of damage, measurement of the locus $\bar{r}_m$ of minimum damage gives a locus of points in the intensity profile where the intensity is just equal to the threshold value for damage. Meyerhofer found that the threshold energy flux was 4.5 W-sec/cm^2 for 10.6-μm radiation incident on foamed polystyrene. The data are reduced by plotting the reciprocal of the total energy deposited in the target against $\bar{r}_m$. Resolution appears to be limited by the finite size of the bubbles in the polystyrene foam.

Stovell (1967) has used a thin asbestos sheet to examine the mode pattern in a cw CO_2 laser. At low laser powers, the sensitivity could be improved by heating the asbestos to bias it at a high temperature, where the differential heating due to the laser flux would be most noticeable.

Inaba *et al.* (1967) have demonstrated the feasibility of direct photography of the intensity distribution in a cw CO_2 laser beam using Kalver film. The film is first exposed to uv light in the 3400–4400 Å region and is then developed by the heating effect of absorbed laser radiation. For exposing in the uv, an energy flux of 0.2 W-sec/cm^2 is required at 43°C. Development occurs when the film is heated to 110°C for about 1 sec. An infrared laser intensity of about 0.12 W/cm^2 is needed to effect development.

Perhaps the most versatile method of studying the spatial variation of cw laser radiation involves the thermal quenching of visible luminescence from a ZnCdS phosphor excited continuously with uv light (McGee and Heilos, 1967; Bridges and Burkhardt, 1967; Condas and Brown, 1970). Suitable surfaces are prepared by coating a thin Mylar film with a lacquer containing the phosphor. The Mylar film is then backed by a massive aluminum heat sink. Irradiation with a 6-W "black light" produces a bright yellow fluorescence over the surface of the phosphor. This fluorescence is quenched in regions subjected to heating by the incident laser radiation, which then appear dark. The sensitivity was reported to be $\simeq$300 mW/cm^2 and the response time was $\simeq$0.1 sec (Bridges and Burkhardt, 1967). Units of this type are commercially available.

Two similar devices were later reported by Condas (1971). One system based on a phosphor of Zn_2SiO_4 : 0.5% Mn used the thermoluminescence induced by incident radiation to enhance the emission intensity in the irradiated region. In the other, heating produced a change in the wavelength of the emitted light.

An even simpler thermal detector useful for pulsed CO_2 lasers has been described by Robinson *et al.* (1971). In an application involving the determination of wavelengths emitted from a pulsed TEA laser, it was found that a graphite block placed at the exit plane of a spectrometer allowed visual observation of the oscillating wavelengths. Each laser line gave rise to a bright flash of visible radiation when dispersed and allowed to fall on the graphite block.

Laser calorimeters based on the evaporation of a known quantity of liquid nitrogen (Bayer and Schaack, 1969) and on the pressure change produced by the absorption of 10.6-μm radiation in a gas (Quel *et al.*, 1969) have also been reported in the literature.

Spinak *et al.* (1968) discuss the use of an infrared image convertor and a closed-circuit television system to view the mode distribution in a cw CO_2 laser.

3.4.5 The Photon Drag Detector

A novel detector for measuring the time dependence of high peak power CO_2 laser pulses based on the momentum transfer between photons and electrons and holes in a suitable semiconductor was first reported by Gibson *et al.* (1970) and Danishevskii *et al.* (1970). The momentum carried by a single photon is $h\nu/c$, where c is the speed of light. A flux of n photons/sec will carry momentum at the rate $nh\nu/c = P/c$, where P is the total power in the beam. When this beam is passed through an attenuating material and partially absorbed, the rate of momentum transfer to the absorbers per unit volume will be (for p-type material)

$$(P\alpha_h/Ac)\exp(-\alpha x)$$

where α is the absorption coefficient of the material, α_h the absorption coefficient due to holes, x the path length in the material, and A the cross-sectional area of the beam. In germanium and some other semiconductors, part of this absorption arises because of the presence of free carriers, which consequently receive momentum in the direction of the beam. Carriers are therefore swept or "dragged" along with the photon beam and an emf can be observed that opposes this motion. The field that opposes the electron motion can be estimated by equating the force produced on an electron by this field to its rate of change of momentum, i.e., for a p-type material

$$eE = (P\alpha_h/AcN)\exp(-\alpha x)$$

where E is the opposing field and N the density of free carriers. The open circuit voltage V_{oc} is obtained by integrating this expression over the length of the sample (Gibson *et al.*, 1970; Bishop *et al.*, 1973):

$$V_{oc} = (\mu r\alpha_h/c)\int_0^L F(x)\,dx$$

where $F(x) = P(x)/A$, $N_e = 1/r\mu$, μ is the mobility of the majority carrier, r the resistivity, and L the length of the rod:

$$F(x) = F(0)\exp[-(\alpha_p + \alpha_h)x]$$

where α_p is the absorption coefficient due to phonons. Integrating, one obtains

$$V_{oc} = \frac{F(0)\mu r}{c}\left(\frac{\alpha_h}{\alpha_h + \alpha_p}\right)\{1 - \exp[-(\alpha_p + \alpha_h)x]\} \qquad (16)$$

Values of the ratio V_{oc}/Pr (which is called the responsivity) were found (Gibson *et al.*, 1970) to lie in the range 10^{-6}–10^{-7} V/W-Ω-cm for n-type germanium with $N \simeq 10^{17}/\text{cm}^2$. The responsivity decreases with N as the electron concentration decreases, to become $\simeq 10^{-9}$ V/W-Ω-cm for $N \simeq 10^{14}/\text{cm}^3$. In p-type germanium with $r = 0.1$ Ω-cm, the responsivity is again 10^{-6}–10^{-7} V/W-Ω-cm. We see from Eq. (16) that the voltage output should be linearly dependent on incident laser intensity. In fact, the photon drag detector has a linear response over several orders of magnitude of $F(0)$, but a tendency has been observed for the response to exhibit nonlinearities at very high incident intensities (Kamibayashi *et al.*, 1973; Bishop *et al.*, 1973). This effect has been treated theoretically and experimentally by Bishop *et al.* (1973). Most detectors studied were found to be linear up to incident intensities of $\gtrsim 10$ MW/cm^2. The nonlinearities that exist above this intensity are due to a decrease in the absorption coefficient (Gibson *et al.*, 1972) and the resistivity due to a reduction in the hole density. However, Bishop *et al.* show that these effects may be taken into account using the simple theory given above modified to allow for the change in the absorption coefficient and the resistivity that occurs at high incident intensities. The complete expression for the open circuit voltage is

$$V_{\mathrm{oc}} = \frac{\mu r_0}{c} \alpha_0 \int_0^L \frac{F(x)[1 + F(x)/F_{\mathrm{s}}(r)]}{[1 + F(x)/F_{\mathrm{s}}]} dx \tag{17}$$

where α_0 is the absorption coefficient at low $F(0)$, r_0 the resistivity at low $F(0)$, and F_{s} the saturation intensity (usually $\simeq 10$ MW/cm^2). $F(x)$ is obtained from the expression

$$(\alpha_{\mathrm{p}} + \alpha_0)x = \ln\left[\frac{F(0)}{F(x)}\right] + \frac{\alpha_0}{\alpha_{\mathrm{p}}} \ln\left[\frac{\alpha_{\mathrm{p}} F(0) + F_{\mathrm{s}}(\alpha_0 + \alpha_{\mathrm{p}})}{\alpha_{\mathrm{p}} F(x) + F_{\mathrm{s}}(\alpha_0 + \alpha_{\mathrm{p}})}\right] \tag{18}$$

The photon drag detector, while having a low responsivity, is capable of extremely high-frequency response. It has been suggested (Kimmitt *et al.*, 1972) that the response time may be limited only by the time required for light to traverse the detector (<1 nsec). Table 3.2 lists the properties of some photon drag detectors developed by Kimmitt *et al.* (1972).

Photon drag detectors exhibiting higher sensitivity have been developed by Panyakeow *et al.* (1972) and Ribakovs and Gundjian (1974). These

Table 3.2

Response of Photon Drag Detectors[a]

Detector						
Diameter (cm)	Length (cm)	Resistivity (Ω-cm)	Responsivity[b] (μV/W)	Absorption (%)	Response time (nsec)	*NEP* (W/Hz$^{1/2}$)
0.5	2.0	20	100	25	<10	10[c]
1.0	2.0	20	25	25	<1	140[d]
2.5	3.0	25	6	30	<1	600[d]

[a] After Kimmitt *et al.* (1972). [b] With 100X amplifier. [c] For 10-nsec response.
[d] For 1-nsec response.

detectors use p-type tellurium instead of germanium. Increased sensitivity appears to be due in part to the higher absorption coefficient in tellurium at 10.6 μm. The band structure (Panyakeow *et al.*, 1972) also appears to be particularly advantageous in this material. A responsivity of 5×10^{-6} V/W was obtained by cooling the detector to 77°K. This value appears, however, to exceed considerably that expected from the theory as discussed by Ribakovs and Gundjian (1974).

The photon drag detector forms the basis of a method proposed by Patel (1971a) to detect subnanosecond 10.6-μm pulses. This experiment is shown schematically in Fig. 3.9. Since the photon drag process is a directional process, i.e., the momentum transfer vector and hence the polarity of the induced voltage depends on the direction in which light passes through the detector, pulses passing in opposite directions will give rise to voltage pulses of opposite polarity. Two short pulses that do not pass through the detector simultaneously will give the voltage pulses shown in Fig. 3.9b. When they coincide spatially while passing through, no output voltage will be seen (Fig. 3.9c). Patel suggests that the full-wave rectifier circuit shown in Fig. 3.9d should enable measurements of this overlap (or lack of overlap) to be made with a simple low-frequency voltmeter. When the pulses are rectified, two noncoincident pulses will add to give an output voltage (Fig. 3.9e) and a reading on the voltmeter. When they coincide, no voltage will be generated and the voltmeter will indicate a null. By changing the overlap between the pulses in the detector, the pulsewidth

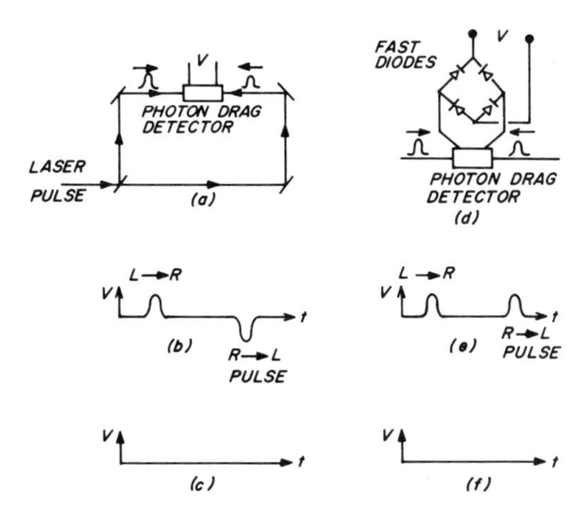

Fig. 3.9. System for measuring the profile of short pulses at 10.6 μm as suggested by Patel (1971a). (a) Experimental apparatus, (b) $V(t)$ for no pulse overlap in photon drag detector, (c) $V(t)$ for perfect overlap, (d) full-wave rectifier circuit, (e) $V(t)$ for no overlap, (f) $V(t)$ for overlap.

can be measured. Pulsewidths of <100 psec might be measured using this technique.

The above approach is not the only one suggested to overcome the difficulty of measuring psec pulses at 10.6-μm. Baumhacker *et al.* (1973) and Gibson *et al.* (1972) have proposed a method based on the optical Kerr effect in CS_2. Alcock and Walker (1973) have used infrared upconversion (Section 3.4.8) to visible light to detect nsec pulses at 10.6 μm.

3.4.6 Photoconductive and Photovoltaic Detectors

High-sensitivity photoconductive and photovoltaic detectors are available with wavelength responses throughout the near- and far-infrared regions of the spectrum. These detectors are all based on the generation of free carriers in semiconductor materials by the absorption of infrared photons and as such are exclusively photon- or quantum-type detectors. In photoconductive detectors operating in the vicinity of 10 μm a change in conductivity of a semiconductor is produced by the absorption of photons, which either transfer electrons from a donor level to the conduction band or from the valence band into low-lying acceptor levels. The long-wavelength cutoff for these devices depends on the energy difference between, in the first case, the donor level and the bottom of the conduction band, and in the second case, the top of the valence band and the acceptor level. Since this energy difference is only $\simeq$0.1 eV for a detector with a cutoff at $\lambda \simeq 10$ μm the detector must be cooled to a cryogenic temperature to avoid thermal population or depletion of the acceptor or donor levels. Typically, detectors of this sort are cooled to temperatures in the range 4–77°K. The need for liquid helium or liquid nitrogen coolants is to some extent a disadvantage and provides some limitation in the use of these detectors with CO_2 lasers.

Photovoltaic detectors generate a voltage when exposed to radiation by the creation of carriers in one material that diffuse across a junction formed between this material and another that is doped with different impurities. This charge separation produces a voltage across the junction. Two advantages of photovoltaic detectors are that usually no biasing is needed and that the resistance of the unbiased detector element is low so that they lend themselves to incorporation in high-speed circuitry. A disadvantage that the photovolatic detectors share with photoconductive devices is that they are easily damaged by intense laser radiation. Use of these detectors in the monitoring of high-power CO_2 lasers requires a provision for attenuating the incident radiative intensity.

Table 3.3 summarizes the performance of a number of photoconductive and photovoltaic detectors at a wavelength of 10 μm. It can be seen that

Table 3.3

Detectivity and Response Time of Photoconductive (PC) and Photovoltaic (PV) Detectors at a Wavelength of 10 μm

Detector	Type	D^* (10 μm)[a]	Response time (nsec)	Temperature (°K)	Cut-off wavelength[b] (μm)	Reference
Ge:Au	PC	6×10^8 (900)	$<10^3$	65	6.9	Heard (1968)
Ge:Zn	PC	3×10^9 (800)	<10	4.2	39.5	Heard (1968)
Ge:Zn, Sb	PC	2×10^9 (900)		50	15	Heard (1968)
Ge:Cu	PC	1.5×10^{10} (900)		4.2	27	Heard (1968)
Ge:Cd	PC	9×10^9 (500)		4.2	21.5	Heard (1968)
Ge–Si:Au	PC	3×10^9 (90)	100	50	10.1	Heard (1968)
Ge–Si:Zn, Sb	PC	10^{10} (100)	100	50	13.3	Heard (1968)
Si:Al	PC	3×10^9 (15 kHz)	1	20		Soref (1966)
Cd, Hg:Te	PV	7×10^9 (900)		77	14	Cohen-Solal and Riant (1971)
Cd, Hg:Te	PV	10^{10} (1.8 kHz)	<1	77		Verie and Serieix (1972)
Ge:Cu	PC		1.6	4		Bridges *et al.* (1968)
Ge:Hg	PC		1–8	4		Bridges *et al.* (1968)
Ge:Au	PC		30	77		Bridges *et al.* (1968)
Ge:Cu, Sb	PC		1.6	4		Bridges *et al.* (1968)
Te	PC		<100	83		Miura and Tanaka (1968)
$Pb_{1-x}Sn_xTe$	PC	10^{10} (900)[c]	15	4.2–77	11–20	Melngailis and Harman (1968)
HgCdTe	PV	10^{10} (800)		77	12	Fiorito *et al.* (1973)
HgCdTe	PV	7.3×10^{10}	1	77	9–13	Marine and Motte (1973)

[a] Modulation frequency in brackets.
[b] The cut-off wavelength is that at which the observed D^* decreases to 50% of its peak value.
[c] Peak value.

in some cases the $D^*(10\ \mu m)$ of these detectors approaches the limit for BLIP detectors in this wavelength range. BLIP D^*'s at 10 μm are 4×10^{10} and 6×10^{10} cm-Hz$^{1/2}$/W for PC and PV detectors, respectively, viewing a 290°K background through a solid angle of 2π steradians. Commercial versions of most of these detectors are available.

3.4.7 Heterodyne Detection

A considerable increase in the sensitivity of detectors can be accomplished using the technique of optical heterodyning. We can see how this increase comes about by using the following simple analysis (Heard, 1968). If the optical field at the surface of the detector due to the received signal is

$$e_1(t) = E_1 \cos \omega_1 t$$

and that due to a local oscillator is

$$e_2(t) = E_2(\cos \omega_2 t + \psi)$$

where ψ is the difference in phase between the two fields at a given point on the surface of the detector, then the output of the detector

$$i(t) \propto e^2(t) = (E_1 \cos \omega_1 t)^2 + [E_2 \cos(\omega_2 t + \psi)]^2 + 2E_1E_2 \cos \omega_1 t \cos(\omega_2 t + \psi) \tag{19}$$

where $e(t) = e_1(t) + e_2(t)$. The first two terms in this equation represent fields that are oscillating at optical frequencies. Since the detector does not respond to these frequencies (10^{13}–10^{15} Hz), these terms give rise to two dc components, I_1 and I_2, respectively. The last term in this equation represents fields oscillating at the sum and difference frequencies $\omega_1 + \omega_2$ and $\omega_1 - \omega_2$. The detector will not follow oscillations at $\omega_1 + \omega_2$ but may produce an output that does vary at the difference frequency. The output would be

$$i_{\text{if}} \propto E_1E_2 \cos[(\omega_1 - \omega_2)t - \psi] = 2(\overline{I_1 I_2})^{1/2} \cos[(\omega_1 - \omega_2)t - \psi] \tag{20}$$

Then by using a strong local oscillator (I_2 large) a weak incident signal may be amplified in an if amplifier and detected with greater sensitivity. One significant advantage of heterodyne detection is that only the incident coherent radiation is amplified: background radiation that is incoherent is rejected. Thus, the D^* of a detector operated in the optical heterodyne mode can be larger than that obtained under BLIP conditions. Of course the detector must be of the "square-law" type.

Leiba (1969) was the first to demonstrate optical heterodyne detection with pyroelectric detectors. Soon after, Abrams and Glass (1969) reported optical heterodyne detection with SBN-type pyroelectric material and some fundamental limitations in the use of pyroelectric detectors in this mode were pointed out. The experiment is as shown in Fig. 3.10. The "signal" is obtained from 10.6-μm radiation scattered from a rotating wheel while a beam splitter allows a large local oscillator power to be directed into the detector ($\simeq$1 W). One advantage of the pyroelectric detector is that this amount of power can be relatively easily dissipated. The scattered light is shifted in frequency by $\simeq$1 MHz by the Doppler effect off the rotating wheel and amplification occurs at this frequency. The minimum detectable power is theoretically predicted to be $\simeq 8 \times 10^{-16}$ W/Hz for the SBN detector operated in this mode. However, in practice the amplifier introduces a noise component that limits this minimum detectable power to 1.5×10^{-11} W/Hz. This is still an improvement of a factor of 10^3 over the minimum detectable power for the same detector operated in the conventional mode.

A similar experimental arrangement was used by Contreras and Gaddy (1971) in the evaluation of the minimum detectable power of a thin bismuth bolometer operated as an optical heterodyne detector. Here the minimum detectable power was observed to be close to the theoretical limiting value (3.8×10^{-11} W/Hz).

Arams *et al.* (1967), Vérié and Sirieix (1972), and Peyton *et al.* (1972) have studied optical heterodyne detection with photoconductive (Ge : Cu) and photovoltaic (HgCdTe) detectors. An *NEP* as low as 8×10^{-20} W/(Hz)$^{1/2}$ was reported (Verie and Sirieix, 1972) using HgCdTe. A comprehensive study of design requirements for heterodyne detection at intermediate frequencies into the gigahertz range using photoconductive detectors was given by Abrams *et al.* (1967). Abrams and White (1972) have shown that difficulties encountered in practical optical heterodyne detector systems due to the drift of local and received frequencies can be overcome

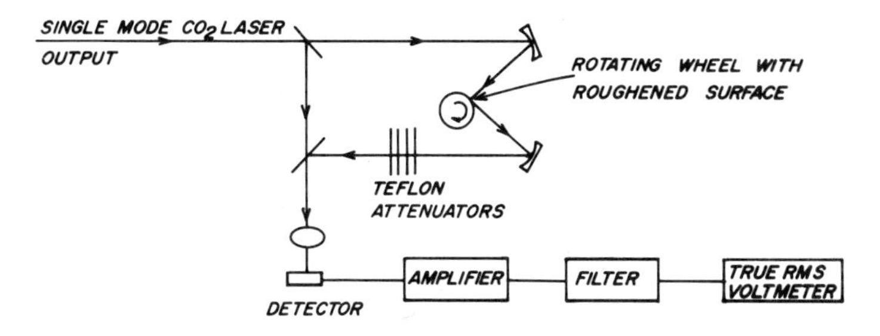

Fig. 3.10. System for laboratory experiments on optical heterodyne detection. Radiation scattered from the rotating wheel is Doppler shifted (after Abrams and Glass, 1969).

by the use of three-frequency detection. In this method, which may be useful in the detection of Doppler-shifted signals, two frequencies ω_1 and ω_2 are mixed with the local oscillator frequency ω_L in a photodetector. Two sidebands, one with $\omega = \omega_1 - \omega_L$ and the other with $\omega = \omega_2 - \omega_L$ are formed. These signals are then passed into a square law detector, which gives an output at $\omega_1 - \omega_2$. Since this output no longer depends on ω_L, frequency drift due to changes in ω_L (or ω_1 and ω_2) is no longer important.

Minimum detectable powers in the 10^{-14}–10^{-13} W/Hz range are possible (Abrams and Gandrud, 1970) using metal–insulator–metal point contact diodes operating at room temperature in the optical heterodyne detection mode. However, these devices are fragile and are not easily constructed. Further studies on point contact diodes as radiation detectors are given by Hocker *et al.* (1968), Daneu *et al.* (1969), Evenson *et al.* (1970a,b), and Twu and Schwarz (1974).

3.4.8 Infrared Up-Conversion

There has been considerable interest in recent years in the possibilities offered by infrared up-conversion as a new type of detector for infrared radiation. The theory of this type of device has been given by Yariv (1968), Kleinman and Boyd (1969), and Lucy (1972). Infrared and visible radiation are mixed in a nonlinear optical mixing material to produce a signal at the sum of the infrared and visible frequencies. This signal can be detected by any of a number of fast-sensitive short-wavelength detectors, obviating the need for a separate infrared detector.

Proustite (Ag_3AsS_3) has been found to satisfy the requirements for up-conversion of 10.6-μm laser radiation to visible light (Hulme *et al.*, 1967; Warner, 1968a,b; Voronin *et al.*, 1971; Alcock and Walker, 1973). This crystal has high values of its nonlinear coefficients, good power-handling capabilities, and low absorption in the 0.6–13 μm region. The photon conversion efficiency of this and other mixer crystals is, however, quite low ($\simeq 10^{-6}$; Warner, 1968a,b) and this may limit some applications of the up-conversion method. Alcock and Walker (1973) have shown in an elegant experiment that up-conversion in Ag_3AsS_3 can be used in the detection of nanosecond pulses from a TEA CO_2 laser, synchronized with pulses from a Nd : YAG laser. This method offers the possibility of using a variety of techniques developed to measure picosecond light pulses in the visible for similar measurements on short infrared pulses. Synchronously pulsed CO_2 and Nd : YAG lasers have been used in a real-time infrared image up-conversion by Tseng (1974) using proustite. With a pulse repetition frequency of 130 Hz it was possible to view the up-converted image of a source illuminated with 10.6-μm laser radiation on an image intensifier tube operating at visible wavelengths.

Investigations of other nonlinear materials as parametric infrared up-converters have been reported. $ZnGeP_2$ was shown (Boyd *et al.*, 1971) to have an up-conversion efficiency some 140 times greater than that of proustite and a theoretical performance as an infrared detector that was comparable to that of the Ge : Hg photoconductive detector. The conversion quantum efficiency for 10.6-μm radiation in HgS was found to be 0.4×10^{-9} (Boyd *et al.*, 1968) using a 1-mW He–Ne laser as the pump, and it was concluded that, without a significant improvement in material properties, HgS would be of little use as a sensitive detector.

3.5 WINDOWS AND MIRRORS

With the rapid development of high-power cw and pulsed CO_2 lasers practical laser systems are limited more and more by such considerations as the susceptibility of windows and mirrors to damage. In this section we will discuss some materials commonly used for windows in high-power laser systems as well as some materials useful for high-power reflectors. Since rapid development in solid state and multilayer film technology is still continuing, the latest information on high-power window materials and reflecting optics is best obtained by consulting one of the journals that carry advertisements for these elements (*Laser Focus, Optical Spectra, Optics and Laser Technology*, etc.).

The ideal high-power laser window material would have the following characteristics:

(i) low absorption coefficient at the laser wavelength
(ii) high thermal conductivity
(iii) high heat capacity
(iv) low coefficient of thermal expansion
(v) chemical stability, i.e., nonhydroscopic
(vi) excellent polishing properties
(vii) suitability for dielectric coatings
(viii) refractive index independent of temperature

There are no ideal window materials in the sense defined by these criteria, but many materials have been found that adequately satisfy enough of these requirements to make them useful transmitters of high-power 10.6-μm laser radiation. Table 3.4 lists some of these parameters for the most commonly used window materials at 10.6 μm. We see that KBr has the lowest absorption at 10.6 μm, but some of the semiconductors (e.g., CdTe, ZnSe,

Table 3.4

Some Properties of Infrared Window Materials[a,b]

Material	Thermal expansion coefficient ($\times 10^6$/°C)	Thermal conductivity ($\times 10^{-2}$ W/cm°C)	Heat capacity (J/cm³)	Absorption coefficient at 10.6 μm (cm⁻¹)	Chemical stability
NaCl	38.9	6.5	1.845	1.34×10^{-3}	−
KCl	36	6.5	1.347	4.83×10^{-4}	−
KBr	43	4.8	1.197	5×10^{-5} (estimated)[c]	−
CsBr	47	0.96	1.171	4.4×10^{-3}	−
CsI	47	1.13	0.9094	1.3×10^{-3}	−
KRS-5 (TlBr–TlI)	58	0.54		5×10^{-3}	+
ZnS	6.7	26		0.38	+
ZnSe	7.7	13	2.646	6×10^{-3} (estimated)	+
CdTe	4.5	7	1.224	1.2×10^{-3}	+
GaAs	5.7	37	1.420	1.2×10^{-2}	+
Si	4.2	120	1.58	2.5	+
Ge	6	59	1.652	(3.6×10^{-2})[d]	+

[a] After Sparks (1971).
[b] The minus signs denote materials that are hydroscopic, while plus signs denote those materials that are stable in moist air.
[c] Residual absorption in the alkali halides may be due to impurities (Patten *et al.*, 1971).
[d] For all semiconductors, the absorption coefficient is dependent on resistivity and temperature.

and GaAs) have relatively low absorption together with enhanced thermal conductivity and coefficients of thermal expansion that are lower than those of the alkali halides by an order of magnitude. In addition, the semiconductor materials can usually be polished for a finer finish than the alkali halides and will retain this finish even in moist atmospheres. Although plastic coatings have been suggested (Ferrar, 1969) for alkali halide optics to protect them against water damage, these coatings are effective only at low incident intensities. Multilayer dielectric films can enhance the resistance of alkali halide window materials to attack by moist air.

One problem that occurs with semiconductor windows is that heating produces an increase in absorption coefficient (Bishop and Gibson, 1973). This yields an unstable situation above a critical temperature that can lead to thermal runaway. Thermal runaway has been studied experimentally in germanium by Young (1971) and in general terms for germanium and silicon window materials by Johnston and O'Keefe (1972). Single-crystal germanium disks 40 mm in diameter and 6 mm thick with a resistivity of 50 Ω-cm were cooled over an area of 760 mm^2 on the face nearest the laser discharge. Young's data are as follows:

No cooling except by convection:	$F_c = 26\ W/cm^2$
Cooled by a 3-m/sec flow of air at 20°C:	$F_c = 31\ W/cm^2$
Cooled by 10-cm^3/sec water flow at 20°C:	$F_c = 42\ W/cm^2$
Cooled by N_2 gas at −40°C:	$F_c = 87\ W/cm^2$

where F_c is the critical incident laser intensity. Thermal runaway was found to occur when the germanium temperature reached about 50°C. The values of F_c depend, of course, on the detailed cooling mechanism and must be regarded as conservative since cooling was not optimized. A general rule of thumb is that with efficient edge cooling, windows in this size range can tolerate incident intensities of up to 100 W/cm^2. Other semiconductor materials (notably GaAs and CdTe) do not "run away" until higher temperatures are reached and hence can be subjected to higher incident laser intensities. The temperature dependence of the absorption coefficient at 10.6 μm in GaAs and ZnSe has recently been investigated by Skolnik *et al.* (1974). Chemical-vapor-deposited ZnSe was found to have an absorption coefficient that was independent of temperature for temperatures $\lesssim 500°K$. This indicated that the absorption in this material may be due mainly to surface losses or to impurities. Similar measurements on the absorption of KCl window material have been made by Deutsch (1974). Horrigan *et al.* (1969) have surveyed CO_2 laser windows suitable for use in high-power conventional laser systems.

The low reflection coefficient of the alkali halides at 10.6 μm can be increased (or lowered) by coating with single or multilayer films of other ir materials. Gaver and Seguin (1970) have discussed one method of preparing these coatings, which uses a triode sputtering source. A $\lambda/4$ (at 10.6 μm) layer of Ge on NaCl yielded a reflectivity of 65% at the CO_2 laser wavelength, while 97% reflectivity was obtained from $5 \times \lambda/4$ coatings of Ge and CdS in alternating layers. Coatings of this sort can be produced in the laboratory after some trial and error. Most commercially available window materials can be coated to yield any desired reflectivity. Some considerations in the preparation of beam splitters at 10.6 μm by coating NaCl with ZnSe have been discussed by Davis and Cathey (1969). Comprehensive data on the design and performance of antireflection coatings for ZnSe have been presented by Rudisill *et al.* (1974). A two-layer coating of ThF_4 and ZnSe on ZnSe yielded an attenuation due to reflection and absorption $<0.1\%$ at the coated surface.

There have been many studies of pulsed laser damage in transparent media (see Ready, 1971, Chapter 6 and references therein). The main processes involved in the generation of damage are

(i) stimulated Brillouin scattering to produce photons,
(ii) intrinsic or dielectric breakdown initiated perhaps by a multiphoton process, and
(iii) localized breakdown at defects and inclusions in the material.

Most of these processes will be sensitive to the laser wavelengths, which makes a comparison between experiments performed at visible wavelengths and results expected at 10.6 μm somewhat unreliable. A quantitative comparison of damage effects at 10.6, 1.06, and 0.69 μm has been reported by Fradin and others. Agarbiceanu *et al.* (1969) have examined the effect of high-power CO_2 laser radiation on NaCl. Emmony *et al.* (1973) show that the damage to a germanium output window takes the form of coarse surface damage in the region subjected to the highest laser intensity. This damage is, however, overlapped by linear etch channels showing a characteristic periodic structure with the periodicity equal to the laser wavelength (10.6 μm). Emmony *et al.* suggest that this effect occurs because of the presence of surface defects that scatter the incident laser light along the surface. The scattered radiation interferes with incident laser radiation to produce interference fringes with a "wavelength" of 10 μm.

Quantitative studies of damage to window materials at 10.6 μm have been reported by Hanna *et al.* (1972), Braunstein *et al.* (1973), Smith (1973), Davit (1973), Reichelt and Stark (1973), and Posen *et al.* (1973). Some of these data are summarized in Table 3.5.

This and other work (Fradin and Bua, 1974) shows that breakdown can often be attributed to micron-sized inclusions. Damage in ZnSe (Fradin and Bua, 1974) occurred at intensities of $\simeq$340 MW/cm^2 when the laser beam was focused to a diameter of 65 μm and at 260 MW/cm^2 when focusing was to 130 μm. It is interesting that damage due to inclusions is sensitive to focusing conditions for the same total incident intensity, while that due to intrinsic breakdown is not. Damage can also occur due to the melting of small particles of dust on the window surface in the incident beam or to the treatment of the surface with a solvent (Barber, 1969). Care must therefore be taken to ensure that the environment around laser optical components be kept as free from particulate contamination as possible. Occasionally incident damage may not be apparent, but may affect the performance of the optical component. Pappu *et al.* (1972) describe a method that enables this damage to be detected.

In high-power cw systems window heating due to residual absorption of laser radiation has been shown (Sparks, 1971) to lead to a lensing effect. This effect occurs because of nonuniform heating across the window. A radial temperature gradient produces a change in thickness of the window and a radial gradient in the refractive index. Materials that are least sensitive to this distortion are NaCl, KCl, and KBr among the alkali halides and ZnSe and CdTe in the group of semiconductor window materials. Losses introduced in Brewster angle windows by thermal distortion have been discussed by Sinclair (1970).

Mirrors for low-power CO_2 lasers can be made of fused quartz, Pyrex, stainless steel, or brass coated with a vacuum-deposited layer of gold. However, for high-power cw lasers (>200 W) and lasers with high-power pulsed outputs, these materials are generally unsuitable. Polished copper and gold-coated zirconium–copper have been used as mirrors in many high-power CO_2 laser systems. A variety of high-power reflectors are now commercially available. These mirrors are usually water cooled.

Braunstein and Braunstein (1971) have reported some data on coatings suitable for high-power CO_2 laser mirrors. ThF_4 was found to be useful for overcoating silver mirrors to prevent tarnishing. Multilayer coatings of alternate ThF_4 and CdTe layers on Ag, Cu, or Al were predicted to have over 99.8% reflectivity with six layers. Experimentally, 99.1% reflectivity was obtained for two layers coated on Cu and Al substrates.

Studies on laser damage to mirrors have been reported by Bennett (1971), Bliss and Milam (1972), Wang *et al.* (1973), and Apollonov *et al.* (1974). Wang *et al.* (1973) used a uv preionized TEA, TEM_{00} CO_2 laser to evaluate damage thresholds for pure- and coated-metal mirrors. A summary of their results is as follows:

Copper or molybdenum mirror:	35 J/cm^2
Coated with CdTe or ZnTe:	1–2 J/cm^2
Coated with As_2S_3, KCl, or ThF_4:	30–65 J/cm^2

Table 3.5

Representative Damage Thresholds for a Variety of Window Materials at 10.6 μm

Material	Preparation	Number of pulses	Critical intensity or fluence	Laser type	Reference
NaCl		100	>13 J/cm^2	TEA, TEM$_{00}$, 75 nsec	Davit (1973)
		1	17 J/cm^2	TEA, TEM$_{00}$, 75 nsec	Davit (1973)
	Harshaw	1	3 J/cm^2	TEA, TEM$_{00}$, nsec pulse	Reichelt and Stark (1973)
KCl	Hughes HRL B11-11 polished with Linde B		>75 J/cm^2	TEA, TEM$_{00}$, 200 nsec	Braunstein *et al.* (1973)
		100	>13 J/cm^2	TEA, TEM$_{00}$, 75 nsec	Davit (1973)
		1	17 J/cm^2	TEA, TEM$_{00}$, 75 nsec	Davit (1973)
	(100), (110), or (111)	cw	$>3.8 \times 10^4$ W/cm^2	cw	Posen (1973)
	Ge coated	cw	5.1×10^3–1.4×10^4 W/cm^2	cw	Posen (1973)
KBr	(100)	cw	$>3.8 \times 10^4$ W/cm^2	cw	Posen (1973)
Ge	20 Ω-cm	100	>7.5 J/cm^2	TEA, TEM$_{00}$, 75 nsec	Davit (1973)
	n-type	1	17 J/cm^2	TEA, TEM$_{00}$, 75 nsec	Davit (1973)
	AR coated	100	>7.5 J/cm^2	TEA, TEM$_{00}$, 75 nsec	Davit (1973)
		20	13 J/cm^2	TEA, TEM$_{00}$, 75 nsec	Davit (1973)
Te	Cleaved	1	$<43 \times 10^6$ W/cm^2	*Q*-switched, 200 nsec	Hanna *et al.* (1972)

		>30,000	$>30 \times 10^6$ W/cm^2	*Q*-switched, 200 nsec	Hanna *et al.* (1972)
	Mechanical cutting and etching	1000	$\lesssim 10 \times 10^6$ W/cm^2	*Q*-switched, 200 nsec	Hanna *et al.* (1972)
	Mechanical cutting and etching	>30,000	$>30\text{–}43 \times 10^6$ W/cm^2	*Q*-switched, 200 nsec	Hanna *et al.* (1972)
	Chemical cutting and etching	1000	43×10^6 W/cm^2	*Q*-switched, 200 nsec	Hanna *et al.* (1972)
	Chemical cutting and etching	>30,000	$>43 \times 10^6$ W/cm^2	*Q*-switched, 200 nsec	Hanna *et al.* (1972)
GaAs		1	$<107 \times 10^6$ W/cm^2	*Q*-switched, 200 nsec	Hanna *et al.* (1972)
		100	76×10^6 W/cm^2	*Q*-switched, 200 nsec	Hanna *et al.* (1972)
		>30,000	$>63 \times 10^6$ W/cm^2	*Q*-switched, 200 nsec	Hanna *et al.* (1972)
GaAs	Purest, $n_e \lesssim 10^{13}/\text{cm}^3$	1	$30 \pm 10 \times 10^6$ W/cm^2	TEA, 100 nsec	Smith (1973)
CdTe	Hughes HRL 225-4	1	2 J/cm^2	TEA, multimode, 200 nsec	Braunstein *et al.* (1973)
ZnSe	Raytheon 417 heavy inclusions	1	5.6 J/cm^2	TEA, TEM_{00}, 200 nsec	Braunstein *et al.* (1973)
	Raytheon 41, intermediate inclusions	1	41 J/cm^2	TEA, TEM_{00}, 200 nsec	Braunstein *et al.* (1973)
Proustite		1	$<76 \times 10^6$ W/cm^2	*Q*-switched, 200 nsec	Hanna *et al.* (1972)
		100	53×10^6 W/cm^2	*Q*-switched, 200 nsec	Hanna *et al.* (1972)
		>30,000	$>46 \times 10^6$ W/cm^2	*Q*-switched, 200 nsec	Hanna *et al.* (1972)

The equivalent rectangular laser pulse corresponding to the laser output observed in these measurements had a duration of 0.6 μsec. Coatings of wide bandgap dielectrics such as KCl and AsS_3 were found to increase the damage threshold over that attainable from uncoated metallic reflectors.

3.6 OPTICAL RESONATORS

Two mirrors arranged so that light reflected from one is returned by the other constitute an optical resonator. Because of the importance of optical resonators in the design of laser systems the literature on this subject is vast. In this section only a few basic principles associated with the design and use of optical resonators in CO_2 laser systems will be discussed. Full discussions can be found in many books on lasers (for example, Bloom, 1968; Röss, 1969; Siegman, 1971) and in numerous review articles (see Ronchi, 1972, for a bibliography).

An optical resonator will have a number of possible spatial distributions of the electromagnetic field, which correspond to normal modes (or simply "modes") of the resonator. Axial or longitudinal modes contain an integral number of half-wavelengths of the electromagnetic field within the resonator. Certain configurations of the electromagnetic field are also possible transverse to the axis of the resonator. These are transverse modes. Since the transverse dimension in a laser resonator is usually considerably smaller than the longitudinal dimension or separation between the mirrors, transverse and longitudinal modes are essentially independent of each other. Thus one may think of a certain transverse configuration of the electromagnetic field that is maintained as a wave propagates back and forth in the resonator and which always presents the same distribution of electromagnetic field transverse to the optic axis on reaching one of the reflectors.

Axial modes occur at frequencies $\nu_{mnq} = cq/2d$, where q is a large number and d the separation between the mirrors. The integers m and n are usually small for low-loss modes of the resonator and define the transverse mode configuration TEM_{mn}. Simple expressions are available for the distribution of intensity in the TEM_{mn} modes in common resonator configurations. The intensity in the x,y plane perpendicular to the optic axis of the resonator (z axis) is

$$\frac{I_{mn}}{I_0}(x, y) = \left(\left[H_m\left(\frac{\sqrt{2}x}{w}\right)H_n\left(\frac{\sqrt{2}y}{w}\right)\right] \exp\left[-\left(\frac{x^2+y^2}{w^2}\right)\right]\right)^2 \tag{21}$$

where H_m is the Hermite polynomial of order m, w the spot size of the beam defined as the radius (from the z axis) at which the intensity of the TEM_{00} mode decreases by a factor $1/e^2$, and I_0 the intensity on the beam axis. w is given by the expression

$$w = w_0\left[1 + \left(\frac{\lambda z}{\pi w_0^2}\right)^2\right]^{1/2} \tag{22}$$

where λ is the wavelength and w_0 the minimum spot size obtained for the TEM_{00} mode at the point where the wavefront is planar. z is measured from this point. Some Hermite polynomials of low order are

$$H_0(x) = 1, \qquad H_1(x) = x, \qquad H_2(x) = 4x^2 - 2, \qquad H_3(x) = 8x^3 - 12x$$

Photographs of the intensity distribution in several low-order TEM_{mn} modes can be found in Kogelnik and Li (1966) and in most books on lasers. The most interesting solution to Eq. (21) from the point of view of laser machining operations is that with $m = n = 0$. This is the fundamental mode, in which the intensity distribution takes the particularly simple form

$$I_{00}(x, y)/I_0 = \exp(-2r^2/w^2) \tag{23}$$

where $r = (x^2 + y^2)^{1/2}$ is a radial coordinate measured from the z axis. Thus in the fundamental mode, the intensity will decrease, according to the Gaussian distribution, as r increases. This distribution is maintained throughout the beam, i.e., in both the near and far fields. Furthermore, the fundamental mode output has a constant phase across the entire wavefront and thus lends itself to focusing to the minimum possible spot size.

Figure 3.11 shows the propagation of a Gaussian beam away from the

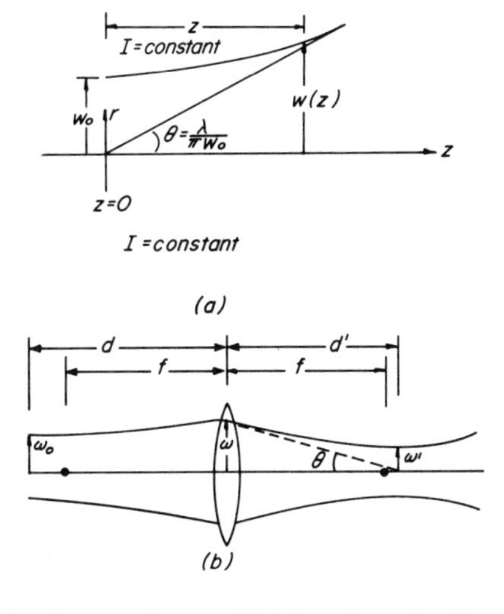

Fig. 3.11. (a) Propagation and (b) focusing of a Gaussian beam.

beam waist, where $w = w_0$ and $z = 0$. The variation of w with z is as given in Eq. (22). The beam divergence in the far field is given by the angle

$$\theta = \lim_{z \to \infty} dw/dz = \lambda/\pi w_0$$

Suppose that a lens is now placed in the beam as shown in Fig. 3.11b. The focal length of this lens is f and it brings the beam to a focus at the point d'. Since the initial divergence of the beam is small, $d' \simeq f$. Also, as before, we have $w' = \lambda/\pi\theta$, but now θ is defined by the beam radius w at the lens, or alternatively by the lens radius. Then $\theta \simeq w/f$ and therefore

$$w' = f\lambda/\pi w \tag{24}$$

If we identify w with the lens radius, i.e., the lens provides the limiting aperture, then Eq. (24) gives the minimum radius of the spot that can be formed by focusing. Since $f/\pi w$ can be made $\simeq 1$, the minimum spot radius is $\simeq \lambda$. It should be remembered that this value is obtained only in the limit of a perfect Gaussian beam propagating through distortionless optics. Some discussion of distortions produced by real optical systems is given by Arata and Miyamoto (1972). The output of a laser oscillating on one or more higher order modes will no longer satisfy the above requirements. With multimode beams the following expression is sometimes used to estimate the minimum focal spot radius:

$$r_{\min} \simeq f\theta \tag{25}$$

where θ is the angular divergence of the beam.

Equation (22) relates the beam "radius" to distance away from the point with $w = w_0$. Since this expression is valid whenever a Gaussian beam is brought to a focus, it may be used to obtain an estimate of the depth of focus of the beam. Defining the depth of focus as the value of $|z|$ for which w/w_0 (ω/ω' in Fig. 3.11b) $= 1.5$,

$$|z| = 1.12\pi w_0^2/\lambda \tag{26}$$

A general relation between the parameters shown in Fig. 3.11 for focusing with a single perfect lens has been given by Dickson (1970):

$$w' = w_0 \frac{d'}{d}\left[1 + \frac{f_F^2}{d^2}\right]^{-1/2} \times \left\{1 + \frac{d^4}{f_F^2}\left(1 + \frac{f_F^2}{d^2}\right)\left[\frac{1}{d'} - \frac{1}{f} + \frac{1}{d(1 + f_F^2/d^2)}\right]^2\right\}^{1/2} \tag{27}$$

where $f_F = \pi w_0^2/\lambda$. When $d = 0$ and $f = \infty$, this expression reduces to that given in Eq. (22) for propagation in the fundamental mode without focusing.

Measurement of the distribution of intensity within a focused high-power laser beam is both difficult and usually inaccurate. Some methods involving the measurement of thermal effects on a sensitive material placed in the beam have already been described in Section 3.4.4. These methods are suitable only for nonfocused beams. Recently, Skinner and Whitcher (1972) have devised a dynamic measurement technique that makes use of the shape of pulses generated in a photodetector when the beam is chopped with a straight-edged chopper. Assuming the beam is Gaussian, the intensity distribution is

$$I_{00}(x, y) = I_0 \exp(-2r^2/w^2) = (2P/\pi w^2) \exp(-2r^2/w^2) \tag{28}$$

where P is the total power in the beam. If a shutter blocks off all points in the beam for which $x \leq a$, then the power transmitted by the remaining part of the beam will be

$$P(a) = \int_{-\infty}^{\infty} \int_{a}^{\infty} I_{00}(x, y)\, dx\, dy = \tfrac{1}{2}P \operatorname{erfc}[a\sqrt{2}/w] \tag{29}$$

With chopping, $a \equiv a(t) = R\alpha t$, where R is the radius of the chopper wheel at the point where it intersects the beam, α the angular velocity of the chopper, erfc the complementary error function, and t the time after the edge of the chopper blade has crossed the center of the beam. Observation of $P(a, t)$ then allows a Gaussian distribution with a given value of w to be fitted to the beam from the observed pulse shape. Skinner and Whitcher were able to obtain the Gaussian beam radius of a 1-kW cw CO_2 laser beam using this technique. The depth of focus can also be measured in this way by repeating the sampling process away from the focal point of the focusing lens or mirror.

Other methods of obtaining the intensity distribution in a beam have also been reported. A pinhole can be moved through the beam monitoring the power transmitted through the pinhole to obtain the intensity distribution as a function of position (Arata and Miyamoto, 1972). A straight-edge may be slowly translated through the beam as described above, but while monitoring the transmitted power on a power meter. An array of small pyroelectric detectors can also give a real-time measurement of the mode structure and intensity distribution. This method is most useful for sampling the output from pulsed lasers.

In the design of optical resonators one has in general five parameters that can be varied to obtain optimization for a particular system. These parameters are d, the separation between the mirrors; r_1 and r_2, the radii of curvature of the two mirrors, and R_1 and R_2, the reflectivities of the two mirrors. Although it is difficult to generalize optimum relationships for all five of these parameters, the first three are subject to some stringent requirements if the optical resonator is to be stable, i.e., if the low-order modes are to be narrowly confined to the optic axis and have low losses due to diffraction around the sides of the resonator. This relationship can be seen most clearly by defining the parameters

$$g_1 = 1 - d/r_1, \qquad g_2 = 1 - d/r_2 \tag{30}$$

Every combination of d, r_1, and r_2 then gives rise to a point in g_1g_2 space. When plotted in this way, the lines $g_1g_2 = 1$ define the boundaries between stable and unstable regimes of operation for the optical resonator. A plot of this sort is shown in Fig. 3.12. The cross-hatched regions correspond to values of g_1 and g_2 that yield stable resonator configurations, while all other regions are unstable (Fox and Li, 1963; Boyd and Kogelnik, 1962).

One disadvantage of the stable resonator configurations given above is that the volume occupied by each mode of the resonator never approaches the volume of the active medium. Thus maintenance of a large-volume high-gain discharge in the resonator will lead to oscillation on many modes of the system. Attempts to overcome this effect and to obtain a single-mode output by aperturing will result in lower overall efficiency, since energy will not be extracted from most of the excited discharge volume. Siegman (1965) was the first to discuss some possible benefits to be derived from operation with an unstable resonator configuration. Subsequent ex-

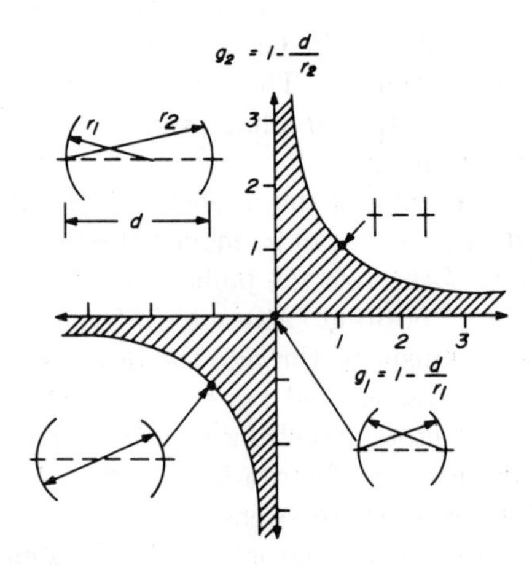

Fig. 3.12. Mode chart plotted in g_1g_2 (cross-hatched) plane, which shows the regions of stable and unstable operation.

perimental and theoretical studies have been reported by Kahan (1966), Barone (1967), Sinclair and Cottrell (1967), Siegman and Arrathoon (1967), Bergstein (1968), Krupke and Sooy (1969), Siegman and Miller (1970), Siegman (1971, 1974), and many others. Advantages of operation with unstable resonators can be summarized as follows:

(1) single transverse-mode operation at high Fresnel numbers $N = a^2/\lambda d$, where a is the radius of the output mirror (not the radius of curvature)
(2) extraction of stored energy from the bulk of the laser medium
(3) elimination of partial reflectors

These advantages have led to the adoption of the unstable resonator configuration in many high-power cw (Hoag *et al.*, 1974) and pulsed (Dyer *et al.*, 1972b) CO_2 laser systems.

An unstable resonator configuration studied by Krupke and Sooy (1969) using a conventional cw CO_2 laser is shown in Fig. 3.13. The output of this resonator when the mirrors are confocal is in the form of a collimated annulus. It was predicted that given uniform excitation, stored energy density, and gain, the total output power should scale linearly with the Fresnel number. This is what makes the unstable resonator configuration so useful for large-volume CO_2 lasers. It is interesting that Dyer *et al.* (1972b) found that using an unstable resonator with a double-discharge TEA laser 60% of the output energy was obtained in the initial sharp pulse, while without

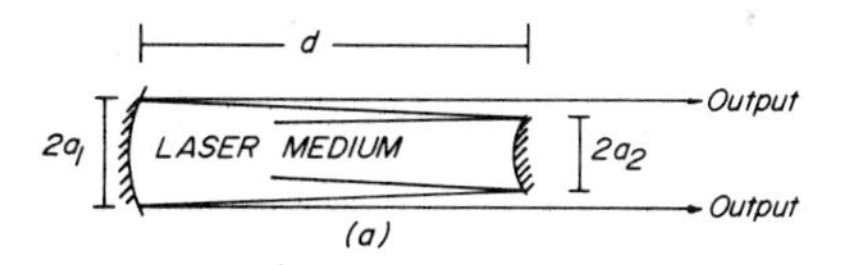

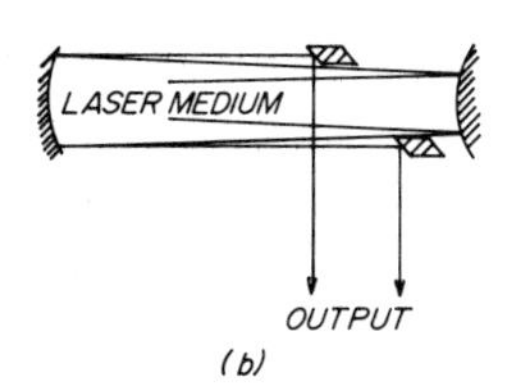

Fig. 3.13. Confocal unstable resonators (after Krupke and Sooy, 1969). (a) Power extraction around edge of smaller mirror. (b) Power extraction using annular coupling mirror within cavity.

this configuration and using a stable cavity, much of this energy was contained in the low-peak-power tail of the output pulse, which lasted for several microseconds.

Wisner *et al.* (1973) have used an unstable resonator of the type shown in Fig. 3.13b with an electric discharge convectively cooled CO_2 laser. Diffraction-limited output was obtained from this system at power levels of up to 1500 W and cavity Fresnel numbers of 5 to 35.

3.7 MODULATORS

Many applications of lasers require that the output of the laser be modulated in some way. Practical communications systems involve amplitude, phase, or frequency modulation of the laser transmitter. Some of the most successful methods of modulating CO_2 lasers have been taken over directly from the technology developed for modulation of visible lasers (electro-optic and acousto-optic devices). Other modulation techniques have been developed primarily for the CO_2 laser (Stark modulation and free carrier absorption). In this section some practical modulation devices for CO_2 lasers will be discussed, but no attempt will be made to cover the physical principles involved in the operation of these devices in any sort of detail. Excellent review articles are available on most of the subjects to be covered in this section and the reader is referred to these articles for fundamental discussions on the physics of practical modulation devices. The topics of some reviews are electro-optic light modulators (Kaminow and Turner, 1966), acousto-optical modulation and deflection devices (Gordon, 1966), and nonlinear optics (Yariv, 1968; Smith, 1970). A summary of methods used to modulate the output of CO_2 lasers is given in Table 3.6.

In certain materials the application of an electric field has the effect of inducing either a birefringence in a normally isotropic material or a change in the birefringence in a material that already possesses this property. This change in birefringence has the effect of inducing a phase retardation for light propagating through the crystal. The phase retardation is therefore proportional to the applied electric field and hence modulation of the electric field yields a modulation in the phase of plane-polarized light transmitted by the crystal. This is the basis for a group of devices known as electro-optic modulators.

A figure of merit for the electro-optic modulator can be obtained from the following (Kamimow, 1968). The phase retardation due to light passed through a modulator of length L, thickness t, and width w is

$$\Gamma = \pi n^3 r V L / \lambda t \tag{31}$$

where n is the refractive index, V the voltage across the element, and r the electro-optic coefficient. The power dissipated by the element is

$$P = (\epsilon_0/2\pi)[wt/L](\epsilon/n^6r^2)\lambda^2\Gamma^2 \Delta f \quad (32)$$

when the element is placed in parallel with an inductance and resistance to form a resonant circuit with bandwidth Δf. ϵ_0 is the permittivity of the crystal, while ϵ is the dielectric constant. The ratio wt/L is limited by diffraction effects to a minimum value $\simeq 4\lambda/n\pi$. Thus

$$P \propto \lambda^3\epsilon/n^7r^2 \quad (33)$$

and the ratio

$$M = n^7r^2/\epsilon \quad (34)$$

is one figure of merit for the material. This definition of M has been used to compare the electro-optic modulator materials listed in Table 3.6. Although the highest value of M is obtained with Se, Kamimow (1968) points out some reasons why this material is actually a less desirable modulator material than GaAs. In fact, most modulators reported in use with CO_2 laser systems utilize either GaAs (Bridges *et al.*, 1968) or CdTe (Kiefer *et al.*, 1972). The bandwidths of these modulators can be extremely large: Kiefer *et al.* (1972) obtained 500 MHz limited by the modulator driver, while McAvoy *et al.* (1972) report a 110-MHz bandwidth using coupling modulation with GaAs. CuCl has been modulated at up to 455 KHz (Sueta *et al.*, 1970). GaAs and CdTe modulators have been operated (Huang *et al.*, 1974) at modulation rates of 1 GHz. The modulation efficiency at this frequency was 0.5% for GaAs and 1% for CdTe.

The modulator can be operated either inside or outside the laser cavity. Usually operation inside the cavity requires less driving power for the modulator and is preferred. However, losses in the modulator may somewhat reduce the laser output power. An intracavity modulator configuration is shown schematically in Fig. 3.14a. Plane-polarized light from the laser is partially converted to light with the plane of polarization rotated by 90° by the modulator. This is coupled out by a plate held at the Brewster angle.

Since the refractive index of the modulator element changes when a voltage is applied, the optical length of the cavity also changes during modulation. The corresponding shift of the output frequency is given by (Kiefer *et al.*, 1972)

$$\Delta\nu = cn^3rLV/2\lambda d \quad (35)$$

where d is the length of the cavity and c the velocity of light. Thus, an intracavity modulator may also be used for frequency modulation.

Table 3.6

Summary of Modulators Used with the CO_2 Laser

Modulator material	Type	Details[a]	Reference
GaAs	Electro-optic	$r_{41} = 1.6 \times 10^{-12}$ m/V $n = 3.3$ $M = 3.5 \times 10^{-21}$ m²/V²	Yariv *et al.* (1966), Walsh (1968), Kaminow (1968), Bridges *et al.* (1968), McAvoy *et al.* (1972), Huang *et al.* (1974)
CdTe	Electro-optic	$r_{41} = 6.8 \times 10^{-12}$ m/V $n = 2.6$ $M = 3.7 \times 10^{-21}$ m²/V²	Kiefer and Yariv (1969), Kiefer *et al.* (1972), Nikolaev and Koblova (1971), Huang *et al.* (1974)
ZnTe	Electro-optic	$r_{41} = 1.4 \times 10^{-12}$ m/V $n = 2.7$ $M = 0.8 \times 10^{-21}$ m²/V²	Kaminow (1968)
CdS	Electro-optic	$r_e = 5.5 \times 10^{-12}$ m/V $n = 2.3$ $M = 1.0 \times 10^{-21}$ m²/V	Kaminow (1968), Nikolaev and Koblova (1971)
Se	Electro-optic	$r_{11} = 2.5 \times 10^{-12}$ m/V $n = 2.8$ $M = 4.2 \times 10^{-21}$ m²/V	Kamimow (1968), Teich and Kaplan (1966)
Ge	Acousto-optic		Abrams and Pinow (1971)

Te	Acousto-optic		Dixon and Chester (1966)
Ge	Free carrier absorption		Melngailis and Tarmenwald (1969), Flynn and Schhickmann (1968), de Cremoux and Leiba (1969), Müller *et al.* (1972)
InSb	Free carrier absorption		Benoit (1970)
NH_3	Stark effect	$\lambda_m = 10.28\ \mu m$	Landman *et al.* (1969)
NH_2D	Stark effect	$\lambda_m = 10.59\ \mu m$	Johnston and Melville (1971)
CH_3F	Stark effect	$\lambda_m = 9.658\ \mu m$	Landman *et al.* (1969)
CH_3Cl		$\lambda_m = 9.604\ \mu m$	
CH_3Br		$\lambda_m = 10.612\ \mu m$	
CH_3I		$\lambda_m = 10.532\ \mu m$	
NF_3		$\lambda_m = 9.586\ \mu m$	
CH_3CHF_2	Stark effect	Many lines modulated	Jensen and Tobin (1972)
CH_3CF_3			
CH_3CH_2F			
CH_3OH			
CH_3SH			
CH_3NH_2			
C_2HCl_3			
1,1-difluoroethylene	Stark effect	Many lines in 10.4-μm band modulated	Hall and Pao (1971)
1,2-difluoroethane			
Vinyl chloride			
Methyl fluoroform			

[a] See text for notation.

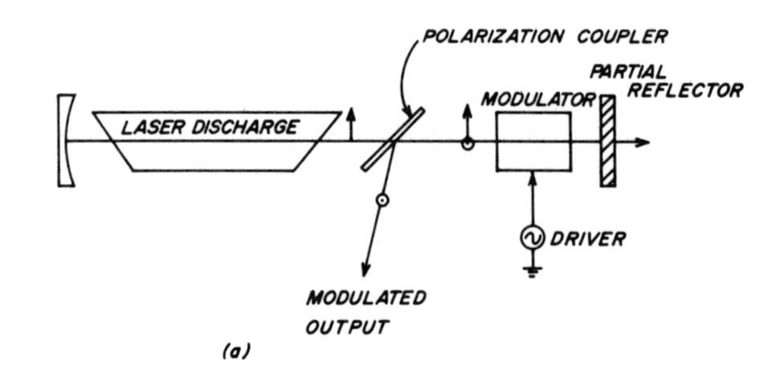

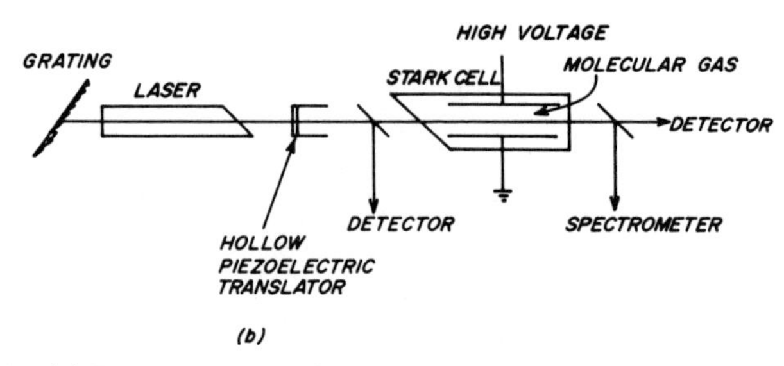

Fig. 3.14. (a) Intracavity modulator using an electro-optic modulator (after Kiefer *et al.*, 1972). (b) Modulation of output by Stark effect in a molecular gas (after Jensen and Tobin, 1972).

Some design requirements for guided-wave electro-optical modulators using GaAs or CdTe have been discussed by Chang and Loh (1972).

Application of an electric field to a molecular gas results in the splitting of rotational levels with rotational quantum number J into $2J + 1$ sublevels (see Section 8.4). The splitting of a particular sublevel from the position of the unperturbed rotational level depends on the strength of the applied electric field. If monochromatic laser radiation is passed through a gas whose molecules have a vibration–rotation line close to the laser frequency, one of the sublevels of this transition may sometimes be brought into coincidence with the laser frequency by application of the appropriate electric field. When the gas is in this state, the laser radiation will be absorbed; when the electric field is removed, the resonance will be destroyed and the incident radiation will be transmitted by the gas. Unfortunately, chance resonances between vibration–rotation lines of simple stable molecular gases and CO_2 laser frequencies occur quite rarely, and this limits the range of laser lines that can be modulated. Furthermore, even when a resonance can be produced with reasonable values of the electric field strength, the resonance is not always with one of the strong lines of the laser [$P(18)$, $P(20)$, $P(22)$ lines of the 10.4-μm band]. Nevertheless, the Stark modulation method has been shown in certain cases to be competitive with electro-optic modulation (Landman *et al.*, 1969; Claspy and Pao, 1971; Johnston and Melville, 1971; Jensen and Tobin, 1972; Hall and Pao, 1971).

Figure 3.14b shows a system used by Jensen and Tobin (1972) for the experimental investigation of Stark modulation of the output of a CO_2 laser by a variety of molecular gases. The grating was used for selection of a particular output wavelength and the cavity length was adjusted using the piezoelectric translator to yield oscillation on the center frequency of the selected line. The Stark cell consisted of two flat aluminum bar electrodes, 0.85 m long and separated by 1 cm. Typically, the gas pressure in the Stark cell was $\simeq$1 Torr and the applied voltage was in the range 600–700 V/cm. Under these conditions, modulation depths of several percent were obtained. Much larger modulation depths have, however, been obtained with NH_2D. Johnston and Melville (1971) report a modulation depth of 40% for the $P(20)$ line at 10.6 μm using a 19.7-cm column of gas and an rms field of 200 V/cm. Similarly, the CO_2 laser line at 9.604 μm has been modulated to a depth of 20% using a field of 1.5 kV/cm applied to methyl chloride (Landman *et al.*, 1969). Some advantages of Stark modulation have been discussed by Claspy and Pao (1971) and a detailed study of the mechanisms involved in modulation with several polyatomic gases has been presented by Martin *et al.* (1974).

A variety of modulation devices based on the interaction between 10.6-μm laser radiation and current carriers in semiconductors have been reported in the literature. One simple device developed by de Cremoux and Leiba (1969) is shown schematically in Fig. 3.15. Holes injected into n-type Ge from a pn junction absorb 10.6-μm radiation and make a transition between two subbands in the valence level. The cross section for this pro-

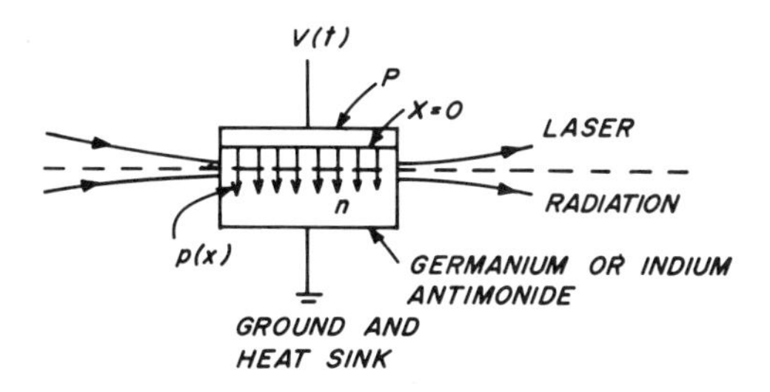

Fig. 3.15. Modulator using free carrier absorption in n-type Ge or n-type InSb (after de Cremoux and Leiba, 1969).

cess is $\sigma_h = 6.5 \times 10^{-16}$ cm². A competing process, due to the excitation of electrons, has the cross section $\sigma_e = 1.5 \times 10^{-17}$ cm² and thus the total absorption coefficient for 10.6-μm radiation, in the absence of lattice absorption, is (Bishop and Gibson, 1973)

$$\alpha = 1.5 \times 10^{-17}n + 6.5 \times 10^{-16}p/\text{cm} \tag{36}$$

where n is the electron density and p the hole density. By artificially increasing p in the n-type material through injection of holes from a pn junction, the value of α can be made large. Since p is a function of time with an ac field applied to the diode, the absorption at 10.6 μm is also time dependent and modulation of the transmitted beam is possible.

The spatial distribution of hole density within the n-type material is given by

$$p(x) = p_0 \exp(-x/L^*)$$

where, in the case of ac modulation of hole density, $p_0(t) = p_0 \exp(j\omega t)$, and

$$L^* = \text{diffusion length} = [D\tau/(1 + j\omega\tau)]^{1/2}$$

where D is the diffusion coefficient for holes and τ the minority carrier lifetime. For $\tau \simeq 1$ μsec and $\omega > 1$ MHz, $L^* \simeq 30$ μm. Then this type of device requires focusing to an area that is almost equal to the diffraction-limited spot size for high-frequency operation. This places quite severe limitations on the maximum power that can be dissipated and an effective means of cooling the semiconductor must be provided. de Cremoux and Leiba (1969) discuss these limitations and predict that a device of this sort should be capable of modulating a 10-W CO_2 laser beam at frequencies of up to 10 MHz. A subsequent study by Benanti and Jacobs (1972) using a p–i diode showed that the variation in $p(x)$ was far from exponential. Near the p–i junction, dp/dx = const, while farther into the bulk material near the ohmic contact $dp/dx = 0$. This has the effect of extending the region of useful modulation farther away from the p–i junction.

In another report on this subject, Benoit (1970) found that a modulation efficiency of almost 100% could be obtained by hole injection into n-type InSb at 77°K. The laser power was 2 W focused to a spot 50 μm in diameter. The limitation on modulation frequency is provided in this, as in the above devices, by the lifetime of holes in the n-type material. With n-type InSb, $\tau \simeq 1$ μsec and modulation frequencies are limited to a few megahertz. Some improvement in response due to a decrease in τ with an applied magnetic field was predicted. Modulation due to free carrier absorption in intrinsic Ge under crossed magnetic and electric fields has been reported by Flynn and Schlickman (1968). Müller *et al.* (1972) have shown that when the modulation is accomplished with energetic carriers, the relaxation time dominates the time response. Since this is short (10^{-12} sec), broad-band modulation is possible.

Long-wavelength (200 μm–2 mm) laser outputs have been modulated by free carriers released by impact ionization in samples cooled to 4.2°K (Melngailis and Tannenwald, 1969). Here, under quiesent conditions, carriers are trapped in shallow levels below the conduction band or above the valence band, and the sample does not absorb long-wavelength radiation. Application of an electric field causes these carriers to be ejected into the corresponding band and contribute to the absorption. Some studies of the interaction of CO_2 laser radiation with semiconductors that are of general interest can be found in Klein and Rudko (1968), Danishevskii *et al.* (1969), Behrendt *et al.* (1970), Müller and Nimtz (1971), Hongo *et al.* (1971), Kazanskii *et al.* (1972), Panyakeow *et al.* (1972), Herrmann and Vogel (1972), and Malz *et al.* (1973).

The acousto-optic modulation of laser output has been treated theoretically by Gordon (1966a,b) and Maydan (1970) and experimentally by Dixon and Chester (1966), Abrams and Pinnow (1971), and Bogdanov *et al.* (1971). When an acoustic wave propagates through a solid it is accompanied by localized changes in solid density. This change in density yields a varying refractive index, and hence a beam of light traversing the sample in the region subjected to acoustic excitation may suffer a deflection. The deflection may more accurately be thought of as the result of energy and momentum transfer from acoustic phonons to optical photons. Energy and momentum conservation are given by

$$\omega_s = \omega \pm \Omega, \qquad \bar{k}_s = \bar{k} \pm \bar{K} \tag{37}$$

where ω_s and ω are the angular frequencies of the scattered and incident photons respectively, $\bar{k}_s$ and $\bar{k}$ are the wavevectors of the scattered and incident photons, and Ω and $\bar{K}$ are the angular frequency and wavevector, respectively, of the scattering phonons. Since $\Omega \ll \omega$, ω_s, the scattered light will be of nearly the same wavelength as the incident light. Furthermore, $k_s \simeq k$, although the angle between $\bar{k}_s$ and $\bar{k}$ is

$$\theta = \sin^{-1}[K/2k] \tag{38}$$

and is not always small. The deflection of the beam may be used to effect modulation either by increasing the cavity loss in an intracavity modulation configuration or by removing the beam from the normal propagation direction when the modulator is outside the laser.

3.8 OTHER OPTICAL COMPONENTS

The measurement of power and energy in a high-power laser beam with a sensitive detector often requires that the intensity of the incident radiation be attenuated by many orders of magnitude before it is allowed to fall onto the detector surface. This prevents damage to the detector and also ensures that the detector response may be kept linear. With CO_2 as with other laser light, the problem lies not in the attenuation of the beam, but in accomplishing this attenuation in a standardized and reproducible manner. For example, it is not much use to measure the intensity in a high-power beam by attenuation if the attenuation factor at the intensity level of the incident beam is unknown or known only with low accuracy.

The simplest method of reducing the intensity of a laser beam is to bring the beam to a focus with a short-focal-length lens or mirror and then to sample the transmitted beam at a distance far removed from the focus. This is practical only when the intensity of the initial beam is small and is impossible at high-intensity levels, where breakdown may occur in the focal region.

Pulsed CO_2 laser beams may be effectively attenuated by absorption in one or more layers of Teflon or some other plastic material. Alternatively, thin interference films on transmitting substrates or even absorption in a bulk absorber such as germanium or one of the other semiconductors may be used. It is important, however, to ascertain that all regions of the beam are attenuated by the same amount, which requires that the attenuator exhibit intensity-independent attenuation since most laser outputs have localized areas within the beam profile with enhanced intensity.

The scattering of laser radiation off roughened metal surfaces or even off a roughened piece of NaCl or KCl can also be used as an effective means of sending a small flux toward a detector from a high-intensity beam. Care must be taken to ensure that the surface is a true Lambertian scatterer, i.e., that it provides only a diffuse reflectance. Grinding and sandblasting of metal surfaces has been shown to be effective (Voronkov, 1971) but at high incident intensities, the heating of the surface may cause the erosion of the small irregularities responsible for the diffuse reflectance, resulting in an intensity-dependent reflection coefficient. It is important that such a scatterer be calibrated at the intensity levels actually encountered in a particular experiment if the attenuation factor is to be relied upon.

A more sophisticated attenuator for 10.6-μm radiation has been reported by Abrams and Gandrud (1969). This device, which is illustrated in Fig. 3.16 relies on the rotation of the plane of polarization of linearly polarized light by a CdS quarter-wave plate in conjunction with a KCl window

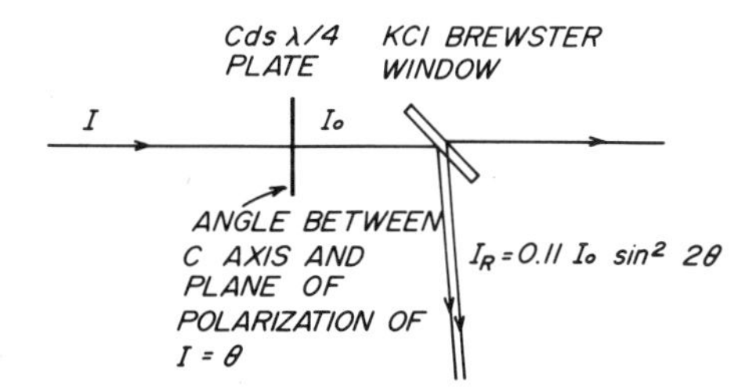

Fig. 3.16. Variable 10.6-μm attenuator (after Abrams and Gandrud, 1969).

mounted at the Brewster angle. When the KCl window is oriented to pass the polarized laser light without the quarter-wave plate, incorporation of the quarter-wave plate in the beam with its *c* axis at an angle θ with respect to the plane of polarization of the laser output will result in a reflected intensity of

$$I_R = 0.11 I_0 \sin^2 2\theta \tag{39}$$

where I_0 is the intensity transmitted by the quarter-wave plate and the factor 0.11 comes from the reflectivity of the KCl window. The maximum attenuation of this device is limited by scattering from the KCl window and was observed to be 43 dB.

Absorption in a flowing gas has been used by Gebhardt *et al.* (1969) to obtain distortionless attenuation of cw CO_2 laser radiation. A mixture of propylene, SF_6, or propane with N_2 is circulated in the closed system shown in Fig. 3.17. The flow speed in the prototype system described by Gebhardt *et al.* was as high as 370 cm/sec at atmospheric pressure and the path length for radiation through the flow was about 7 cm. With a 12.5-W laser power, the attenuation could be varied from 0.5 to 19 dB with no change in the radial profile of the beam after attenuation. Forced convection prevents the development of thermal blooming (see Section 10.3). At

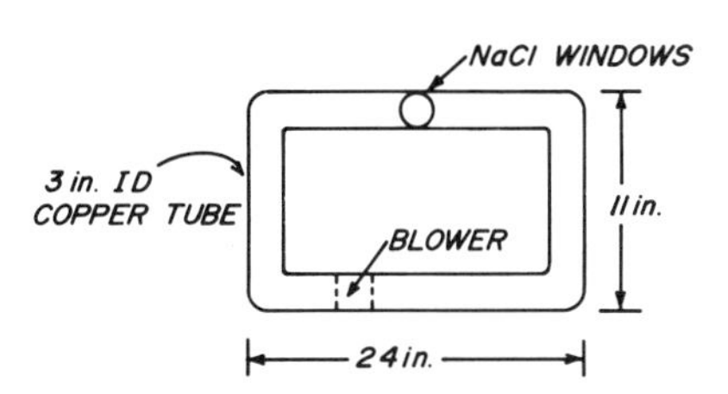

Fig. 3.17. Variable attenuator based on fast flow of absorbing gas (after Gebhardt *et al.*, 1969).

higher flow speeds (10^3 cm/sec) Gebhardt *et al.* predict that incident intensities of up to 10^3 W/cm^2 could be attenuated without distortion.

The problem of sampling energy and power in high-power pulsed CO_2 laser systems during laser–solid interaction studies has been discussed by O'Neil *et al.* (1974). A transmission grating formed by tightly stretched BeCu wires spaced 2.5 mm apart was shown to provide dispersal of the incident radiation into several orders while providing high transmission (with a wire diameter of 0.025 cm, fully 90% of the radiation incident on the grating was transmitted). The advantage of this method is that it allows simultaneous monitoring of energy and power without using beam splitters. Since the intensity in high orders of the diffraction pattern can be less than 0.1% of that in zero order, the measurement does not affect the laser intensity available for surface interaction studies. Furthermore, since the only elements inserted into the beam are metallic (i.e., the wires of the diffraction grating) measurements can be made at high laser intensities without the uncertainties provided by changes in optical transmission due to surface or bulk damage in transmitting optics. In the particular system developed by O'Neil *et al.*, the grating wires were estimated to rise in temperature by only $\simeq$100°C when the laser peak power reached 10^8 W during a 20-μsec pulse.

Massive attenuation of CO_2 laser radiation, as needed, for example, in goggles designed to protect the eyes from stray 10.6-μm reflections, can be obtained from several millimeter thickness of many plastics and glasses. A good review of requirements for this application as well as a list of commercially available eye protectors is given by Carr (1972).

High-power CO_2 laser systems often require that one part of the system be effectively isolated from radiation generated in another part of the system. This requirement is found, for example, in the isolation of a radar receiver from a transmitter and in the isolation of low-power oscillator from an amplifier in a tandem amplifier/oscillator system. Dennis (1967) and later Boord *et al.* (1974) found that this can be accomplished by the use of a Faraday isolator, which rotates the plane of polarization of light transmitted or reflected through a suitable semiconductor. The first isolation device of this type using n-type InSb is shown in Fig. 3.18. The study by Boord *et al.* (1974) showed that n-type InSb was, in fact, the best material available for this application. Isolation properties of this device for signals injected in any of the directions (1)–(4) and detected in other directions (or back out the same beam) may be understood by realizing that the InSb plate produces a 45° rotation in plane-polarized light transmitted. Ports (1) and (3) were isolated by 30 dB in the initial experiments of Dennis (1967). Similar results using ferromagnetic $Cd_2Cr_2S_4$ as an optical isolator

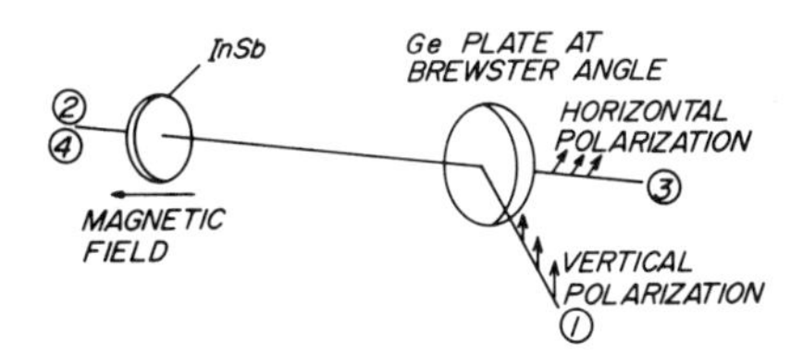

Fig. 3.18. Isolator for use at 10.6 μm. 2, Polarization +45° to horizontal; 4, polarization −45° to horizontal (after Dennis, 1967).

at 10.6 μm have been reported by Jacobs *et al.* (1974). EuO (Dimmock *et al.*, 1969) and $CdCr_2Se_4$ (Bongers and Zanmarchi, 1968) have also been considered.

10.6-μm radiation can be polarized by a stack of transparent plates such as NaCl at the Brewster angle. A more convenient method involves diffraction from or transmission through a wire grid on a nonabsorbing substrate. Cheo and Bass (1971) have developed a method for producing chromium wire grid polarizers on silicon substrates using holographic and photoresist techniques.

Guided-wave propagation of 10.6-μm laser radiation in thin films was first reported by McFee *et al.* (1972) using AgBr coated on NaCl. Radiation was coupled into the thin-film waveguide through a germanium prism. GaAs (Cheo *et al.*, 1973) and GaAs/GaAsP (Finn *et al.*, 1974) optical waveguides at 10.6 μm have been developed. Losses as low as 2 dB/cm have been reported (Finn *et al.*, 1974). A novel parallel-plate waveguide has been discussed by Nishihara *et al.* (1974). Microwave modulation of 10.6-μm radiation propagating in a GaAs waveguide has been reported by Cheo and Gilden (1974).

An interesting optical element based on a saturable absorber such as SF_6 contained in a Fabry–Perot resonator has been described by Szöke *et al.* (1969). One property of this device is that incident light may be either completely reflected or completely transmitted. Szöke *et al.* describe a number of possible applications of this element, including repetitive *Q*-switching, the generation of variable-length pulses, and the possibility of using such a device as a logic element.

Chapter 4

Laser Heating of Solids: Theory

4.1 INTRODUCTION

Some of the first questions that must be answered before it can be estimated whether or not a laser heat source will be suitable for a particular cutting, welding, or drilling requirement are

How much laser power is needed?
How long must this power be applied?
What side effects will be produced in addition to the heating process anticipated?

Finally,

Are these requirements compatible with the specifications of available laser systems?

In many instances, the answers to the first three questions can be obtained by performing a few simple calculations based on classical heat transfer theory. Usually the results of these calculations will suggest an answer to the fourth question.

The purpose of this chapter is to discuss some solutions to the basic heat equation

$$\nabla^2 T - \frac{1}{\kappa}\frac{\partial T}{\partial t} = -\frac{A(x, y, z, t)}{K} \tag{1}$$

which are obtained for laser heating of solids under a variety of conditions that pertain to practical applications. Solutions to this equation can only be obtained in simple analytic form when one is prepared to make a variety of assumptions concerning the spatial and temporal dependence of the impressed laser heat source and the geometry of the sample that is being irradiated. As the description of these boundary conditions becomes more and more rigorous in terms of the actual spatial and temporal dependence of the heat source and the geometry of the workpiece, analytical solutions can no longer be obtained and the resulting expression for $T(x, y, z, t)$ can only be expressed numerically. Solutions to problems of this sort are of little use except in specialized studies and will not be discussed here. We will show that in many cases even quite crude approximations to the actual source and sample boundary calculations are capable of yielding predictions of $T(x, y, z, t)$ that correspond quite closely to actual temperature–time profiles in the solid. Where possible, these predictions have been generalized (i.e., expressed in reduced variable form), so that they may be applied to any material when thermal constants of that material are known.

4.2 HEAT EQUATIONS

The conduction of heat in a three-dimensional solid is given in general by the solution to the equation

$$\rho C \frac{\partial T}{\partial t} = \frac{\partial}{\partial x}\left(K \frac{\partial T}{\partial x}\right) + \frac{\partial}{\partial y}\left(K \frac{\partial T}{\partial y}\right) + \frac{\partial}{\partial z}\left(K \frac{\partial T}{\partial z}\right) + A(x, y, z, t) \tag{2}$$

where the thermal conductivity K, the density ρ, and the specific heat C are dependent both on temperature and position, and heat is supplied to the solid at the rate $A(x, y, z, t)$ per unit time per unit volume. Any temperature dependence of the thermal parameters makes the equation nonlinear, and solutions are very difficult to obtain although numerical solutions are possible in a limited number of cases when the temperature dependence of κ, K, ρ, and C is known. However, since the thermal properties of most materials do not vary greatly with temperature they can often be assumed independent of temperature and can be assigned an average value for the temperature range of interest. In this case, solutions are possible for a number of cases in which thermal properties vary discontinuously (composite solids) or in those cases where a simple analytic expression is available for the spatial variation of K.

If, as will be assumed for the following discussion, the solid is taken to be homogeneous and isotropic, then Eq. (2) reduces to

$$\nabla^2 T - \frac{1}{\kappa}\frac{\partial T}{\partial t} = -\frac{A(x, y, z, t)}{K} \tag{3}$$

where $\kappa = K/\rho C$ is the thermal diffusivity. In the steady state $\partial T/\partial t = 0$ and this equation becomes

$$\nabla^2 T = -A(x, y, z)/K \tag{4}$$

Equations (3) and (4) can be solved in a large number of cases. If no heat is applied to the material, then $A = 0$ and Eqs. (3) and (4) become

$$\nabla^2 T = \frac{1}{\kappa}\frac{\partial T}{\partial t} \qquad \text{(time-dependent case)} \tag{5}$$

$$\nabla^2 T = 0 \qquad \text{(steady-state case)} \tag{6}$$

In practice, cases in which heat sources are present or absent are usually solved by imposing on the solutions of Eqs. (5) and (6) the appropriate boundary conditions of applied heat flux and heat transfer across the surfaces of the solid.

4.3 BASIC DATA

4.3.1 Thermal Constants

In matching experimental heat transfer data to theoretical calculations one must have information on the following thermal parameters of the material or materials under consideration:

(i) K, the thermal conductivity (units, W/cm°C),
(ii) κ, the thermal diffusivity (units, cm^2/sec),
(iii) C_p (or C) the heat capacity (units, J/gm°C) or ρC (units, J/cm^3 °C).

Extensive tabulations of these parameters exist for most materials of engineering interest (see, for example, volumes in the series "Thermophysical Properties of Matter," IFI/Plenum). The practical problem that arises in choosing values of these parameters for a given material is that all depend on temperature. On the other hand, the differential equation for the conduction of heat is not usually soluble in analytic form when these temperature variations are taken into account. Furthermore, other approximations in the form of the boundary conditions, which are often made to permit a simple solution to the heat equation, may introduce inaccuracies in the solution that can be greater than those introduced by neglecting the temperature variation of the thermal parameters.

In some instances it may be expedient to modify the general heat equation (2) by introducing the variable

$$\theta = (1/K_0) \int_0^T K\, dT \tag{7}$$

where K_0 is the value of K at $T = 0°C$. This takes into account the temperature variation of K. Then Eq. (2) becomes

$$\nabla^2\theta - \frac{1}{\kappa}\frac{\partial\theta}{\partial t} = -\frac{A}{K_0} \tag{8}$$

where A and κ now depend on θ. The conditions under which this equation may be easily solved are given in Carslaw and Jaeger (1959, pp. 11, 89).

More commonly, the approximation is made that Eq. (3) can be used with averaged values of the thermal constants over the temperature range of interest. Then (3) becomes

$$\nabla^2 T - \frac{1}{\kappa_{av}}\frac{\partial T}{\partial t} = -\frac{A(x, y, z, t)}{K_{av}} \tag{9}$$

where both κ_{av} and K_{av} are independent of temperature. The average values of these parameters over the temperature range from 0 to T°C are

$$K_{av} = (1/T) \int_0^T K(T)\, dT \tag{10}$$

$$\kappa_{av} = (1/T) \int_0^T \kappa(T)\, dT \tag{11}$$

These integrals may be evaluated numerically when K and κ are not simple functions of T.

In dynamic laser heating processes, it may not be appropriate to use (10) and (11) since these equations give equal weight to all temperatures. In this case, one must examine the time spent by the system at temperatures in the range $0 \to T$ to determine a weighting factor for each $K(T)$ or $\kappa(T)$. On the surface of a material irradiated with a laser beam, the temperature in the vicinity of the focus will usually rise rapidly to within an order of magnitude of the peak temperature and will remain at temperatures within this range for much of the duration of the laser pulse. Equations (10) and (11) may then overestimate the contributions to K_{av} and κ_{av} from $K(T)$ and $\kappa(T)$ in the low-temperature region. It may then be more reasonable to use $K(T_{max})$ and $\kappa(T_{max})$ in Eq. (7) instead of K_{av} and κ_{av} calculated from (10) and (11). So we see that, having decided that K and κ should be assumed to be independent of temperature for the purposes of obtaining a solution to the heat equation, we must still in the outcome assign them a value that faithfully describes heat transfer in the material in the temperature range of interest.

Temperature-dependent values of K for a number of pure metals, alloys, and insulators have been plotted in Appendix A. Data on which these graphs are based were obtained from the recommended values given in Touloukian and Ho (1970a, b) and other volumes in that series. For metals it is apparent that K is usually not a strong function of temperature below the melting point. However, at the melting point, K often changes by a factor of up to two. The temperature variation of K for the liquid phase of metals is usually slower than that of the solid below T_m. $K(T)$ for a few materials and various temperatures is given in Table 4.1.

Table 4.1

Thermal Conductivity Data for Some Metallic and Nonmetallic Solids

Material	K (W/cm°C)				
	273°K	500°K	1000°K	2000°K	3000°K
Aluminum	2.36	2.38			
Chromium	0.948	0.85	0.65		
Cobalt	1.04	0.745			
Copper	4.01	3.88	3.56	1.82	1.80
Gold	3.18	3.09	2.78	1.20	1.25
Iron	0.835	0.615	0.325	0.425	0.46
Lead	0.355	0.325	0.215		
Molybdenum	1.39	1.30	1.12	0.88	
Nickel	0.94	0.72	0.72		
Platinum	0.715	0.72	0.785		
Rhodium	1.51	1.40	1.21		
Silver	4.28	4.12	3.74	1.97	1.91
Tantalum	0.574	0.582	0.602	0.64	0.665
Tin	0.682	0.595	0.405		
Titanium	0.224	0.197	0.207		

Table 4.1—(*Continued*)

Material	K (W/cm°C)				
	273°K	500°K	1000°K	2000°K	3000°K
Tungsten	1.82	1.49	1.20	1.0	0.91
Uranium	0.270	0.317	0.44		
Vanadium	0.313	0.33	0.385	0.51	
Zinc	1.22	1.11	0.67		
Zirconium	0.232	0.21	0.236	0.313	
Armcoiron	0.747	0.593	0.323	0.635	
302 Stainless steel	0.13	0.155	0.24		
303 Stainless steel	0.15	0.16	0.25		
304 Stainless steel	0.168	0.186	0.255		
Alumel (94.9% Ni, 2% Mn, 2% Al, 1% Si)	2.9	3.1			
Yellow brass (72% Cu, 22% Zn, 4% Pb, 2% Sn)	1.06				
Inconel	0.15				
Monel	0.213				
Zircaloy 2	0.12				
Beryllium oxide	3.0				
Nickel oxide	0.4				
Thoria (ThO_2)	0.15	0.06	0.03		
Zirconia (ZrO_2)	0.02	0.02	0.02		
Al_2O_3 (polycrystalline)	0.397	0.20	0.078	0.06	
Pyrolytic graphite[a]	22.3	11.3	5.3	2.5	
	0.106	0.054	0.025	0.012	
MgO (polycrystalline)	0.53	0.269	0.097	0.085	
Fused quartz	0.0133	0.0162	0.0287		
TiO_2 (polycrystalline)	0.089	0.0588	0.0346		
Basalt	0.002				
Dolomite		0.012			
Earth (0.15 gm/cm^3)	0.0019				
Granite	0.015				
Limestone	0.01				
Steatite	0.032				
Polyvinyl chloride	0.00155				
Polyethylene	0.00385				
Plexiglass	0.00154				
Hardwood	0.00158				
Pine	0.00138				
Cardboard	0.0015				
Wallboard	0.0005				

[a] Conduction parallel and perpendicular to basal plane, respectively.

Similar data on $C_p(T)$ and $K(T)$ are given in Appendices B and C and in Tables 4.2 and 4.3. Thermal diffusivities have been calculated from K and C_p data using standard values for ρ, the solid density. In this calculation no attempt was made to compensate for the variation of ρ with T.

Table 4.2

Specific Heats for Some Materials

	C_p (J/gm°C)				
Material	273°K	500°K	1000°K	2000°K	3000°K
Aluminum	0.83	1.0			
Chromium	0.5	0.49	0.58		
Copper	0.38	0.417	0.471		
Gold	0.135	0.135	0.151		
Iron	0.42	0.54	0.98		
Lead	0.129	0.136			
Molybdenum	0.245	0.261	0.288	0.39	
Nickel	0.44	0.52	0.56		
Platinum	0.132	0.138	0.152	0.18	
Silver	0.234	0.243	0.272		
Tantalum	0.137	0.144	0.154	0.174	0.237
Tin	0.226	0.264			
Titanium	0.52	0.58	0.74	0.7	
Tungsten	0.132	0.138	0.15	0.175	0.203
Uranium	0.116	0.133	0.178		
Vanadium	0.47	0.51	0.62	0.83	
Zinc	0.378	0.422			
Zirconium	0.28	0.322	0.36		
Brass	0.38				
Inconel	0.41				
Pb–Sn (solder)	0.175				
Monel	0.42				
Zircaloy 2	0.03				
Armco iron		0.8	0.95		
304 Stainless steel	0.37	0.383	0.45		
Beryllium oxide	0.92				
Graphite	0.64	1.17	1.67	2.1	2.1
Nickel oxide (NiO)	0.57	0.84			
Thoria (ThO_2)	0.23	0.26	0.29		
Zirconia (ZrO_2)	0.46	0.54	0.63		
Alumina (Al_2O_3) (polycrystalline)	1.00	1.07	1.22	1.52	
Magnesium oxide (MgO)	0.70	1.12	1.245		
Fused quartz	0.7	0.99	1.15		
Titanium dioxide (TiO_2)	0.70	0.85	0.93	1.0	

Table 4.3

Thermal Diffusivities of Metals and Nonmetals

Material	κ (cm²/sec)				
	273°K	500°K	1000°K	2000°K	3000°K
Aluminum	1.03	0.88			
Chromium	0.27	0.235	0.16		
Copper	1.19	1.04	0.85		
Gold	1.22	1.19	0.93		
Iron	0.28	0.145			
Lead	0.24	0.21			
Molybdenum	0.54	0.49	0.38	0.22	0.13
Nickel	0.2	0.17	0.14		
Platinum	0.255	0.24	0.24	0.27	
Silver	1.74	1.61	1.3		
Tantalum	0.25	0.24	0.235	0.22	0.17
Titanium	0.097	0.075	0.062		
Tungsten	0.70	0.56	0.41	0.295	0.23
Uranium	0.13	0.126			
Vanadium	0.112	0.1085	0.104	0.104	
Zinc	0.45	0.36			
Zirconium	0.124	0.10	0.101		
Al_2O_3 (polycrystalline)	1.0	0.048	0.016	0.012	
MgO	0.16	0.065	0.022	0.02	
Fused quartz	0.0073	0.0062	0.0094		
TiO_2	0.031	0.017	0.009		
ThO_2	0.07	0.02	0.01		
ZrO_2	0.0074	0.0063	0.0053		

4.3.2 Emissivity

Theoretical calculations of the heating effect of high-power laser radiation require that one knows how much of the radiation incident on a target is absorbed and how much is reflected. For transparent or semitransparent materials this requires a measurement of both reflectivity and transmissivity. For opaque materials a measurement of the reflectivity $R_\lambda(T)$ will suffice, since the emissivity $\epsilon_\lambda(T)$ or the fraction of the incident intensity absorbed is given by

$$\epsilon_\lambda(T) = 1 - R_\lambda(T) \tag{12}$$

where λ refers to the wavelength of the incident radiation and T is the target temperature. General rules for the variation of $\epsilon_\lambda(T)$ with λ and T

for insulating materials cannot be easily formulated and direct spectroscopic measurements are usually required. However, $\epsilon_\lambda(T)$ for metals in the infrared spectral region ($\lambda > 2\ \mu$m) can be calculated from data on the temperature-dependent resistivity of the metal. In this section, the results of this calculation will be given and $\epsilon_{10\ \mu m}(T)$ for some common metals will be tabulated. It must be stressed however, that this calculation and the numerical values for $\epsilon_{10\ \mu m}(T)$ actually arrived at will be valid only for metals heated in vacuum without a surface oxide layer. The presence of surface films will greatly increase $\epsilon_{10\ \mu m}(T)$.

The complex refractive index of a metal

$$m = n - in' \tag{13}$$

exhibits common behavior for all metals at wavelengths $\lambda \gtrsim 2\ \mu$m. This common behavior takes the form of an increase in both n and n' and a tendency for $n \simeq n'$. The square of m can be written

$$m^2 = \beta - i\eta \tag{14}$$

and approaches $-i\eta$ as $\eta \gg 1$. Since from theory

$$\eta = 60\lambda/r \tag{15}$$

where λ is the wavelength in meters and r the resistivity of the metal in Ω-m^2/m (the conversion factor of 60 has the dimensions of ohms), the limiting value $m^2 = -i\eta$ is approached at long wavelengths. Then

$$m = (\tfrac{1}{2}\eta)^{1/2}(1 - i), \qquad \eta \gg 1 \tag{16}$$

and since for perpendicular incidence of radiation

$$\epsilon_\lambda(T) = 1 - R_\lambda(T) = 1 - \left|\frac{m-1}{m+1}\right|^2 \tag{17}$$

the emissivity becomes (at long wavelengths)

$$\epsilon_\lambda(T) \simeq (8/\eta)^{1/2} \tag{18}$$

where η is a function of both wavelength and temperature. The absorption coefficient of the metal is given by

$$\alpha = 4\pi n'/\lambda \simeq \tfrac{1}{4}\lambda(2/\eta)^{1/2}, \qquad \eta \gg 1 \tag{19}$$

Following Bramson (1968), Eq. (18) may be expanded to give

$$\epsilon_\lambda(T) = 0.365[r/\lambda]^{1/2} - 0.0667[r/\lambda] + 0.006[r/\lambda]^{3/2} \tag{20}$$

where r is now in the units Ω-cm^2/cm (shortened to Ω-cm) and λ is in cm.

Writing the resistivity r as

$$r = r_{20°C}(1 + \gamma[T - 293]) \tag{21}$$

$\epsilon_\lambda(T)$ becomes

$$\epsilon_\lambda(T) = 0.365[r_{20}(1 + \gamma T)/\lambda]^{1/2} - 0.0667[r_{20}(1 + \gamma T)/\lambda] + 0.006[r_{20}(1 + \gamma T)/\lambda]^{3/2} \tag{22}$$

where it is now understood that T is in °C. For the CO_2 laser wavelength $\lambda = 10.6\ \mu m$, this expression becomes

$$\epsilon_{10.6\ \mu m}(T) = 11.2[r_{20}(1 + \gamma T)]^{1/2} - 62.9[r_{20}(1 + \gamma T)] + 174[r_{20}(1 + \gamma T)]^{3/2} \tag{23}$$

Bramson (1968) gives data on r_{20} and γ that may be used to estimate $\epsilon_{10.6\ \mu m}(T)$ for most simple metals over a moderate range of temperature. Table 4.4 reproduces some of these data, and Fig. 4.1 shows a generalized

Table 4.4

Resistivity at 20°C (r_{20}) and Coefficient of Resistivity Change with Temperature (γ)[a]

Material	r_{20} (Ω-cm)	γ (Ω-cm/°C)
Aluminum	2.82×10^{-6}	3.6×10^{-3}
Brass	8.00×10^{-6}	1.5×10^{-3}
Bronze	8.00×10^{-6}	3.5×10^{-3}
Constantan	4.90×10^{-5}	1.0×10^{-5}
Copper	1.72×10^{-6}	4.0×10^{-3}
Gold	2.42×10^{-6}	3.6×10^{-3}
Invar	7.8×10^{-5}	2.0×10^{-3}
Iron	9.80×10^{-6}	5.0×10^{-3}
Manganese	4.40×10^{-5}	1.0×10^{-5}
Molybdenum	5.60×10^{-6}	4.7×10^{-3}
Nichrome	1.00×10^{-4}	4.0×10^{-4}
Nickel	7.24×10^{-6}	5.4×10^{-3}
Platinum	1.05×10^{-5}	3.7×10^{-3}
Silver	1.62×10^{-6}	3.6×10^{-3}
Steel		
alloy	1.50×10^{-5}	1.5×10^{-3}
mild	1.50×10^{-5}	3.3×10^{-3}
structural	1.20×10^{-5}	3.2×10^{-3}
Tantalum	1.55×10^{-5}	3.1×10^{-3}
Tin	1.14×10^{-5}	4.0×10^{-3}
Tungsten	5.50×10^{-6}	5.2×10^{-3}
Zinc	5.92×10^{-6}	3.5×10^{-3}

[a] From Bramson (1968).

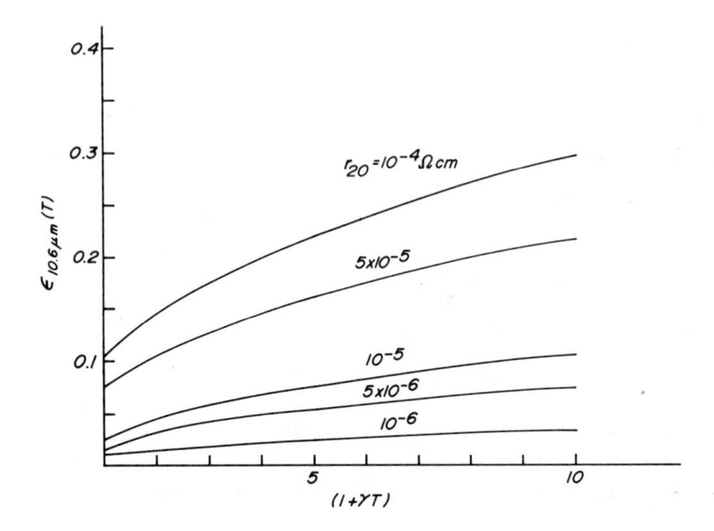

Fig. 4.1. Emissivity at 10.6 μm for metals.

plot of $\epsilon_{10.6\ \mu m}(T)$ versus $(1 + \gamma T)$ for r_{20} in the range 10^{-4}–10^{-6} Ω-cm. $\epsilon_{10.6\ \mu m}(T)$ calculated in this way should be treated with caution, particularly at high temperatures where the approximation for r given by Eq. (21) may not be strictly valid. In any case, the maximum temperature used to evaluate $1 + \gamma T$ should not exceed the melting point of the material.

We see that even metals with high resistivity, such as nichrome, have low values of $\epsilon_{10.6\ \mu m}$ even at high temperatures. Thus, in the absence of surface oxidation or some processing that increases $\epsilon_{10.6\ \mu m}$, most metals will absorb less than 20% of incident 10.6-μm radiation even at elevated temperatures. The increase of $\epsilon_{10.6\ \mu m}(T)$ with temperature means that progressively more incident radiation may be absorbed as T increases. This occasionally leads to a thermal runaway effect, which can help or hinder thermal processing of metallic materials.

Bennett (1971) has published a detailed theoretical and experimental study of the reflectivities and absorptivities of several CO_2 laser mirror materials. Particular emphasis was placed on mirrors formed from evaporated silver or gold films. The method of preparation of these mirror surfaces was found to be critical if highest reflectivity was required. Much of this variation appears to be due to microroughness or changes in the electrical conductivity of the surface layer caused by the presence of dislocations and lattice disorder. Thin dielectric coatings on silver or gold substrates were found invariably to involve an increase in the emissivity of the surface, although some increase in the resistance of silver mirrors to atmospheric corrosion was noted.

Obviously, the emissivities of the surfaces of many metallic and dielectric materials are of fundamental interest in the design of high-power laser windows and reflectors. This subject has been discussed in greater detail in Section 3.5.

4.4 UNIFORM HEATING OVER THE SURFACE BOUNDING A SEMI-INFINITE HALF-SPACE

The simplest heat transfer problem encountered in laser interaction studies is given by the system of a semi-infinite half-space that is heated uniformly over its bounding surface. In discussing this problem, Ready (1971) defines three situations in which the heat transfer equations can be easily solved.

4.4.1 Surface Source, Constant in Time

When laser radiation can be considered to be absorbed in a very thin surface layer and the temporal variation of the pulse is given by

$$F(t) = \begin{cases} F_0, & t > 0 \\ 0, & t < 0 \end{cases}$$

then the variation of temperature with depth is given by (Carslaw and Jaeger, 1959)

$$T(z, t) = (2\epsilon F_0/K)(\kappa t)^{1/2} \operatorname{ierfc}[z/2(\kappa t)^{1/2}] \tag{24}$$

Where ierfc is the integral of the error function erfc,

$$\operatorname{ierfc} x = \int_x^\infty \operatorname{erfc} s \, ds, \qquad \text{and} \qquad \operatorname{erfc} x = (2/\pi)^{1/2} \int_x^\infty e^{-s^2} \, ds \tag{25}$$

The surface temperature $T(0, t)$ is seen to be proportional to $t^{1/2}$:

$$T(0, t) = (2\epsilon F_0/K)[\kappa t/\pi]^{1/2} \tag{26}$$

We see that there is no limiting surface temperature: if the flux were maintained indefinitely at F_0, $T(0, \infty) \to \infty$. Also, for this boundary condition the energy flux $E = F_0 t$, and it is evident that the temperature reached at the surface for a given pulse energy is $\propto (t)^{-1/2}$. To reach a predetermined temperature with given pulse energy, it is more effective to shorten rather than to lengthen the pulse. This shows clearly the importance of the rate of energy input in establishing a final temperature.

If the radiation is applied in the form of a pulse,

$$F(t) = \begin{cases} F_0, & 0 < t < T \\ 0, & t < 0, \quad t > T \end{cases}$$

then $T(z, t)$ is as given by Eq. (24) while the pulse is applied, but the temperature subsequently varies as

$$T(z, t)_{t>T} = \frac{2F_0\kappa^{1/2}}{K}\left\{t^{1/2} \operatorname{ierfc} \frac{z}{2(\kappa t)^{1/2}} - (t - T)^{1/2} \operatorname{ierfc} \frac{z}{2[\kappa(t - T)]^{1/2}}\right\} \tag{27}$$

With this geometry, the transfer of heat is one dimensional and the thermal penetration depth defined by Eq. (24) during the pulse is given by $Z = (4\kappa t)^{1/2}$. The solutions (24) and (27) can therefore be used for uniform surface heating of slabs provided W, the thickness of the slab, is $> (4\kappa t)^{1/2}$.

In addition, these solutions will also be approximately valid for the situation where heating proceeds only over a limited area of the free surface of a semi-infinite slab, provided that l, a characteristic dimension of the heated area, satisfies the condition $l > (4\kappa t)^{1/2}$. Here the z axis should be thought of as extending into the material from the center of the heated region and Eqs. (24) and (27) will give the true temperature of the material only along this axis.

4.4.2 Distributed Source, Constant in Time

The laser pulse is as given above, except that the absorption cannot be considered to be localized in a surface layer, and temperatures are to be estimated within the region of absorption. Defining the absorption coefficient for radiation of the laser wavelength as α cm^{-1}, Ready (1971) obtains

$$\begin{aligned} T(z, t) = {} & \frac{2\epsilon F_0}{K}(\kappa t)^{1/2} \operatorname{ierfc}\left[\frac{z}{2(\kappa t)^{1/2}}\right] - \frac{\epsilon F_0}{\alpha K} e^{-\alpha z} \\ & + \frac{\epsilon F_0}{2\alpha K} \exp(\alpha^2 \kappa t - \alpha z) \operatorname{erfc}\left[\alpha(\kappa t)^{1/2} - \frac{z}{2(\kappa t)^{1/2}}\right] \\ & + \frac{\epsilon F_0}{2\alpha K} \exp(\alpha^2 \kappa t + \alpha z) \operatorname{erfc}\left[\alpha(\kappa t)^{1/2} + \frac{z}{2(\kappa t)^{1/2}}\right] \end{aligned} \tag{28}$$

where erfc and ierfc are the error function and the integral of the error function, respectively. If we take $z = \alpha^{-1}$ and introduce the normalization $\tau = \alpha^2 \kappa t$, then this expression may be rewritten

$$\frac{T(\alpha^{-1}, \tau)K\alpha}{\epsilon F_0} = -e^{-1} + 2\tau^{1/2} \operatorname{ierfc}\left[\frac{1}{2\tau^{1/2}}\right] + e^{(\tau-1)} \operatorname{erfc}(\tau^{1/2} - 0.5\tau^{-1/2}) + e^{(\tau+1)} \operatorname{erfc}(\tau^{1/2} + 0.5\tau^{-1/2}) \qquad (29)$$

From the original boundary conditions, this solution will be valid for all $t > 0$ but not at $t = 0$.

A practical heating situation described by this analysis occurs in the welding of plastic sheets with cw CO_2 lasers. At 10.6 μm the absorption coefficient of many plastics including polyethylene is of the order 10–20 cm^{-1}. Equation (29) plotted in Fig. 4.2 shows that the temperature at a depth $z = \alpha^{-1}$ rises instantaneously to the value $\simeq 0.6\epsilon F_0/K\alpha$ on application of the laser pulse. The low-absorption coefficients of plastics at 10.6 μm require that Eq. (28) be used for a prediction of temperatures in the layer in which laser radiation is absorbed. This layer may be several millimeters in thickness.

4.4.3 Surface Source, Variable in Time

The laser pulse varies with time although the incident intensity is still uniform over the boundary of the semi-infinite half-space. Furthermore,

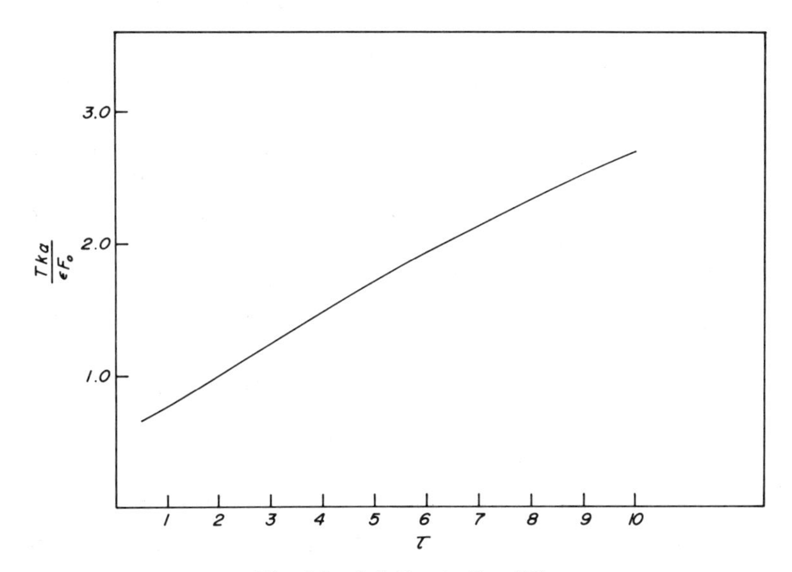

Fig. 4.2. Solution to Eq. (29).

the absorption coefficient is large so that radiation is effectively absorbed at the surface. In this case, which is still an elementary one as far as laser applications are concerned, no simple analytical expression is available for $T(z, t)$. However, the integral

$$T(z, t) = \int_z^\infty \int_0^t \frac{F(s)}{F_0} \frac{\partial}{\partial t} \frac{\partial T'(z', t - s)}{\partial z'} \, dz' \, ds \tag{30}$$

can be evaluated numerically, and Ready (1965, 1971) has plotted $T(z, t)$ for copper subjected to a pulse from a Q-switched laser. In Eq. (30), T' is the solution to the heat equation for the case of a square heat pulse of absorbed intensity F_0.

When the absorption coefficient is large and Eq. (24) can be used for T', this integral simplifies to

$$T(z, t) = \frac{\kappa^{1/2}}{K\pi^{1/2}} \int_0^t \frac{F(t - s) \exp(-z^2/4\kappa s)}{s^{1/2}} \, ds \tag{31}$$

One special example of the boundary conditions that lead to an analytical expression for $T(z, t)$ from Eq. (30) occurs when the flux decreases as $t^{-1/2}$ after $t = 0$ (Carslaw and Jaeger, 1959). In that case,

$$T(z, t) = \frac{F(t) \pi^{1/2} (\kappa t)^{1/2}}{K} \operatorname{erfc}\left[\frac{z}{2(\kappa t)^{1/2}}\right] \tag{32}$$

4.4.4 Surface Source, Pulsed

This problem has been treated by Carslaw and Jaeger (1959), White (1963), and Rykalin *et al.* (1967c). The simplest solution is obtained when the source generates a series of rectangular pulses (Fig. 4.3a). White (1963) has shown that the resulting temperature distribution can be obtained by superimposing single-pulse solutions from Eqs. (24) and (27). Figure 4.3b shows the temperature rise on the surface of a semi-infinite solid irradiated with the pulses in Fig. 4.3a.

Rykalin *et al.* (1967c) have discussed the conditions under which heating with a series of pulses can be considered continuous.

4.5 CIRCULAR SURFACE SOURCE ON SEMI-INFINITE HALF-SPACE

4.5.1 Uniform Source, Constant in Time

Various approximations to the intensity distribution within the focus of a laser beam are possible. In this section, we consider that total laser power

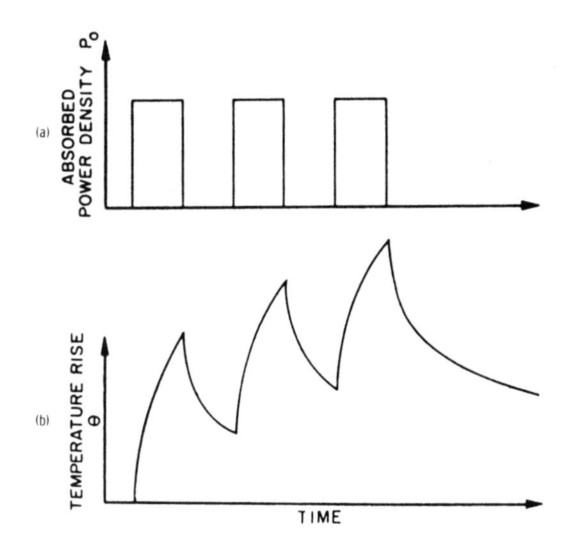

Fig. 4.3. Variation of temperature with time for a semi-infinite half-space on irradiation with a series of pulses (after White, 1963).

P is incident over a circular area πA^2 and that the intensity within this area is constant at the value $P/\pi A^2$. In practice, the distribution of intensity within the focus is a complex function of position and time (Levine *et al.*, 1967; Waynant *et al.*, 1965) but laser-induced thermal effects do not seem to be overly sensitive to this distribution provided that the temperature (i.e., thermal effect) is sampled away from the immediate area in which the interaction occurs. For this reason, it is often convenient to assume as above that all "fine structure" in the intensity distribution is eliminated and that the thermal effect is the same as that which would be produced by absorption of the equivalent total power over a circular area whose radius may be chosen empirically. We will also discuss below the somewhat more refined approximation that the intensity distribution has a Gaussian spatial distribution within the focal area.

Consider the case of heating a large block of material with laser radiation focused onto the surface as shown in Fig. 4.4. The time-dependent temperature distribution in the solid is obtained by solving Eq. (5) for applied power P for $t > 0$ over the circle $x^2 + y^2 = A^2$, $z = 0$, of the semi-infinite region

$$-\infty \leq x \leq +\infty, \qquad -\infty \leq y \leq +\infty, \qquad 0 \leq z \leq +\infty$$

The solution (Carslaw and Jaeger, 1959) at the point whose cylindrical

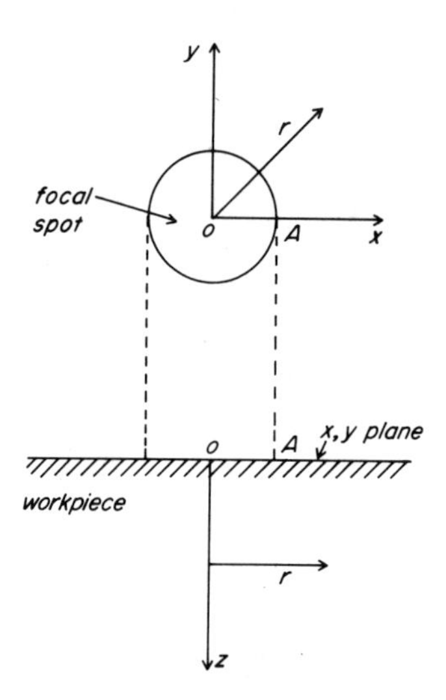

Fig. 4.4. Coordinate system.

coordinates are (r, z) is then

$$T(r, z, t) = \frac{P\epsilon}{2\pi AK} \int_0^\infty J_0(\lambda r) J_1(\lambda A) \left\{ e^{-\lambda z} \operatorname{erfc}\left[\frac{z}{2(\kappa t)^{1/2}} - \lambda(\kappa t)^{1/2} \right] \right.$$

$$\left. - e^{\lambda z} \operatorname{erfc}\left[\frac{z}{2(\kappa t)^{1/2}} + \lambda(\kappa t)^{1/2} \right] \right\} \frac{d\lambda}{\lambda} \tag{33}$$

where ϵ is the fraction of the energy absorbed from the beam, and J_0 and J_1 are Bessel functions of the first kind. This integral can be evaluated numerically to determine the temperature at any point in the solid at any time. Of greater interest is the temperature variation with time for points directly below the focal spot. The temperature at positions along the z axis is given by

$$T(0, z, t) = \frac{2P\epsilon(\kappa t)^{1/2}}{\pi A^2 K} \left[\operatorname{ierfc}\left(\frac{z}{2(\kappa t)^{1/2}} \right) - \operatorname{ierfc}\left(\frac{(z^2 + A^2)^{1/2}}{2(\kappa t)^{1/2}} \right) \right] \tag{34}$$

If we define the dimensionless variables

$$\theta = \frac{TAK\pi}{P\epsilon}, \qquad \Gamma = \frac{2(\kappa t)^{1/2}}{A}$$

for temperature and time, respectively, then Eq. (34) becomes

$$\theta(0, z, \tau) = \Gamma\left[\operatorname{ierfc}\frac{z}{A\Gamma} - \operatorname{ierfc}\frac{(z^2 + A^2)^{1/2}}{A\Gamma}\right] \tag{35}$$

which implies a surface temperature variation given by

$$\theta(0, 0, \tau) = \Gamma\left[\frac{1}{\pi^{1/2}} - \operatorname{ierfc}\frac{1}{\Gamma}\right] \tag{36}$$

or

$$T(0, 0, t) = \frac{2P\epsilon(\kappa t)^{1/2}}{\pi A^2 K}\left[\frac{1}{\pi^{1/2}} - \operatorname{ierfc}\left(\frac{A}{2(\kappa t)^{1/2}}\right)\right] \tag{37}$$

To obtain the steady state values at any depth below or at the center of the focal spot, we let $t \to \infty$ in Eq. (35) and then

$$\theta(0, z, \infty) = \frac{1}{A}\left[(z^2 + A^2)^{1/2} - z\right] \tag{38}$$

This implies that the maximum surface temperature attainable is given by

$$\theta(0, 0, \infty) = 1 \qquad \text{or} \qquad T(0, 0, \infty) = P\epsilon/\pi AK \tag{39}$$

Equation (35) has been plotted in Fig. 4.5 to illustrate the variation of the

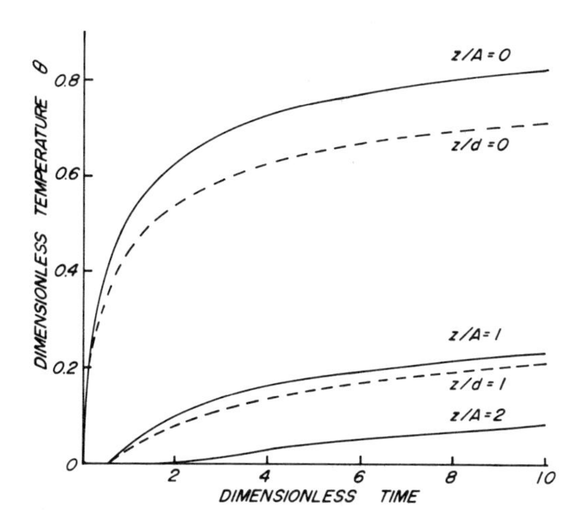

Fig. 4.5. Dimensionless temperature θ vs. dimensionless time $\tau = 4\kappa t/A^2$ or $4\kappa t/d^2$ for various depths when heating with continuous disk (——) and Gaussian (– –) sources.

dimensionless temperature θ with $\tau = \Gamma^2 = 4\kappa t/A^2$ and depth below the focal spot. It can be seen that the temperature rises rapidly at first and approaches 75% of its steady state value within $\tau = 4$ or $t = A^2/\kappa$, after which change in temperature with time proceeds at a progressively decreasing rate. The time $t = A^2/K$ can therefore be associated with the thermal time constant for a heating process of this type. It can also be seen that there is an increasing time delay before the beginning of noticeable temperature increase as one proceeds to greater depths.

If values are substituted for ϵ, K, and A in Eq. (39) and T is set equal to T_m, the melting temperature, then this expression yields a measure of the maximum power that can be applied without damaging the surface of the material, or conversely the minimum power that is required if melting is desired. This quantity is also of importance in a determination of the suitability of materials used as laser mirrors under given focusing conditions. Table 4.5 gives minimum values of P/A for the production of melting at the surface of various metal slabs using the CO_2 laser. The value of ϵ used is that for the melting temperature and wavelength 10.6 μm when heating is done in vacuum. P/A is expected to be smaller for heating done in air if convection losses can be neglected. It is of interest to plot the value of P/A required to produce melting at the center of the focal area as a function of the length of the radiation pulse. A plot of this sort is given in Fig. 4.6 for several different metals. As an example, a power of 50 kW focused at 10.6 μm to a circular area with $A = 0.1$ cm would produce

Table 4.5

Minimum Values of P/A for Melting of an Infinite Slab with 10.6-μm Radiation Focused to a Circular Area of Radius A

Material	P/A ($\times 10^4$ W/cm)
Al	13
Au	26
Mg	6.5
Cu	34
Sn	0.85
Zn	3.1
Pb	0.43
Pt	5.3
Ta	4.9
Ni	4.4
W	8.9
Mo	7.3

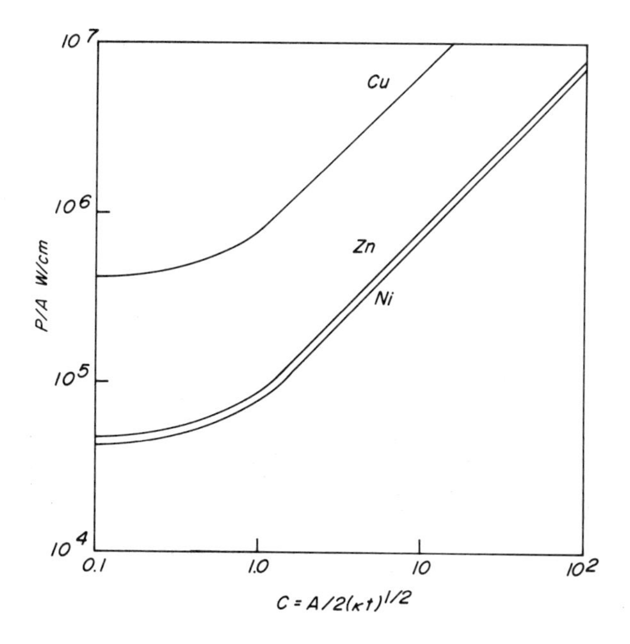

Fig. 4.6. Critical power for melting in vacuum.

melting ($T = 1080°C$) in normalized time $C = 0.4$ or $t = A^2/4\kappa C^2 \simeq 20$ msec when incident on copper in vacuum. On the other hand, a pulsed laser generating a constant power of 3×10^6 W for 1.6 μsec would also produce melting.

Another quantity of interest is the average temperature that can be achieved over the focal spot. Solving the steady state Eq. (6) and averaging over the circle of radius A gives (Carslaw and Jaeger, 1959)

$$T_{\mathrm{av}} = 8P\epsilon/3\pi^2AK = 0.85T(0, 0, \infty) \tag{40}$$

We note that the average temperature does not differ greatly from the maximum temperature and also that $T_{\mathrm{av}}/T_{\max}$ is independent of the material.

Guenot and Racinet (1967) discuss the shape of isotherms in the vicinity of the focal spot in more detail using an instantaneous heat source model.

4.5.2 Uniform Source, Variable in Time

The temperature as a function of time and position in a semi-infinite solid when Q J are instantaneously liberated over a disk of radius A located in the plane $z = 0$ is (Carslaw and Jaeger, 1959; Paek and Gagliano,

1972)

$$T(r, z, t) = \frac{Q}{2\rho c\pi A^2(\pi\kappa^3 t^3)^{1/2}} \int_0^A \exp\left[-\frac{(r^2 + r'^2 + z^2)}{4\kappa t}\right] I_0\left(\frac{rr'}{2\kappa t}\right) r'\,dr' \tag{41}$$

where I_0 is the modified Bessel function of order zero. For a time-dependent heat input $Q(t')$ the temperature is found by integrating Eq. (41) over t'. Then

$$T(r, z, t) = \frac{1}{2\rho c\pi^{3/2}\kappa^{3/2}} \int_0^A \int_0^t \frac{Q(t')}{(t - t')^{3/2}} \exp\left[-\frac{(r^2 + r'^2 + z^2)}{4\kappa t}\right] \times I_0\left(\frac{rr'}{2\kappa t}\right) r'\,dr'\,dt' \tag{42}$$

Paek and Gagliano (1972) have used this expression in a consideration of temperature and stress distributions in Al_2O_3 slabs subjected to ruby or CO_2 laser pulses.

4.5.3 Effect of Defocusing from a Circular Area

Occasionally, because of lack of distortionless optics the spot on the material is more elliptical than circular. Here some insight can be gained into the effect of this distortion by approximating the elliptical spot by a rectangle of dimension $(2l, 2a)$. The maximum equilibrium temperature at the surface in this case is (Carslaw and Jaeger, 1959)

$$T(0, 0, \infty) = (P\epsilon/2K\pi la)[a \sinh^{-1}(l/a) + l \sinh^{-1}(a/l)] \tag{43}$$

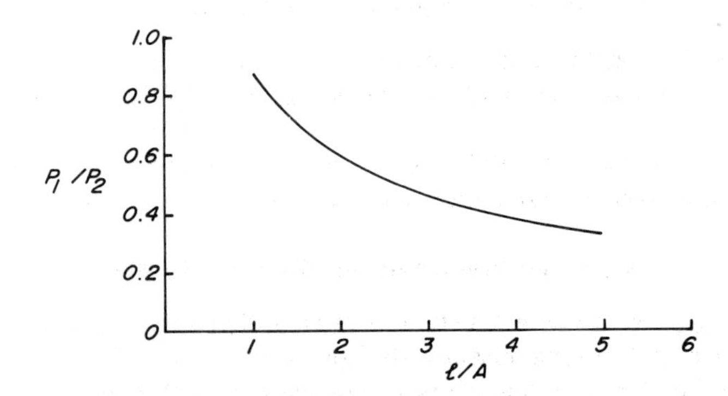

Fig. 4.7. P_1/P_2 vs. l/a for semi-infinite sheet and $A = a$.

If we call P of Eq. (39) P_1, and that of Eq. (43) P_2, then for $A = a$,

$$P_1/P_2 = (1/2l)[a \sinh^{-1}(l/a) + l \sinh^{-1}(a/l)] \tag{44}$$

The ratio P_1/P_2 is plotted versus l/a in Fig. 4.7, assuming as above $A = a$. It is evident that even a slight defocusing of the laser spot on the material can significantly increase the power required to reach a given T at the focus. Thus we see that defocusing by a factor of three ($l/a = 3$) must be compensated by an increase in P of a factor of two to reach the same equilibrium temperature at the focus.

4.6 GAUSSIAN SURFACE SOURCE ON SEMI-INFINITE HALF-SPACE

4.6.1 Constant in Time

We will now consider the case where the intensity distribution in the focal area can best be described by a Gaussian function. This is the situation in the case of a laser operating in the TEM_{00} mode and focused with distortionless optics. The intensity on the surface of the material can be written

$$F(r) = F_0 \exp(-r^2/d^2) \tag{45}$$

where F_0 is the intensity at the center of the spot and d the Gaussian beam radius. In doing the analysis we use the technique adopted by Ready (1971). The temperature distribution due to an instantaneous ring source at the surface of a semi-infinite solid is given by (Carslaw and Jaeger, 1959)

$$T_{\text{inst ring}}(r, z, t) = \frac{Q}{4\rho c(\pi\kappa t)^{3/2}} \exp\left[\frac{-r^2 - r'^2 - z^2}{4\kappa t}\right] I_0\left(\frac{rr'}{2\kappa t}\right) \tag{46}$$

where Q is the total energy generated over the ring, r' the radius of the ring, I_0 the modified Bessel function of order zero, and r the radial distance from the origin. For a Gaussian source,

$$Q = 2\pi r' q_0 \exp(-r'^2/d^2)\, dr' \tag{47}$$

where q_0 is the energy per unit area at the origin. Substituting for Q in Eq. (47) and integrating we obtain

$$T_{\text{inst Gauss}}(r, z, t) = \frac{q_0}{2\rho c(\pi\kappa^3 t^3)^{1/2}} \exp\left[-\frac{r^2 + z^2}{4\kappa t}\right] \times \int_0^\infty \exp\left[-r'^2\left(\frac{1}{4\kappa t} + \frac{1}{d^2}\right)\right] I_0\left(\frac{rr'}{2\kappa t}\right) r'\, dr' \tag{48}$$

Ready (1971) has evaluated this integral and gives

$$T_{\text{inst Gauss}}(r, z, t) = \frac{q_0 d^2}{\rho c(\pi\kappa t)^{1/2}(4\kappa t + d^2)} \exp\left[\frac{-z^2}{4\kappa t} - \frac{r^2}{4\kappa t + d^2}\right] \tag{49}$$

For a noninstantaneous source we set $q_0 = \epsilon F(0, t')\,dt'$ and integrate to get

$$\begin{aligned} T_{\text{noninst Gauss}}(r, z, t) &= \frac{d^2}{\rho c(\pi\kappa)^{1/2}} \int_0^t \frac{\epsilon F(0, t')\,dt'}{(t - t')^{1/2}[4\kappa(t - t') + d^2]} \\ &\quad \times \exp\left[\frac{-z^2}{4\kappa(t - t')} - \frac{r^2}{4\kappa(t - t') + d^2}\right] \\ &= \frac{\epsilon F_{\max} d^2}{K}\left(\frac{\kappa}{\pi}\right)^{1/2} \\ &\quad \times \int_0^t \frac{r(t - t')\,dt'}{t'^{1/2}(4\kappa t' + d^2)} \exp\left[\frac{-z^2}{4\kappa t'} - \frac{r^2}{4\kappa t' + d^2}\right] \end{aligned} \tag{50}$$

where $\epsilon F(0, t)$ is the absorbed intensity (W/cm^2) at the center of the Gaussian spot and $\epsilon F_{\max}$ its greatest value. $F(0, t)/F_{\max} = p(t)$ is the temporal shape of the laser pulse normalized to its maximum value. If we introduce dimensionless variables

$$\tau = 4\kappa t/d^2, \qquad \zeta = z/d, \qquad \xi = r/d, \qquad \phi = 2K\pi^{1/2}T/d\epsilon F_{\max}$$

Eq. (50) becomes

$$\phi(\xi, \zeta, \tau) = \int_0^\tau \frac{p(\tau - \tau')\exp[-\xi^2/(\tau' + 1)]\exp(-\zeta^2/\tau')\,d\tau'}{\tau'^{1/2}(\tau' + 1)} \tag{51}$$

A set of generalized curves can be determined from this equation for any given laser pulse shape. For a cw laser, $p(\tau - \tau') = 1$ and Eq. (51) reduces to [with $F(0, t) = F_{\max} = F_0$]

$$\phi(\xi, \zeta, \tau) = \int_0^\tau \frac{\exp[-\xi^2/(\tau' + 1)]\exp(-\zeta^2/\tau')\,d\tau'}{\tau'^{1/2}(\tau' + 1)} \tag{52}$$

The temperature at the center of the focal spot is given by

$$\phi(0, 0, \tau) = \int_0^\tau d\tau'/\tau'^{1/2}(\tau' + 1) = 2\tan^{-1}(\tau)^{1/2} \tag{53a}$$

or

$$T(0, 0, t) = (\epsilon F_0 d/K\pi^{1/2}) \tan^{-1}(4\kappa t/d^2)^{1/2} \tag{53b}$$

and the equilibrium value for continuous heating is

$$\phi(0, 0, \infty) = \pi, \qquad \text{or} \qquad T(0, 0, \infty) = \epsilon F_0 d\pi^{1/2}/2K \tag{54}$$

Figure 4.8 shows a plot of reduced temperature $\phi(0,0,\tau)$ versus τ for most times of interest in laser interaction studies. This graph is linear for times $\tau \lesssim 1$. Note that $F_0 = P'/\pi d^2$, where P' is the total power incident on the target. To compare this result with that obtained for focusing with a constant intensity $P/\pi A^2$, $\theta = \phi(0, 0, \tau)/2\pi^{1/2} = TdK\pi/P'\epsilon$ is plotted versus $\tau = 4\kappa t/d^2$ in Fig. 4.5, together with the solution to Eq. (35) (Gonsalves, 1973). Note that if we set the Gaussian radius d equal to the radius of the circular source A and $P = P'$ then the time and temperature scales on the two plots will coincide and we see that both models exhibit the same basic behavior. Points below the surface show the time delay noticed in the case of the circular source. With $d = A$, comparison of the equilibrium temperatures as given by Eqs. (35) and (53) shows that a higher temperature is produced by the circular source

$$\theta_{\text{Gaussian}}/\theta_{\text{circular}} = \pi^{1/2}/2 = 0.885$$

In practice, however, if the intensity distribution in the output of the laser is Gaussian due to operation in the fundamental mode, then focusing to much smaller spot sizes is possible. The comparative analysis given above

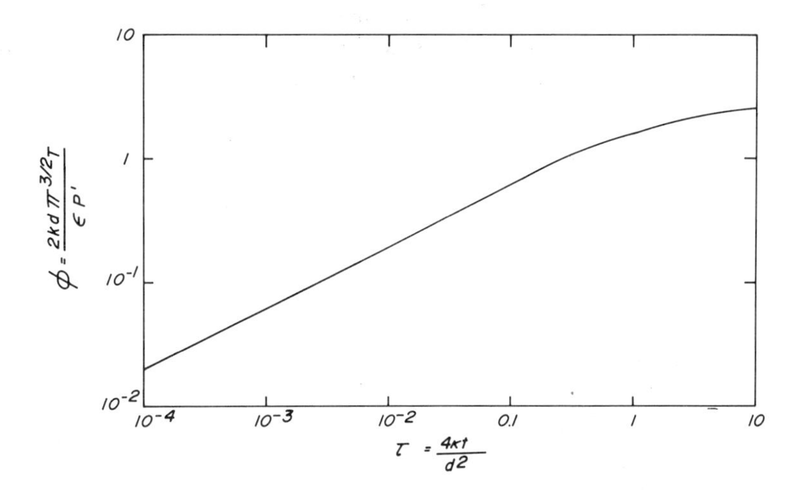

Fig. 4.8. $\phi(0, 0, \tau)$ vs. τ from Eq. (53a).

would then not be valid even if the total power generated were such that $P = P'$. Because of the smaller spot size attainable with Gaussian beams, a low-power laser operating in the fundamental mode will often produce the same thermal effect as a laser of much higher power running in a multimode regime. Furthermore, with smaller spot sizes, the heating effect can be more closely regulated and the heat-affected region can be kept small.

4.6.2 Variable in Time

The analysis given in the previous section may be extended to the situation in which the pulse shape is time dependent simply by defining $p(t)$ for pulse shapes of interest. Ready (1971) has shown that the normalized pulse shape plotted in Fig. 4.9 is representative of pulses obtained from a number of different types of lasers. In this plot, t_p is the duration of the pulse. The laser pulse reaches its maximum power in a time $\simeq 0.2\ t_p$. Ready gives generalized time–temperature plots for several boundary conditions of interest in the use of a laser as a heat source. These plots can be used together with the appropriate thermal constants for a given material to predict the time-dependent temperature at various positions within the irradiated solid.

As an example of the detailed predictions that can be made from Ready's generalized plots, Fig. 4.10 shows $T(t)$ for two depths in a molybdenum target irradiated with a 100-nsec pulse and absorbing 10 MW/cm^2 at the center of a Gaussian focal area with $d = 0.035$ cm. It can be seen that the surface temperature peaks slightly after the peak of the laser pulse and then decreases slowly as heat stored in the surface diffuses into the material. The temperature at a depth $z = 1.4 \times 10^{-4}$ cm does not reach its maximum value until about 50 nsec after the peak of the laser pulse.

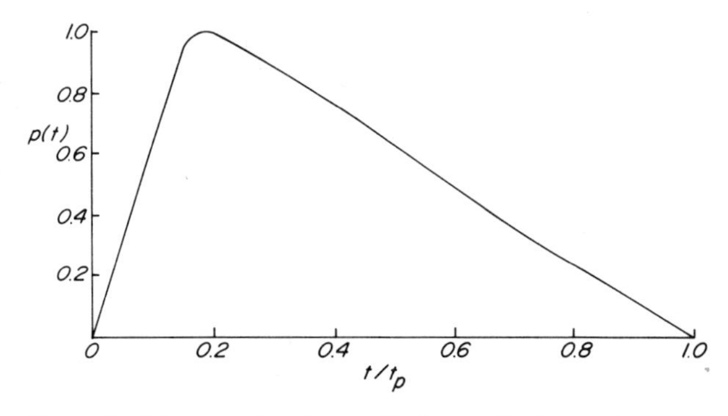

Fig. 4.9. Generalized laser pulse shape $p(t)$ (normalized to unity) as a function of time t, expressed as a fraction of the total pulse length t_p (Ready, 1971).

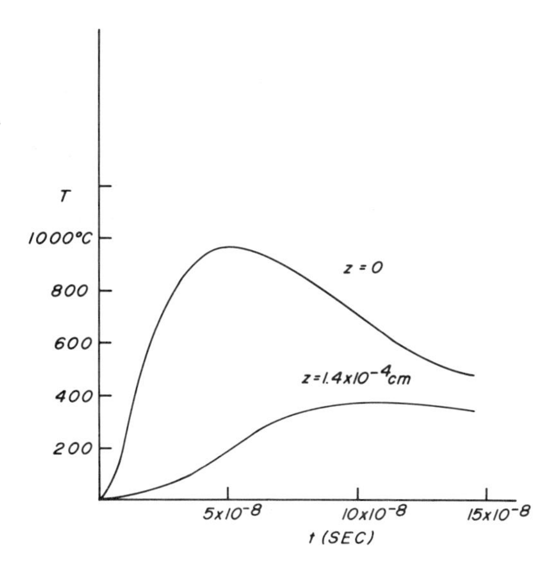

Fig. 4.10. Temperature at surface and at $z = 1.4 \times 10^{-4}$ cm inside Mo target on irradiation with 100-nsec pulse. Absorption, 10 MW/cm^2; $d = 0.035$ cm.

To see how very simple expressions can often be used to estimate heating effects roughly, we can use the formula $l \simeq (\kappa t)^{1/2}$ to estimate how far heat will diffuse in the 50 nsec after the temperature on the surface maximizes. As $\kappa \simeq 0.38$ cm^2/sec, for molybdenum $l \simeq (0.38 \times 5 \times 10^{-8})^{1/2} \simeq 10^{-4}$ cm. Thus, the temperature at this depth should reach its maximum value about 50 nsec after the peak of the pulse. This prediction is compatible with the lower curve in Fig. 4.10.

The temperature can be estimated roughly as follows: in the length of the pulse (100 nsec) heating will occur to a depth $l \simeq 10^{-4}$ cm, as noted above; the heated volume is then approximately $V \simeq \pi \times d^2 \times l \simeq 3.9 \times 10^{-7}$ cm^3. Since the specific heat per unit volume $\rho c = K/\kappa \simeq 3.0$ J/cm^3/°C, the heat capacity of V is $\rho c V = 1.2 \times 10^{-6}$ J/°C. The laser delivers 10^7 W/cm^2 of absorbed power at the peak of the pulse and because of the shape of the pulse we can say very approximately that

$$E = (\text{energy flux at } r = 0) = \int_0^{t_p} F(0, t)\, dt \simeq 0.5\, F_{\max} t_p \simeq 0.5 \text{ J/cm}^2$$

Then the total energy delivered to the area $\pi d^2 \simeq E\pi d^2 \simeq 2 \times 10^{-3}$ J. The average temperature rise in the volume V in 100 nsec is then $\Delta T = E\pi d^2/\rho c V \simeq 1700$°C. Although this calculation is very approximate we can see that it is capable of yielding an order of magnitude estimate of the temperature rise produced. In view of the approximations that are still present in the exact solution (e.g., lack of consideration of temperature dependence of thermal constants, uncertain time and temperature dependence of the emissivity) a simple calculation of the sort outlined above may often be preferred even when an exact solution can be obtained.

The solution to the heat equation can be simplified even more and expressed in analytical form if the laser pulse is represented to be triangular in time. For the time-dependent pulse,

$$F(0, t) = F_m t/t_1, \qquad t \leq t_1 \tag{55}$$

The temperature at the point $z = 0$, $r = 0$, can be obtained from

$$\theta = \frac{1}{\tau_1}[(\tau + 1)(\tan^{-1}\tau^{1/2}) - \tau^{1/2}], \qquad 0 \leq t \leq t_1 \tag{56}$$

where $\theta = KT\pi^{1/2}/F_m d$, $\tau = 4\kappa t/d^2$, and $\tau_1 = 4\kappa t_1/d^2$.

Similarly for the pulse

$$F(0, t) = F_m[1 - t/t_2], \qquad 0 \leq t \leq t_2 \tag{57}$$

the temperature is

$$\theta = \frac{1}{\tau_2}[(\tau_2 - \tau - 1)\tan^{-1}\tau^{1/2} + \tau^{1/2}], \qquad 0 < t < t_2 \tag{58}$$

where $\tau_2 = 4\kappa t_2/d^2$. θ from Eq. (56) is plotted in Fig. 4.11.

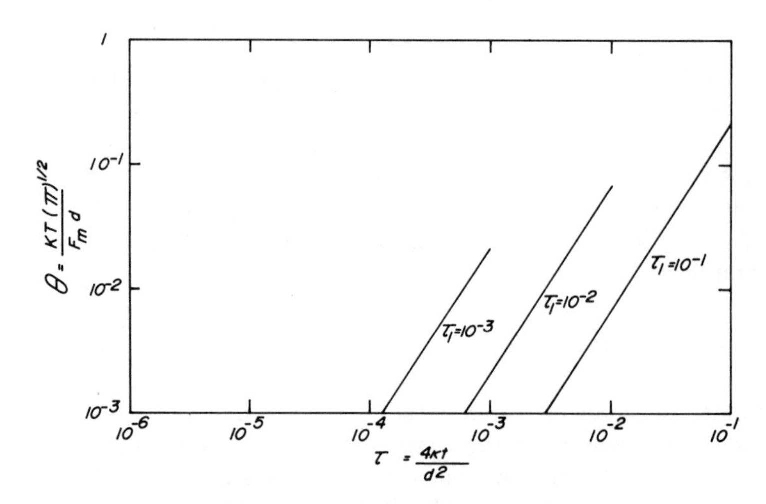

Fig. 4.11. Solution to Eq. (56) for various τ_1.

Once again, taking our example of molybdenum excited with a 100-nsec pulse of peak intensity $F_m = 10^7$ W/cm^2 focused to a Gaussian spot with $d = 0.035$ cm, we get $T(t_1) = 810$°C if the pulse is represented by Eq. (56) with $t_1 = 20$ nsec. Although calculations based on these formulas obviously grossly simplify the time dependence of the laser pulse and are not at all accurate when the detailed time dependence of surface temperature is required, it is possible to obtain a quick estimate of one very important parameter: the maximum surface temperature. This quantity may suffice when it is desired to obtain an approximate value for the laser power and intensity required to produce a given temperature rise in a workpiece.

Since the depth heated by a pulse of duration t is $\simeq(\kappa t)^{1/2}$, the expressions given in this section may be used for laser heating of sheets of finite thickness, provided the sheet thickness is several times larger than this scale depth. Furthermore, if $d \gtrsim (\kappa t)^{1/2}$ the surface of the sheet removed from the focal area will not be heated significantly during the laser pulse. These expressions can therefore be used to estimate the temperature rise in sheets of finite lateral extension provided the above condition is satisfied.

4.7 SURFACE HEATING OF A SEMI-INFINITE SLAB OF FINITE THICKNESS

4.7.1 Uniform Surface Source, Constant in Time

In the absence of focusing of the laser output we suppose that laser radiation is incident over the surface $z = l$ and that the surface $z = 0$ is insulated. The temperature distribution is therefore only dependent on the coordinate z, and for absorbed laser intensity ϵF_0, is (Carslaw and Jaeger, 1959)

$$T(z, t) = \frac{\epsilon F_0 t}{\rho c l} + \frac{\epsilon F_0 l}{K}\left[\frac{3z^2 - l^2}{6l^2} - \frac{2}{\pi^2}\sum_{n=1}^{\infty}\frac{(-1)^n}{n^2} \times \exp\left(-\frac{\kappa n^2\pi^2 t^2}{l^2}\right)\cos\frac{n\pi z}{l}\right] \qquad (59)$$

We see that the first term in this equation corresponds to a linear increase in temperature with time that is the same for all points in the sheet. The second term takes into account the fact that heat is reflected from the front and back surfaces after being absorbed at $z = l$. Figure 4.12 shows a plot of $T(0, t)$ and $T(l, t)$ in terms of the normalized temperature $KT/F_0 l$ for dimensionless time $\kappa t/l^2$. The effect of the second term in Eq. (59) is

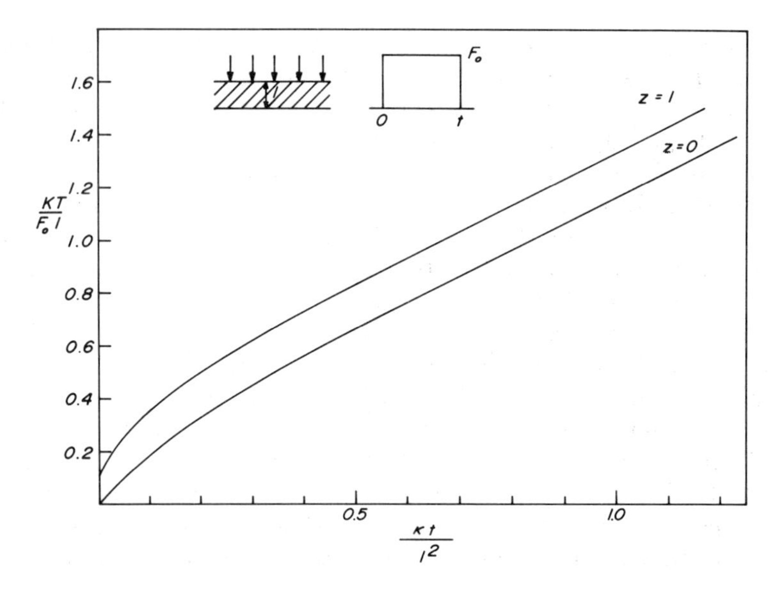

Fig. 4.12. $T(0, t)$ and $T(l, t)$ from Eq. (59).

seen to be greatest for $\kappa t/l^2 < 0.5$. In the limit as $t \to \infty$, the temperature of all points in the slab is proportional to t.

It is of some interest for welding applications to examine the ratio of temperatures at the front and back surfaces as a function of time. This ratio is most conveniently plotted as $\beta = 1 - T(0)/T(l)$ as shown in Fig. 4.13. The temperature difference between front and back surfaces of the slab is seen to decrease rapidly at first and then to decline more gradually at higher values of $\kappa t/l^2$.

As an example of the type of simple calculation that can be performed using the graphs of Figs. 4.12 and 4.13, consider the welding of a 0.1-cm thick nickel slab. The melting and boiling temperatures of nickel are 1430 and 2810°C, respectively. If the heat pulse is to be terminated when $T(l) = 2810$°C and $T(0) = 1430$°C, then Fig. 4.13 shows that $\beta = [T(l) - T(0)]/T(l) = 0.49$ at $\tau = 0.08$. Since $\kappa \simeq 0.16$ cm²/sec, this implies a time $t = 0.08 \times (10^{-1})^2/0.16 = 0.5 \times 10^{-2}$ sec. The absorbed intensity of laser radiation would then have to be (from Fig. 4.12) $F_0 \simeq K \times 2810/0.32 \times 10^{-1}$. With $K = 0.72$ W/cm/°C, $F_0 = 6.3 \times 10^4$ W/cm². A laser pulse giving constant absorbed intensity of 6.3×10^4 W/cm² for 5 msec would then produce the desired effect.

Although the solutions to the heat equation given above were obtained with the assumption that flux is applied uniformly over one entire surface

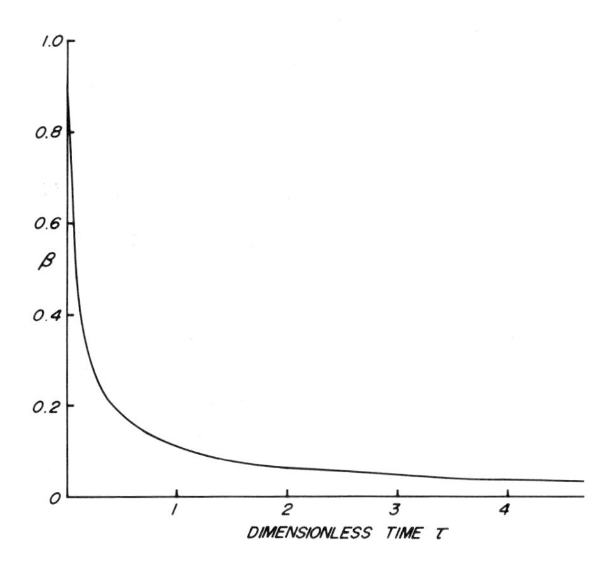

Fig. 4.13. The difference β between front and back surface temperatures of a slab normalized to the front surface temperature vs. time $\tau = \kappa t/l^2$.

of the slab, the formulas arrived at may also be used with some confidence for certain other boundary conditions. We expect, for example, that on focusing to a circular spot, Eq. (59) will still be valid for predicting temperatures along the optical axis of the system when the condition $A > l$ is satisfied.

Brugger (1972) has considered the problem of the uniform heating of an infinite slab with a beam whose intensity decays exponentially with distance into the sheet as

$$F = F_0 \exp(-\alpha z)$$

When the source is constant in time, the temperature distribution is given by

$$T(z, t) = \frac{\epsilon F_0}{2\kappa\alpha\rho c} \sum_{n=-\infty}^{\infty} A_n + \frac{\epsilon F_0}{\rho c}\left(\frac{t}{\kappa}\right)^{1/2} \sum_{n=-\infty}^{\infty} B_n - \frac{\epsilon F_0}{\kappa\alpha\rho c} e^{-\alpha z} \tag{60}$$

where

$$A_n = \exp(\kappa\alpha^2 t \pm \alpha[z - 2nl])\left\{\operatorname{erfc}\left[\alpha(\kappa t)^{1/2} \pm \frac{(z - 2nl)}{(4\kappa t)^{1/2}}\right]\right.$$

$$\left. - \operatorname{erfc}\left[\alpha(\kappa t)^{1/2} \pm \frac{(z - 2nl)}{(4\kappa t)^{1/2}} + \frac{l}{(4\kappa t)^{1/2}}\right]\right\} \tag{60a}$$

$$B_n = 2\,\mathrm{ierfc}\left[\frac{|z - 2nl|}{(4\kappa t)^{1/2}}\right] - \exp(-\alpha l)\;\mathrm{ierfc}\left[\frac{|z - (2n \pm 1)l|}{(4\kappa t)^{1/2}}\right] \tag{60b}$$

4.7.2 Circular Surface Source, Constant in Time

We now consider the solution to the heat equation that is obtained when total power P is focused to a circular area πA^2 on the surface of an infinite sheet. The intensity is constant within the focal area and is given by $F = P/\pi A^2$. A fraction ϵ of this intensity is absorbed. The absorbed radiation is now assumed to uniformly heat a right circular cylinder of area πA^2 and height l. This cylinder is assumed to have infinite thermal conductivity so that the absorbed power is dissipated uniformly into the surrounding sheet with intensity $\epsilon P/2\pi Al$. Defining a radial coordinate r that measures perpendicular to the axis of the cylinder, the general solution for $T(r,t)$ valid for all $r \geq A$ is (Carslaw and Jaeger, 1959)

$$T(r, t) = \frac{-P\epsilon}{\pi^2 AKl}\int_0^\infty (1 - \exp[-\kappa u^2 t]) \times \left[\frac{J_0(ur)Y_1(uA) - Y_0(uA)J_1(uA)}{u^2[J_1^2(uA) + Y_1^2(uA)]}\right] du \tag{61}$$

where J and Y are Bessel functions of the first and second order, respectively. When the condition $A^2/\kappa t \ll 1$ is satisfied, this integral simplifies and

$$T(r, t) = \frac{P\epsilon}{4\pi Kl}\left[\ln\left(\frac{4\kappa t}{Cr^2}\right) + \frac{A^2}{2\kappa t}\ln\left(\frac{4\kappa t}{Cr^2}\right) + \frac{1}{4\kappa t}\left(A^2 + r^2 - 2A^2\ln\frac{A}{r}\right)\right] \tag{62}$$

where $C = 1.781$. For short times or $A^2/\kappa t$ large, another analytical approximation to this integral is possible:

$$T(r, t) \simeq \frac{P\epsilon}{\pi KlA^{1/2}}\left(\frac{\kappa t}{r}\right)^{1/2}\left[\mathrm{ierfc}\left(\frac{r - A}{2(\kappa t)^{1/2}}\right) - \frac{(3r + A)(\kappa t)^{1/2}}{4Ar} \times \mathrm{i}^2\mathrm{erfc}\left(\frac{(r - A)}{2(\kappa t)^{1/2}}\right) + \cdots\right] \tag{63}$$

where

$$\mathrm{i}^2\mathrm{erfc}\,x = \tfrac{1}{4}[\mathrm{erfc}\,x - 2x\,\mathrm{ierfc}\,x]$$

This solution is valid for small times, provided the condition $l < (\kappa t)^{1/2}$ is satisfied. When t is small enough to make $l > (\kappa t)^{1/2}$, then the cylindrical source approximation is no longer valid, as heat absorbed at the surface cannot be thought of as uniformly heating the cylindrical source of length l in the time available.

For drilling of thin sheets, one requires a knowledge of the temperature internal to the cylindrical source. Since the cylinder has infinite thermal conductivity, the temperature at its surface ($r = A$) gives the temperature of the cylinder as a whole and hence of the volume $0 < r \leq a$, $0 \leq z \leq l$. This temperature is

$$T(A,t) \simeq \begin{cases} \dfrac{P\epsilon}{4\pi Kl}\left[\ln\left(\dfrac{4\kappa t}{CA^2}\right) + \dfrac{A^2}{2\kappa t}\ln\left(\dfrac{4\kappa t}{CA^2}\right) + \dfrac{A^2}{2\kappa t}\right], & A^2/\kappa t \ll 1 \quad (64) \\[2ex] \dfrac{P\epsilon}{\pi KlA}(\kappa t)^{1/2}\left[\dfrac{1}{\pi^{1/2}} - \dfrac{(\kappa t)^{1/2}}{4A} + \cdots\right], & A^2/\kappa t \gg 1 \quad (65) \end{cases}$$

Equation (64) has been found to describe adequately the relation between P_m and t_m, the critical power for the production of melting and the length of the drilling pulse, respectively, in studies of cw CO_2 laser drilling of thin stainless steel sheets (Asmus and Baker, 1969; Gonsalves and Duley, 1971).

Equation (64) is plotted in Fig. 4.14 in terms of the normalized temperature $4\pi KTl/\epsilon P$ for various values of κ/A^2. The use of this graph and its limitations are best illustrated by an example. Suppose we have a sheet of material whose thermal diffusivity $\kappa = 0.1$ cm^2/sec and 0.1 sec is available for the production of a heat effect at temperature T directly in the area of the focus. If we take $A = 10^{-2}$ cm as the radius of the focal spot on the target, then $\kappa/A^2 = 10^3$. From the graph this yields $T = 5.5\,\epsilon P/4\pi Kl$. Assuming values for the emissivity ϵ and thermal conductivity K, this ratio gives a value for P/l, the critical power per unit sheet thickness. We now make two tests to determine the validity of the solution obtained. First, we require $A^2/\kappa t \ll 1$. With $A = 10^{-2}$, $\kappa = 0.1$ cm^2/sec, and $t = 0.1$ sec, it is evident that this condition is satisfied. The second requirement is $l < (\kappa t)^{1/2}$. This implies that for a 0.1-sec pulse l must be less than 0.1 cm for the prediction of P/l to be valid. With these constraints in mind, P can now be found for given sheet thickness l.

Heating in air is usually accompanied by convective losses, which have not been taken into account in the above model. Gonsalves and Duley (1971) found that these losses can be incorporated into the theory by the replacement of P in Eqs. (62) and (64) by $P - P_c$, where P_c is the power

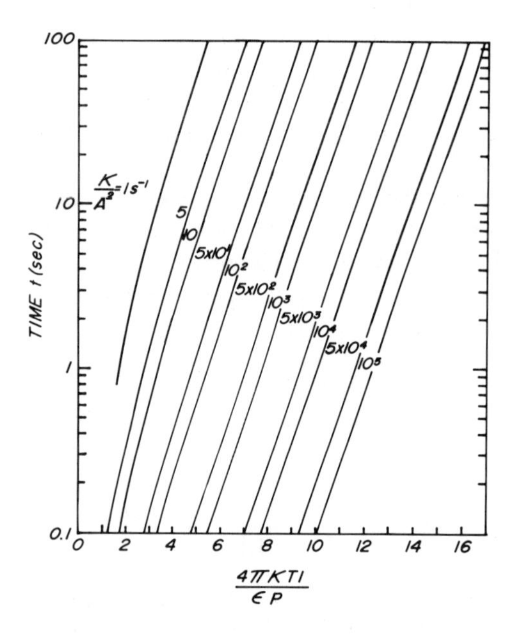

Fig. 4.14. Theoretical curves for the prediction of P or t for thin metal sheets. These curves are valid for thicknesses in the range $l < (\kappa t)^{1/2}$. Temperature T is measured at $r = A$.

needed to balance the convective losses. P_c may be found empirically or calculated for a particular geometry and temperature difference (Carslaw and Jaeger, 1959).

Lin (1967) and Brugger (1972) have calculated the temperature at the center of the irradiated spot on the target without the assumption that heat is dissipated only over the surface $r = A$ of a cylindrical source. The sheet is still assumed to be thermally thin, however, so that temperature depends only on the coordinate r. Their result is

$$T(r = 0) = \frac{\epsilon P}{4\pi Kl}\left\{\frac{4\kappa t}{A^2}\left(1 - \exp\left[-\frac{A^2}{4\kappa t}\right]\right) - \mathrm{Ei}(-A^2/4\kappa t)\right\} \tag{66}$$

where Ei is the exponential integral and

$$\mathrm{Ei}(-A^2/4\kappa t) = \int_{-\infty}^{-A^2/4\kappa t} (e^u/u)\, du$$

This temperature is plotted in normalized form in Fig. 4.15. When $A^2/\kappa t \ll 1$, the temperature predicted from this model is always slightly higher

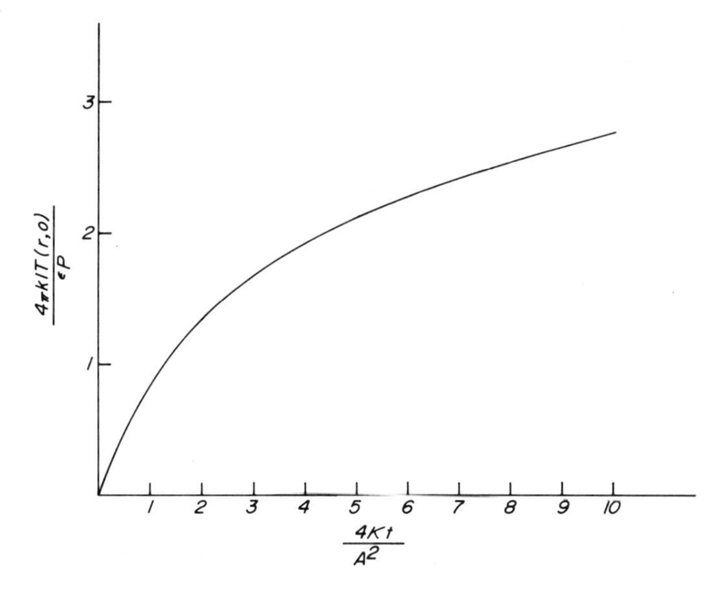

Fig. 4.15. Solution to Eq. (66).

than that predicted from Eq. (62). Lin (1967) has also discussed the incorporation of a radiative loss term into this analysis.

Brugger (1972) has obtained a more general solution, which does not require that the sheet be thermally thin:

$$T(r = 0,z) = \frac{P\epsilon}{\pi A^2} \frac{(4\kappa t)^{1/2}}{K} \sum_{n=-\infty}^{\infty} \left(\operatorname{ierfc} \frac{|z - 2nl|}{(4\kappa t)^{1/2}} - \operatorname{ierfc} \frac{[(z - 2nl)^2 + A^2]^{1/2}}{(4\kappa t)^{1/2}} \right) \tag{67}$$

The shape of isothermal curves in a slab heated by a circular surface source has been discussed by Guenot and Racinet (1967).

4.7.3 Gaussian Surface Source, Constant in Time

In order to develop an expression for the cw heating of a thin sheet with a beam of Gaussian spatial distribution, we start (Carslaw and Jaeger, 1959; Ready, 1971) with an expression for the temperature produced by a point source at the surface of a semi-infinite medium,

$$T_{\text{inst pt}}(r, t, k^2) = \epsilon Q \exp(-\kappa k^2 t - r^2/4\kappa t)/4\pi K l t \tag{68}$$

where l is the sheet thickness as before, Q the total heat liberated, and k a convective term given by

$$k^2 = 2H/Kl$$

where H is the surface conductance of the material (Carslaw and Jaeger, 1959). For free convection, H is a function of geometry and the temperature difference between the material and its surroundings, but a typical value for a plane surface in air is 5×10^{-4} W-cm^2/°C. An expression can be obtained for a circular ring source of radius r' by integrating

$$T_{\text{inst circ}}(r, t, k^2) = \frac{\epsilon Q' \exp(-\kappa k^2 t)}{4\pi K l t} \times \int_0^{2\pi} \exp[-(r^2 + r'^2 - 2rr' \cos\theta')4\kappa t] r'\, d\theta'$$

$$= \frac{2\pi\epsilon Q' \exp(-\kappa k^2 t) \exp[-(r^2 + r'^2)/4\kappa t] r'}{4\pi K l t} I_0\left(\frac{rr'}{2\kappa t}\right) \tag{69}$$

where Q' is now the heat incident per unit length along the ring and I_0 the modified Bessel function of order zero. Substituting

$$Q' = Q_0 \exp(-r'^2/d^2)$$

and integrating from zero to infinity, we obtain the expression for a Gaussian distribution of radius d:

$$T_{\text{inst Gauss}}(r, t, k^2) = \frac{2\pi\epsilon Q_0 \exp(-\kappa k^2 t)}{4\pi K l t} \int_0^\infty r' \exp(-r'^2/d^2) \times \exp[-(r^2 + r'^2)/4\kappa t]\, I_0\left(\frac{rr'}{2\kappa t}\right) dr' \tag{70}$$

which gives on evaluation

$$T_{\text{inst Gauss}}(r, t, k^2) = \frac{\epsilon Q_0 \exp(-\kappa k^2 t) \exp(-r^2/4\kappa t)}{4 K l t} \left[\frac{1}{1/d^2 + 1/4\kappa t}\right] \times \exp\left[\frac{r^2/16\kappa^2 t^2}{1/d^2 + 1/4\kappa t}\right] \tag{71}$$

Doing a time integration gives an expression for a continuous Gaussian source:

$$T_{\text{const Gauss}}(r, t, k^2) = \frac{\epsilon F_0 \kappa d^2}{Kl} \int_0^t \frac{dt'}{(4\kappa t' + d^2)} \times \exp\left[-\kappa k^2 t' - \frac{r^2}{4\kappa t'} + \frac{r^2 d^2}{4\kappa t'(d^2 + 4\kappa t')}\right] \quad (72)$$

where F_0 is the incident intensity at $r = 0$. Substituting dimensionless parameters

$$\zeta = r/d, \qquad \sigma = k^2 d^2/4, \qquad \tau = 4\kappa t/d^2, \qquad \tau' = 4\kappa t'/d^2$$

$$\theta(\xi, \tau, \sigma) = (4Kl/\epsilon F_0 d^2) T(r, t, k^2)$$

we obtain

$$\theta(\xi, \tau, \sigma) = \int_0^\tau \frac{d\tau'}{\tau' + 1} \exp[-\sigma\tau' - \xi^2/(\tau' + 1)] \quad (73)$$

Generalized plots of the dimensionless temperature versus dimensionless time can be made from this equation from which predictions can be made for special situations. Ready (1971) and Lin (1967) have published some results on the variation of θ with τ, ζ, and σ.

For experiments done in vacuum, $k = 0$ since convection losses are zero. In this case, Eq. (73) reduces to

$$\theta(\zeta, \tau, 0) = -\text{Ei}\left(-\frac{\zeta^2}{1 + \tau}\right) + \text{Ei}(-\zeta^2) \quad (74)$$

where Ei is the exponential integral function. Figure 4.16 shows a plot of θ versus ζ for various τ. When τ is small, the temperature profile closely approximates the profile of the incident intensity distribution. From the boundary conditions, these distributions also hold for all $0 \leq z \leq l$ at a particular τ.

In many instances one is interested in temperatures close to the center of the focal spot and hence must consider infinitesimally small r and ζ. For $\zeta \to 0$, Eq. (74) reduces to

$$\theta(0, \tau, 0) = \ln(1 + \tau)$$

and

$$4KlT/\epsilon F_0 d^2 = \ln(1 + 4\kappa t/d^2) \quad (75)$$

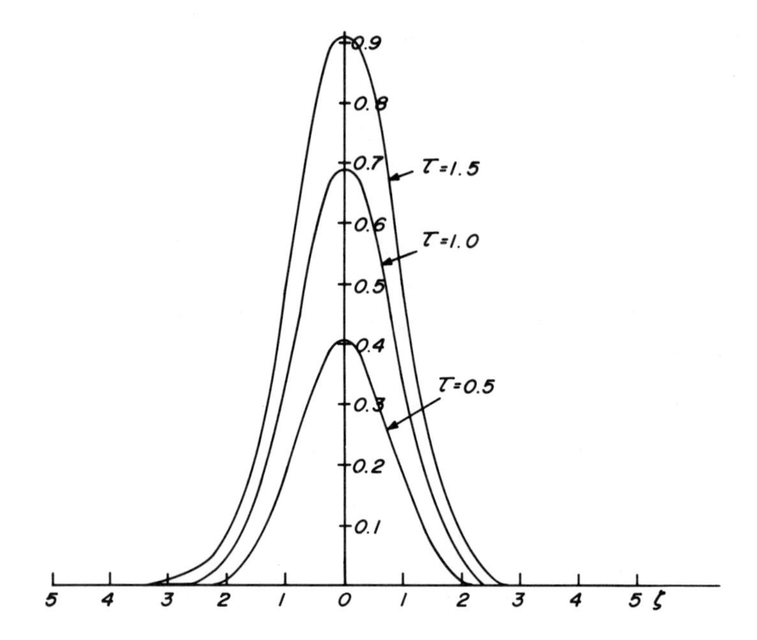

Fig. 4.16. θ vs. ζ for various τ, from Eq. (74).

For comparison between the results of this model and those for the cylindrical model discussed previously we have the following:

Cylindrical source model

$$\frac{4\pi KTl}{P\epsilon} = \ln\left(\frac{4\kappa t}{CA^2}\right) + \frac{A^2}{2\kappa t}\ln\left(\frac{4\kappa t}{CA^2}\right) + \frac{A^2}{2\kappa t} \tag{64}$$

Gaussian source model

$$\frac{4\pi KTl}{P\epsilon} = \ln\left(\frac{4\kappa t}{d^2} + 1\right) \tag{75a}$$

Let

$$4\kappa t/CA^2 = \tau_1, \qquad 4\kappa t/d^2 = \tau_2, \qquad \theta = 4\kappa KTl/\epsilon P$$

Equation (64) reduces to (Gonsalves, 1973)

$$\theta_1 = \ln \tau_1 + \frac{2}{C\tau_1}\ln \tau_1 + \frac{2}{C\tau_1}$$

and (75a) reduces to

$$\theta_2 = \ln(\tau_2 + 1)$$

These two equations have been plotted in Fig. 4.17 for the a range of thermal parameters and heating times of interest for cw lasers. It is evident that the two curves are coincident over almost the entire range, diverging only at lower τ. Therefore, either model can be applied when $\tau \gtrsim 10$. The relation between the two is given by

$$d = C^{1/2}A = 1.33A$$

As a numerical example, consider the heating of a thin sheet with $\kappa = 0.5$ cm^2/sec to temperature T with a 10^{-6}-sec pulse of laser radiation having a Gaussian spatial distribution with $d = 0.1$ cm and constant temporal distribution. $\tau = 4\kappa t/d^2 = 2 \times 10^{-4}$ and $\theta(0,\tau,0) = 2 \times 10^{-4}$. The absorbed intensity $\epsilon F_0 = 2 \times 10^6$ Klt W/cm^2. This solution will be valid only for sheet thicknesses $\lesssim 0.7 \times 10^{-3}$ cm.

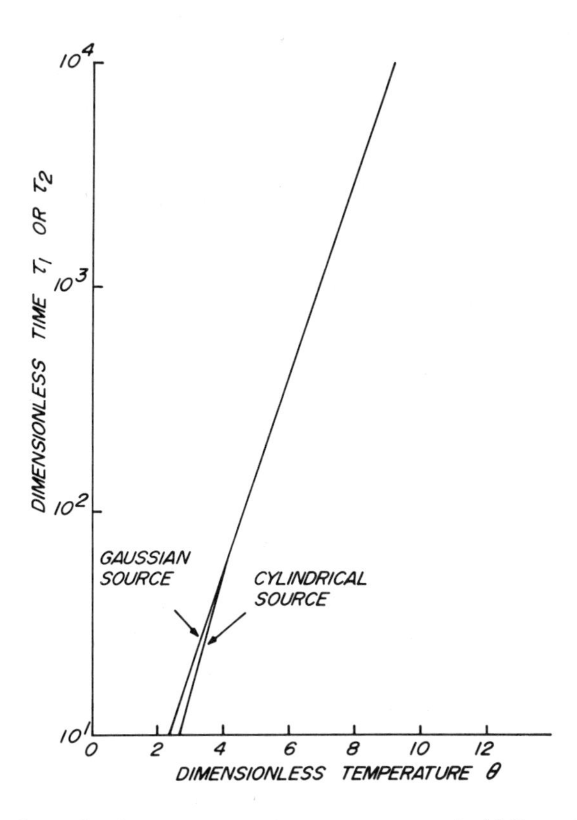

Fig. 4.17. Generalized temperature–time curves, $\tau = 4\kappa'/CA^2$ or $4\kappa t/d^2$ vs. θ for cylindrical and Gaussian heat sources.

For a discussion of heating effects when convective or radiative losses are important the reader is referred to Lin (1967) and Ready (1971).

4.7.4 Time-Dependent Pulse

The system where a slab of finite thickness is heated at one surface by a localized or distributed time dependent source has not been treated extensively in the literature. In principle, when the solution for the temperature distribution is known for a steady source, then $T(r, z, t)$ can be found from Duhamel's theorem (Carslaw and Jaeger, 1959, p. 30). In practice, the resulting solutions involve integrals that can only be evaluated numerically. Complete calculations may occasionally be called for in certain specialized applications but, in general, knowledge of temperature profiles produced by a square heat pulse of the same peak power or the same energy as the true pulse will often suffice for engineering calculations.

Carslaw and Jaeger (1959) have given an example in which a time-varying flux incident uniformly over one surface of a slab yields a temperature distribution that can be expressed analytically. For flux $F(t) = Ft^{m/2}$, where $m = -1, 0, 1, \ldots,$

$$T(z, t) = \frac{2^{m+1}F(t)\kappa^{1/2}t^{1/2}\Gamma(m/2+1)}{K}\sum_{n=0}^{\infty}\left\{\mathrm{i}^{m+1}\mathrm{erfc}\frac{(2n+1)l-z}{2(\kappa t)^{1/2}} + \mathrm{i}^{m+1}\mathrm{erfc}\frac{(2n+1)l+z}{2(\kappa t)^{1/2}}\right\} \tag{76}$$

where Γ is the gamma function and

$$\mathrm{i}^{m+1}\mathrm{erfc}\, x = \int_x^{\infty} \mathrm{i}^m\mathrm{erfc}\, y\, dy$$

4.8 COMPOSITE SLAB

Temperature distributions in two or more slabs of different thermal properties heated by radiative fluxes at one surface are of interest in laser welding applications. Calculations have been performed for a uniform constant flux incident on one surface of a two-layer slab (Matricon, 1951), the steady state temperature on heating a thin film on a highly conductive substrate (Morrison and Morgan, 1966), the temperature $T(r, z, t)$ in a sheet heated with constant flux focused to a Gaussian distribution with heat transfer from the other side (Rykalin and Uglov, 1966), $T_1(r, z, t)$ and $T_2(r, z, t)$ in a two-layer slab heated with constant flux in a Gaussian spatial distribution (Rykalin *et al.*, 1967a), T_1 and T_2 under the above conditions when the thermal contact between the slabs is less than perfect (Rykalin *et al.*, 1967b), and $T(z, t)$ in a slab on a substrate with radiation penetration according to the expression $F = F_0 e^{-\alpha z}$ (Brugger, 1972; Maydon, 1971).

Brugger's solution for the temperature distribution in the slab is

$$T(z, t) = \frac{\epsilon F_0}{2\alpha\kappa_1\rho c} \sum_{n=-\infty}^{\infty} \xi^{|n|} A_n + \frac{\epsilon F_0}{\rho c}\left(\frac{t}{\kappa_1}\right)^{1/2} \sum_{n=-\infty}^{\infty} \xi^{|n|} B_n - \frac{\epsilon F_0}{\alpha\kappa_1\rho c} e^{-\alpha z} + \frac{\epsilon F_0}{2\alpha\kappa_1\rho c} e^{-\alpha l}(1 - \xi) \sum_{n=0}^{\infty} \xi^n C_n \tag{77}$$

where A_n and B_n are as given previously [Eqs. (60a), (60b)] with $\kappa = \kappa_1$,

$$C_n = \operatorname{erfc}\left\{\left[\frac{(2n+1)l \pm z}{(4\kappa_1 t)^{1/2}}\right]\right\}$$

A simpler solution is obtained if the incident radiation is assumed to be absorbed on the surface of the slab (Matricon, 1951; Brugger, 1972). Then

$$T_1(z, t) = \frac{\epsilon F_0}{K_1} [4\kappa_1 t]^{1/2} \sum_{n=-\infty}^{\infty} \xi^{|n|} \operatorname{ierfc}\left[\frac{|z - 2nl|}{(4\kappa_1 t)^{1/2}}\right] \tag{78}$$

where

$$\xi = [K_1(\kappa_2)^{1/2} - K_2(\kappa_1)^{1/2}]/[K_1(\kappa_2)^{1/2} + K_2(\kappa_1)^{1/2}]$$

T_1 is the temperature in the slab; z is measured from the irradiated surface; κ_1 and K_1 are constants for the slab; and κ_2 and K_2 are those for the substrate. This solution has also been obtained by Stern (1973). Stern also gives the following expression for the temperature profile in the substrate when the slab is heated by a surface source at its free surface:

$$T(z', t) = [2T_L/(\Lambda + 1)] \sum_{n=0}^{\infty} \xi^n [I_1(Z^*)] \tag{79}$$

where z' is measured from the slab–substrate interface into the substrate, and

$$T_L = \frac{2\epsilon F(\kappa_2 t)^{1/2}}{K_2(\pi)^{1/2}}, \qquad \Lambda = \frac{K_1}{K_2}\left(\frac{\kappa_2}{\kappa_1}\right)^{1/2}$$

$$Z^* = \frac{z'}{(4\kappa_2 t)^{1/2}} + \frac{(2n+1)l}{(4\kappa_2 t)^{1/2}}, \qquad I_1(x) = \sqrt{\pi}\operatorname{ierfc}(x)$$

Similarly, if the slab is uniformly heated throughout its depth, Stern (1973) gives

$$T(z = 0, t) = T_A[1 - b \sum_{n=0}^{\infty} \xi^n I_2[(2n + 1)l^*]] \tag{80}$$

$$T(z',t) = T_A \left[\frac{\Lambda}{\Lambda + 1}\right] \Big\{ I_2(z'^*) - b \times \sum_{n=0}^{\infty} \xi^n I_2[z'^* + 2(n + 1)l^*] \Big\} \tag{81}$$

where

$$T_A = (\epsilon Ft/K_2 l)\kappa_1, \qquad b = 2/(\Lambda + 1), \qquad l^* = l/(4\kappa_1 t)^{1/2}$$

$$z'^* = z'/(4\kappa_2 t)^{1/2}, \qquad I_2(x) = 4\ \mathrm{i}^2\mathrm{erfc}(x)$$

These temperatures are plotted against time for $\Lambda^2 = 10$, 1, and 0.1 in Stern's article.

Solutions to the more complex problem of the temperature distribution in a thin film on a substrate heated by a constant heat source with a Gaussian spatial distribution have been obtained by Paek and Kestenbaum (1973). Simplifying assumptions were that the temperature was the same across the thickness of the film and that heat was generated only in the film. With these assumptions the temperature distribution becomes

$$\theta_1 = \exp(-\bar{r}^2)U_{11}(\tau) + \epsilon\theta_{12} + \epsilon^2\theta_{13} + \cdots \tag{82}$$

$$\theta_2 = \exp(-\bar{r}^2)U_{21}(\tau,\bar{z}) + \epsilon\theta_{22} + \epsilon^2\theta_{23} + \cdots \tag{83}$$

where

$$\theta_1 = T_1/T_v, \qquad \theta_2 = T_2/T_v, \qquad \bar{r} = r/d$$

$$\bar{z} = z/l, \qquad \tau = \kappa_1 t/l^2, \qquad \epsilon = (l/d)^2$$

and θ_{1i} and θ_{2i}, $i = 1, 2, \ldots, n$, indicate the ith-order perturbed solutions of θ_1 and θ_2, respectively, while U_{1i} is the ith-order nonradial solution in the film or substrate. T_v is the vaporization temperature of the film. Subscripts 1 and 2 refer to film and substrate, respectively, while z is a depth measured from the film–substrate interface into the substrate and r is measured radially from the optical axis. The source intensity distribution is of the form $F = F_0 \exp(-r^2/d^2)$. This shows that, to first order, the temperature distribution in the film will have a Gaussian distribution for times such that radial conduction of heat is unimportant. At longer times, radial conduction will change this distribution as the terms θ_{12} and θ_{13} become important in the expansion. For short times then, the solution for the temperature distribution in the film becomes

$$\theta_1 \simeq \theta_{11} = \exp(-r^{-2}) \left[\frac{(\pi\sigma)^{1/2}}{\beta} S\tau^{1/2} - \frac{\sigma\pi S}{2\beta^2} \ln\left(1 + \frac{2\beta\tau^{1/2}}{(\pi\sigma)^{1/2}}\right)\right] \tag{84}$$

where

$$\sigma = \kappa_2/\kappa_1, \qquad \beta = K_2/K_1, \qquad S = \alpha F_0 l/K_1 T_v$$

and α is the absorption coefficient for the laser light. The second-order solution θ_{12} (which is always negative) was also calculated by Paek and

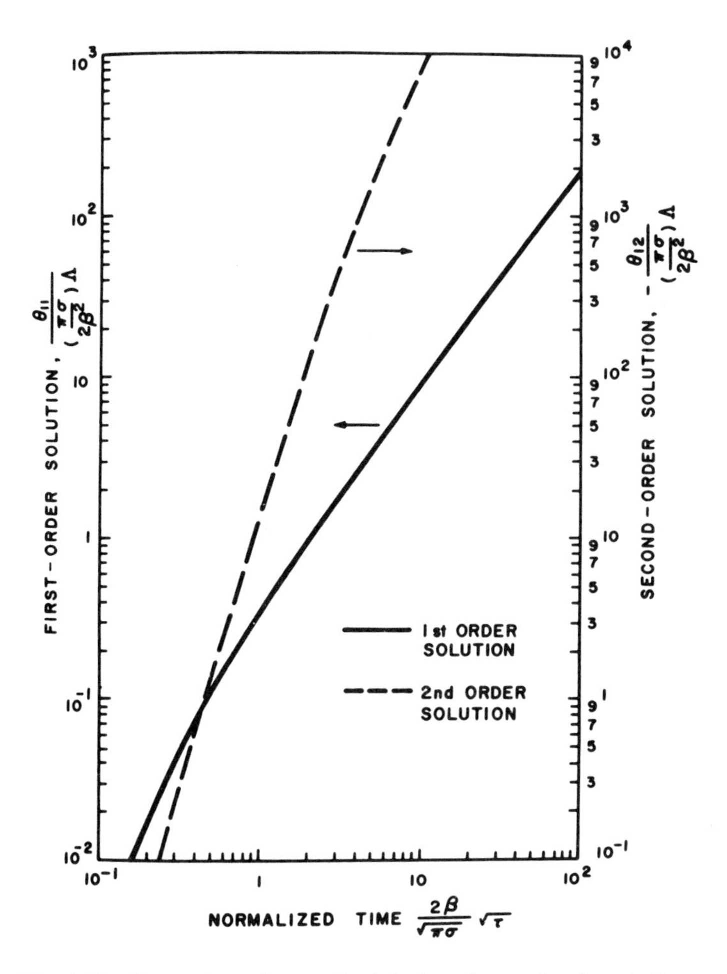

Fig. 4.18. Comparison of normalized first- and second-order solutions.

Kestenbaum and turns out to be much larger than θ_{11}. The factor ϵ, however, is typically 10^{-2}–10^{-8} for systems of interest. The normalized first- and second-order solutions for the temperature are shown in Fig. 4.18.

4.9 HEATING IN THE PRESENCE OF A LIQUID PHASE

We will now consider a group of problems of interest to laser welding of materials. On warming the surface of a material rapidly with a laser of moderate intensity, the surface temperature rises at first in accordance with the predictions of the theory of previous sections. As the melting temperature T_m is reached, an isotherm with $T = T_m$ will propagate into the workpiece with a speed that depends on the initial laser flux distribution time and the thermal constants of both solid and liquid phases. In welding applications, one is interested in the maximum depth of penetration of this isotherm in the time it takes for the surface exposed to the incident laser beam to reach the vaporization temperature. For times greater than this, significant vaporization will occur and the weld area will be depleted of material. As a result, maximum welding depths are obtained only for long laser pulses of low to moderate intensity. With short pulses of high intensity, the vaporization temperature is reached rapidly, precluding stable propagation of the melt into the target. Problems of this sort have been discussed by Masters (1956), Crank (1957), Bahun and Engquist (1963), Fairbanks and Adams (1964), Kaplan (1964), Cohen (1967), Cohen and Epperson (1968), and Ready (1971). In order to make the problem tractable, it is usually assumed that the solid is in the form of a semi-infinite sheet and that it is heated uniformly with a constant flux at its free surface. The geometry with a liquid phase present is shown in Fig. 4.19. The boundary conditions describing this problem are (Cohen, 1967)

$$\begin{aligned}
K_2 \frac{\partial T_2}{\partial x} - K_1 \frac{\partial T_1}{\partial x} &= L\rho \frac{dX(t)}{dt}, && x = X(t) \\
-K_1\, \partial T/\partial x &= F, && x = 0 \\
\partial T_i/\partial t &= \kappa_i\, \partial^2 T_i/\partial_x{}^2, && i = 1, 2 \qquad (85) \\
T_1 = T_2 &= T_m, && x = X(t), \quad t>0 \\
\lim_{x\to\infty} T_2(x, t) &= 0, \\
T_2(x, 0) &= T_s(x), && X(0) = 0
\end{aligned}$$

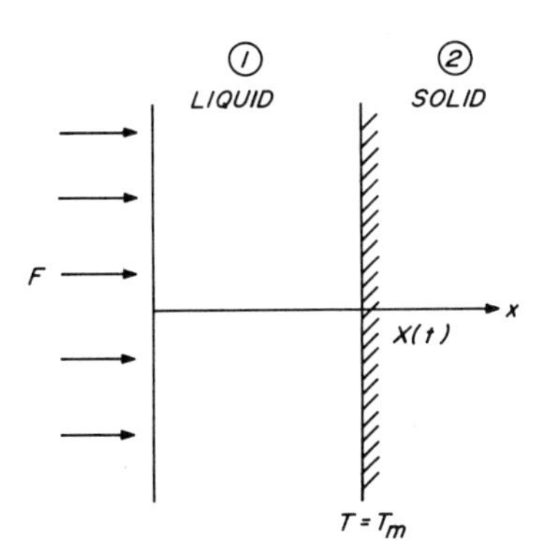

Fig. 4.19. Heating of a semi-infinite solid in the presence of a liquid phase.

where L is the latent heat of fusion. These boundary conditions are initiated at the instant when the surface temperature reaches the normal melting temperature of the material, and thus t is measured from zero time $t = t_m$. In the one-dimensional model considered here, this occurs when [Eq. (26)]

$$t_m = \pi K_2^2 T_m^2 / 4\kappa_2 F^2$$

At this time, the temperature distribution within the solid is given by the function $T_s(x)$. This can also be calculated from Eq. (24). Cohen (1967) has solved this problem for the simplified case where $K_1 = K_2$ and $\kappa_1 = \kappa_2$. It was found that for most metals the depth of penetration of the fusion front is simply given by

$$X(t) = (0.16F/\rho L)(t - t_m) \tag{86}$$

where t here is measured from the start of the laser pulse. The maximum useful penetration depth occurs when $t = t_b$, the time when the boiling temperature T_b is reached at the front surface of the slab. Then from Cohen (1967),

$$t_b - t_m = 4.76 t_m[(T_b/T_m) - 1] \tag{87}$$

The maximum depth of penetration is then given by

$$X_{max} = (1.2K/F) T_m[(T_b/T_m) - 1] \tag{88}$$

where we have made use of the fact that L/CT_m for most metals is $\simeq 0.5$. The product FX_{max}, which is a constant for a given material, is given for several metals in Table 4.6. As expected, maximum depth of penetration is facilitated by K large and a large value for the ratio T_b/T_m. This correla-

Table 4.6

FX_{max} from Eq. (88) for a Semi-Infinite Metal Sheet Heated with Uniform Flux on the Bounding Surface

Metal	FX_{max} ($\times 10^3$)
Ag	2.97
Al	4.77
Au	2.29
Cu	3.25
Ni	1.19
Pb	0.37
Pt	1.95
Ti	0.39
Zn	0.39
Zr	0.66

tion says nothing, of course, about the pulse length required to produce melting to maximum depth. The pulse length must be tailored to equal t_b if maximum penetration with no vaporization is desired. In practice, with all but cw lasers, alteration of the pulse length to match the above conditions may not always be feasible and it is often preferable to change the incident intensity until vaporization is reduced and the maximum depth of penetration is produced.

It is of interest to compare these predictions with those made on the basis of the single-phase heating model of Section 2.1. Equations (24) and (26) can be written

$$T(z, t)/T(0, t) = \pi^{1/2}\,\mathrm{ierfc}[z/Z]$$

where $Z = 2(\kappa t)^{1/2}$. Putting $T(z, t) = T_m$ and $T(0, t) = T_b$, the maximum depth of penetration of the melting isotherm can be found (Fig. 4.20). Horizontal lines on this graph show the appropriate ratios T_m/T_b for different metals. The intercept of a horizontal line with the graph occurs at (z_m/Z_m), where Z_m is here $2(\kappa t_m)^{1/2}$. Since $T(0, t_m) = T_b = 2F(\kappa t_m)^{1/2}/K\pi^{1/2}$, we have

$$Fz_{max} = KT_b\pi^{1/2}(z_m/Z_m)$$

As an example, we have for copper $z_m/Z_m = 0.45$ and $Fz_{max} = 3.7 \times 10^3$ W/cm. The more exact theory would give $FX_{max} = 3.25 \times 10^3$ W/cm. It is apparent that the neglect of a liquid phase makes only a small difference in the predicted penetration depth for given absorbed intensity F.

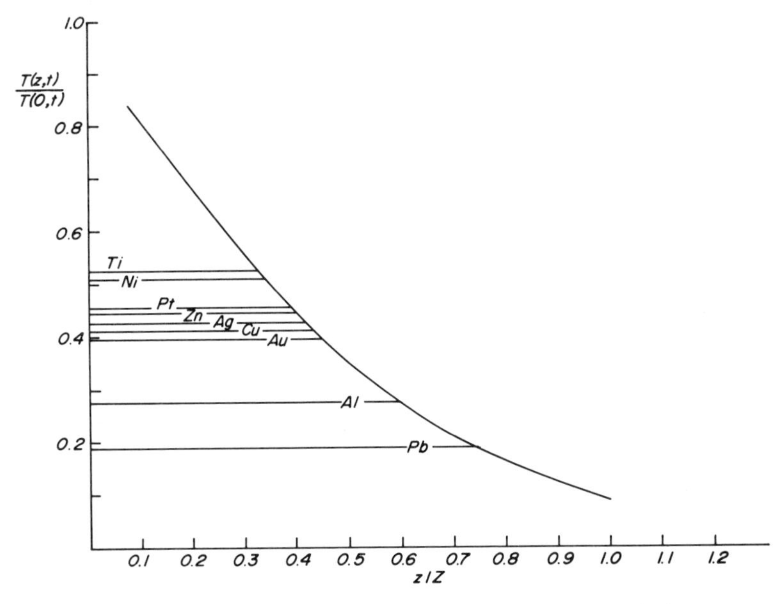

Fig. 4.20. $T(z, t)/T(0, t)$ vs. z/Z from Eqs. (24) and (26).

We can now examine the maximum penetration depth of the melting isotherm for some other focusing conditions neglecting the presence of a liquid phase. The results, while not exact, will give some indication of the welding depths attainable with a given geometry.

Table 4.7

Maximum Depth of Melting z_m/A for Representative Metals (Semi-Infinite Sheet)

Metal	T_m (°C)	T_b (°C)	T_m/T_b	z_m/A
Ag	930	2190	0.425	0.95
Al	630	2300	0.274	1.7
Au	1040	2630	0.396	1.05
Cu	1060	2570	0.413	0.98
Mg	620	1090	0.569	0.6
Ni	1430	2810	0.510	0.7
Pb	330	1740	0.189	2.6
Pt	1740	3800	0.458	0.85
Ti	1700	3250	0.524	0.7
Zn	390	880	0.444	0.9
Zr	1825	3600	0.506	0.7

Assuming that total laser power P is incident on a circular area A^2 on the surface of a semi-infinite sheet (Section 4.5) the limiting temperatures at points along the z axis and at the center of the focal spot are

$$T(z, \infty) = (P\epsilon/\pi A^2 K)[(z^2 + A^2)^{1/2} - z], \qquad T(0, \infty) = P\epsilon/\pi AK$$

Then with $T(z_m, \infty) = T_m$ and $T_b = P_m\epsilon/\pi AK$,

$$T_m = (T_b/A)[(z_m^2 + A^2)^{1/2} - z_m] \tag{89}$$

and

$$\lim_{t\to\infty} \frac{z_m}{A} = \frac{1}{2}\left[\frac{T_b}{T_m} - \frac{T_m}{T_b}\right] \tag{90}$$

gives the maximum penetration depth of the melting isotherm. z_m/A is plotted as a function of T_m/T_b in Fig. 4.21 and some representative values of z_m/A are given in Table 4.7. For most metals, the ultimate penetration depth z_m is limited to $\simeq A$, the radius of the focal spot. The relation between penetration depth and absorbed laser intensity is

$$Fz_m = 0.5KT_b\left[\frac{T_b}{T_m} - \frac{T_m}{T_b}\right] \tag{91}$$

This gives for copper

$$Fz_m = 3.29 \times 10^3 \text{ W/cm}$$

The increased depth of penetration occurs because the surface temperature approaches T_b asymptotically in this model, while in the previous model the boiling temperature is approached more rapidly ($\propto t^{1/2}$). Here the pulse length would have to be $\gtrsim 10\tau = 40\kappa t/A^2$ in order to maximize the penetration depth.

To find the penetration depth for finite times, Eqs. (35) and (36) are used, putting $T(0, 0, \tau) = T_b$ and $T(0, z, \tau) = T_m$.

For thin sheets we can use the cylindrical source model of Section 4.7.2. With

$$\theta_b = (4\pi Kl/P\epsilon)T_b \qquad \text{and} \qquad \theta_m = (4\pi Kl/P\epsilon)T_m$$

one can show that

$$\theta_b - \theta_m = \left[2 + \frac{1}{\tau}\right]\ln\left(\frac{R}{A}\right) + \frac{1}{2\tau}\left[1 - \left(\frac{R}{A}\right)^2\right] \tag{92}$$

when the condition $A^2/\kappa t \ll 1$ is satisfied. τ is $2\kappa t/A^2$ and R is the radial distance at which melting first appears when the cylinder with $r = A$ reaches its boiling temperature. As an example, consider the melting of

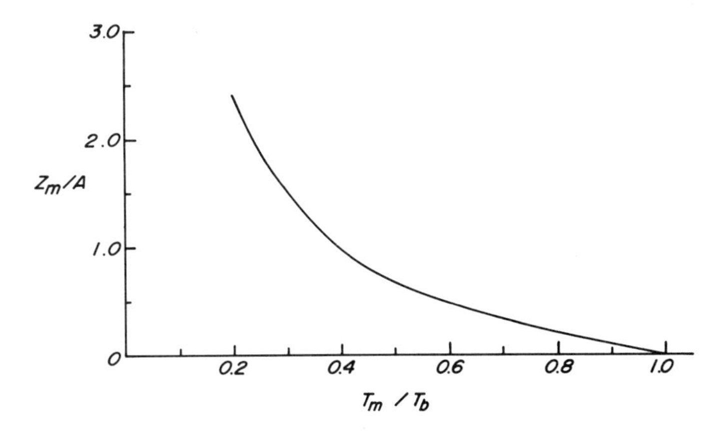

Fig. 4.21. Depth of melting z_m as a function of focal radius A and T_m/T_b for the semi-infinite slab.

copper sheet with a beam focused to $A = 10^{-2}$ cm. Suppose melting is desired over an area with $R = 10^{-1}$ cm in a sheet with $l = 10^{-2}$ cm. A cw CO_2 laser will be used shuttered to produce a pulse of 10-sec duration and the melting will proceed in vacuum. Then $\tau \simeq 1.6 \times 10^5$ using $\kappa = 0.8$ cm²/sec and

$$\theta_b - \theta_m \simeq 2 \ln (R/A) = 4.6$$

The power required, using $\epsilon = 0.04$ and $K = 3.5$ W/cm°C is 3.9 kW.

With constant energy input, Guenot and Racinet (1967) show that an optimum pulse length exists for weld penetration into a slab of finite thickness. They point out that if the pulse length is fixed, an optimum energy exists for maximum weld penetration. Any increase in this energy will result only in an increase of the lateral extent of the weld with little further increase in penetration. They present some experimental data on the welding of thin sheets in support of their conclusions.

When the laser radiation can be considered to generate a line heat source at $r = 0$ in the sheet, a simple analytic expression exists for the temperature distribution and radial extent of the melt puddle. The result is (Carslaw and Jaeger, 1959; Brugger, 1972)

$$T_1(r, t) = T_M + \frac{q}{4\pi\kappa_1}\left[\mathrm{Ei}\left(\frac{r^2}{4\kappa_1 t}\right) - \mathrm{Ei}(\lambda^2)\right], \qquad r \leq r_M \qquad (93)$$

$$T_2(r, t) = \frac{T_M \, \mathrm{Ei}(r^2/4\kappa_2 t)}{\mathrm{Ei}(\beta\lambda^2)}, \qquad r \geq r_M \qquad (94)$$

where r_M is the radius of the melt region. T_M is the melting temperature and T_1, κ_1 refer to the liquid, while T_2, κ_2 refer to the solid metal.

$$\lambda^2 = r_M{}^2/4\kappa_1 t \qquad \text{and} \qquad \beta = \kappa_1/\kappa_2$$

are found from the relation

$$\frac{K_2 T_M}{\mathrm{Ei}\,(\kappa_2\lambda^2)} \exp(-\kappa_2\lambda^2) - \frac{q}{4\pi} \exp(-\lambda^2) = \kappa_1 L\lambda^2 \tag{95}$$

where q is the strength of the line source, while L is the heat of fusion (J/cm^3) and K_2 the thermal conductivity of the solid.

The results of Lin (1967) can be used to estimate the maximum lateral extension of the melt area in a thermally thin sheet heated with a constant beam of Gaussian distribution. The temperatures are

$$T(r, t) = \frac{F_0 d^2}{4Kl} \left[\mathrm{Ei}\left(-\frac{r^2}{d^2}\right) - \mathrm{Ei}\left(-\frac{r^2}{d^2}\,\frac{1}{(1 + 4\kappa t/d^2)}\right)\right] \tag{96}$$

$$T(0, t) = \frac{F_0 d^2}{4Kl} \ln\left(1 + \frac{4\kappa t}{d^2}\right) \tag{97}$$

Putting $T(R, t) = T_m$ and $T(0, t) = T_b$, these equations can be combined to give

$$\theta_m = \mathrm{Ei}\left(-\frac{R^2}{d^2}\right) - \mathrm{Ei}\left(-\frac{R^2}{d^2} \exp(-\theta_b)\right) \tag{98}$$

where $\theta_m = 4\kappa l T_m/F_0 d^2$. Depending on whether the intensity F_0 or the time of pulse t_m is fixed, θ_b is calculated from

$$\theta_b = \begin{cases} \dfrac{4Kl}{F_0 d^2} T_b, & F_0 \ \text{known} \\[2ex] \ln\left(1 + \dfrac{4\kappa t_m}{d^2}\right), & t_m \ \text{known} \end{cases}$$

the unknown quantity F_0 or t_m being obtained from the other equation. θ_b can then be inserted in Eq. (98), and R/d can be found graphically. This equation can be used only when $l < (\kappa t_m)^{1/2}$.

Some discussion of the temperature distribution under the above conditions but including a liquid phase has been given by Lin (1967), while Cohen and Epperson (1968) report the results of a calculation of the time to propagate a melt puddle completely through a ribbon of finite thickness.

Calculations on the time required to melt a thin film on a substrate heated uniformly over its free surface have been made by Stern (1973). The energy retained by the thin film at time t is the difference between the total energy absorbed and that passed to the substrate in time t. This is in toto for complete melting of the film

$$(t_2 - t_1)F' = Ll + H(t_2) - H(t_1) \tag{99}$$

where t_1 is the time at which the surface of the film first melts, t_2 the time at which the melt has completely penetrated the film, F' the flux absorbed, L the latent heat of fusion per cm^3, l the thickness of film, and $H(t)$ the energy supplied to the substrate in time t.

For rapid (adiabatic) heating, no heat is transferred to the substrate and

$$\Delta t = t_2 - t_1 = Ll/F'$$

is the time interval for complete melting. When the temperature in the film is some constant fraction f of that expected for uniform heating of the substrate* and $F' = \epsilon F$, Δt can be obtained from

$$hx - h + f - \frac{2f}{\pi}\left[x \sin^{-1}\left(\frac{1}{x}\right)^{1/2} + (x - 1)^{1/2}\right] = \frac{Ll}{Ft_1} \tag{100}$$

where $x = t_2/t_1$ and $h = F'/\epsilon F$. This solution is valid when the film is thermally thin, so that most of the absorbed heat is conducted to the substrate. Stern (1973) gives plots of $\Delta t/t_1$ versus Ll/Ft_1 for various h and $0 \leq f \leq 1$. h takes into account the change in absorption that occurs when the surface turns from a solid to a liquid. It may therefore be >1.

4.10 VAPORIZATION AND DRILLING

4.10.1 General

The rate at which material is removed in the vicinity of the laser focus becomes significant only when the incident flux and the duration of the pulse are such that the temperature can be brought to the boiling temperature of the material in a time shorter than the pulse length. When these conditions are satisfied, then a vaporization front is established, which has

* This is

$$T(0, t) = \frac{2\epsilon F}{K_2}\left[\frac{\kappa_2 t}{\pi}\right]^{1/2}$$

where K_2 and κ_2 are thermal constants of the substrate.

as its limiting speed (Carslaw and Jaeger, 1959; Landau, 1950)

$$v = \epsilon F/(\lambda + \rho c T) \tag{101}$$

where F is the incident intensity ($\mathrm{W/cm^2}$), λ the heat of vaporization ($\mathrm{J/cm^3}$), ρ the density ($\mathrm{g/cm^3}$), c the specific heat ($\mathrm{J/g°C}$), T the vaporization temperature, and ϵ the emissivity at laser wavelength. This equation assumes that flux F is incident uniformly over the free surface of a semi-infinite sheet and that all material vaporized is completely removed from the solid. In practice, Eq. (101) can also be used to describe the vaporization that occurs in drilling with a focused laser on a finite slab, provided the pulse length is less than the smallest thermal time constant for a particular set of boundary conditions. It can also usually be assumed that a vaporization equilibrium is reached in a time short compared with any fluctuations in the absorbed intensity and therefore that the speed of the vaporization front follows the time-varying absorbed intensity through Eq. (101). Thus, usually to a good approximation,

$$v(t) = \epsilon F(t)/(\lambda + \rho c T) \tag{102}$$

and

$$d(t) = \int_0^t v(t)\, dt = [1/(\lambda + \rho c T)] \int_0^t \epsilon F(t)\, dt \tag{103}$$

where $d(t)$ is the depth of penetration of the vaporization front at time t. This distance can be equated to the drilling depth. As we will discuss below, the temperature T is also a function of $F(t)$ and tends to rise as $F(t)$ increases.

When convective and radiative losses are neglected, the use of available energy is divided between bulk heating of the material and vaporization of material below the focal spot. If drilling is to be done with relatively low intensities, long irradiation times are needed and the fraction of available energy used for bulk heating is very significant, especially when drilling metals. If short, high-power pulses are to be used, then a large fraction of the available energy can be used in the actual drilling process. One can estimate the energy lost to bulk heating of the material by comparing the drilling time to the thermal time constant τ of the material or alternatively by comparing the characteristic distance of heat penetration $(\kappa t)^{1/2}$ to the drilling depth. Assuming that the applied power is sufficient to achieve the boiling temperature, then the contribution from conductive losses will be negligible if the duration of the pulse is small compared to τ.

Kato and Yamaguchi (1968) in a comparative study of the drilling of copper and stainless steel with a normal focused ruby laser pulse noted that at high laser output a greater depth of drilling was obtained in copper, while the reverse was true at low laser output. In their experiment the length of the pulse was kept constant and the pulse energy varied. The pulse duration was comparable to the thermal time constant so that conduction was important. At low pulse energies then, most of the incident energy is lost by conduction to the bulk of the material. Since copper has a higher thermal conductivity than stainless steel, this means that less energy is available for vaporizing the copper and the drilling depth is smaller. As one goes to higher pulse energies the solid becomes unable to conduct away the input energy quickly enough and the major portion of the energy is used for vaporization. Since the energy $(\lambda + \rho c T)$ required for vaporization of unit mass of copper is less than that for stainless steel, greater drilling depths can be achieved in copper.

The regime of intensity that separates the two situations may be estimated if we consider the case where the energy input is equally divided between bulk heating and vaporization. Equating the drilling depth produced by half the flux to the characteristic distance of penetration of heat into the solid, we have

$$(\kappa t_p)^{1/2} = v t_p = \epsilon (F/2) t_p / (\lambda + \rho c T_{vap})$$

and therefore,

$$F = \frac{2}{\epsilon} \left(\frac{\kappa}{t_p} \right)^{1/2} (\lambda + \rho c T_{vap})$$

If t_p is taken to be 10^{-6} sec, then values of F for metals where ϵ is typically 0.1 are in the range 10^6–10^7 W/cm^2, while for insulators where ϵ can usually be taken to be 1.0, it is approximately 10^5 W/cm^2. For $t_p = 10^{-2}$ sec these values decrease to 10^4–10^5 W/cm^2 for metals and 10^3 W/cm^2 for insulators. It is therefore easy to obtain high drilling efficiencies with insulators for both cw and pulsed lasers, while with metals conductive losses are always significant if a typical cw laser is used and often when a typical pulsed laser is used. Note that for the estimations of Eqs. (101)–(103) to be valid, F must be sufficiently high to permit the surface temperature to reach T_{vap} in the pulse length t_p.

4.10.2 Drilling with Low-Intensity Pulses

Let us now consider drilling metals with laser pulses in the range of intensities below 10^6 W/cm^2. As we have seen, in this region conductive losses can be substantial and must be taken into account. We will assume a constant spatial and temporal distribution with focusing to a spot of radius A on the surface of a semi-infinite sheet. For simplicity, and because the heat of fusion is small compared to the heat of vaporization, we neglect the liquid phase. However, the last assumption is more difficult to justify when one observes that the thermal conductivity of most metals changes by a factor of two on transition to the liquid phase (American Institute of Physics Handbook, 1963). Also, experiments indicate that in the drilling process material is often ejected in the molten state by pressure from the vapor inside the hole (Anisimov *et al.*, 1967). The vaporization temperature will be taken to be the normal boiling point of the metal, an approximation that will be justified later.

The minimum power required in order to achieve vaporization is obtained by setting $T = T_b$, the boiling temperature in the steady state Eq. (39), so that

$$P = \pi AKT_b/\epsilon(T_b) \tag{39a}$$

Table 4.8 gives some typical values of P/A for a number of metals when a CO_2 laser is used. In the absence of emissivity data for the boiling temperature at 10.6 μm the value used is the extrapolated value derived from Eq. (23). For low-intensity pulses the duration of irradiation will be large compared to the thermal time constant, so that the power calculated from this equation is a good measure of the conductive loss P_c in a low-intensity drilling process. The time to onset of vaporization t_{vap} will usually be of the order of the thermal time constant or less, depending on the applied power, and it can be determined from Eq. (36) or from Fig. 4.5.

Table 4.8

Minimum Values of P/A for the Production of Boiling on the Surface of an Infinite Slab with 10.6-μm Radiation Focused to a Circular Area of Radius A

Material	P/A ($\times 10^4$ W/cm)
Al	29
Au	48
Mg	9.2
Cu	56
Sn	3.8
Zn	5.3
Pb	1.2
Pt	8.9
Ta	6.8
Ni	6.3
W	12
Mo	11

After the onset of boiling, the rate at which drilling proceeds is determined by the conservation of energy Eq. (101), where we set $T = T_b$, $P = P - P_c$, and $\epsilon = \epsilon(T_b)$:

$$v = \epsilon(P - P_c)/\pi A^2(\lambda + \rho c T_b) \tag{104}$$

Figure 4.22 shows the variation of v with $(P - P_c)/\pi A^2$ for some metals when drilling is done with 10.6-μm radiation. Using this equation to predict v and knowing the duration of the pulse t_p, the depth of drilling can be predicted from the expression

$$d = v(t_p - t_{vap}) = \epsilon(P - P_c)(t_p - t_{vap})/\pi A^2(\lambda + \rho c T_b) \tag{105}$$

where t_{vap} can be determined as outlined above or can often be neglected. For lasers with a varying temporal pulse distribution the depth is given by

$$d = \int_{t_{vap}}^{t_p} \epsilon(P - P_c)/\pi A^2(\lambda + \rho c T_b)\, dt \tag{106}$$

where $P = P(t)$.

As one proceeds to intensities where the pulse duration is comparable to the time constant, Eq. (39a) becomes a progressively less accurate measure of the conductive loss and a more exact calculation must be made for P_c.

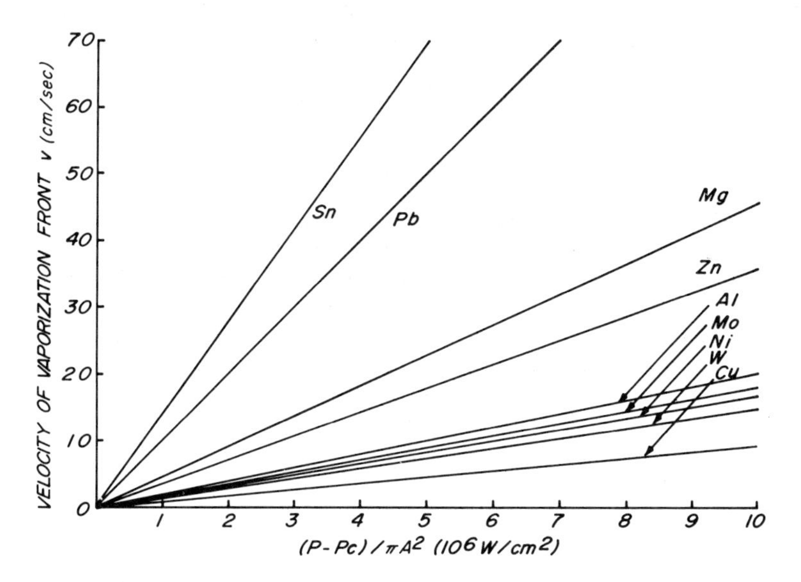

Fig. 4.22. Velocity of vaporization v of some metal surfaces under 10.6-μm radiation as a function of the intensity $(P - P_c)/\pi A^2$ (Gonsalves, 1973).

4.10.3 Drilling with High-Intensity Pulses

Complications in the analytical model due to conductive losses are avoided when we consider the high-intensity regime. Adding the assumption that conductive losses are zero to those of the last section, we proceed to discuss a model.

For short irradiation times Eq. (37) reduces to

$$T = (2P\epsilon/\pi^{3/2}A^2K)(\kappa t)^{1/2} \tag{107}$$

In this case one can predict the time t_{vap} to onset of vaporization if T is set equal to T_b:

$$t_{vap} = \pi^3 A^4 K^2 T_b^2 / 4P^2\epsilon^2\kappa \tag{108}$$

t_{vap} varies inversely as the square of the intensity and is typically in the millisecond region for kilowatt cw lasers and much less for a normal pulsed laser, but varies greatly from one metal to another. Values of t_{vap} for different metals are given in Table 4.9, where ϵ used is that for vacuum at 10.6 μm. For drilling in air ϵ is likely to be greater and t_{vap} would therefore be smaller. For irradiation times approaching the thermal time constant, predictions made from Eq. (108) are inaccurate because of the importance of conduction losses.

After the surface has reached the vaporization temperature, removal of material is governed by the conservation of energy equation

$$v = \epsilon P/[\pi A^2(\lambda + \rho c T_{vap})] \tag{109}$$

Table 4.9

Time t_{vap} to Onset of Vaporization of Metal Surfaces for Incident Intensities F of 10.6-μm Radiation

Metal	$F = 10^6$ W/cm², t_{vap} (m-sec)	$F = 10^8$ W/cm², t_{vap} (μsec)
Cu	31	3.1
Al	9.4	0.94
Ni	2.1	0.21
Mo	5.3	0.53
W	4.6	0.46
Zn	0.69	0.069
Ta	1.5	0.15
Pb	0.068	0.0068
Sn	0.35	0.035

and the thermodynamic equation

$$v = C \exp(-\lambda Z/\rho NkT_{\mathrm{vap}}) \tag{110}$$

where C is the velocity of sound in the material, λ the heat of vaporization (energy/unit volume), Z the atomic number, ρ the density, N Avogadro's number, and k Boltzmann's constant. This equation establishes the rate at which particles can leave a surface at temperature T. Equating (109) and (110), we get

$$P/\pi A^2 = (C/\epsilon)(\lambda + \rho c T_{\mathrm{vap}}) \exp(-\lambda Z/\rho NkT) \tag{111}$$

Anisimov *et al.* (1967) using similar equations have plotted the dependence of temperature and velocity on absorbed intensity. Figures 4.23 and 4.24 show the variation of dimensionless temperature $\rho NkT/Z$ and speed of the vaporization front v with incident intensity $P/\pi A^2$ for some metals when a CO_2 laser is used.

It can be seen from Fig. 4.24 that at low intensities the temperature T remains almost constant. Values of T calculated in this intensity range are close to the normal boiling temperature T_b. Our assumption of the previous section that $T = T_b$ for the low-intensity range is therefore justified. At higher intensities such as those obtained with Q-switched and mode-locked lasers, the temperature changes rapidly with intensity. The

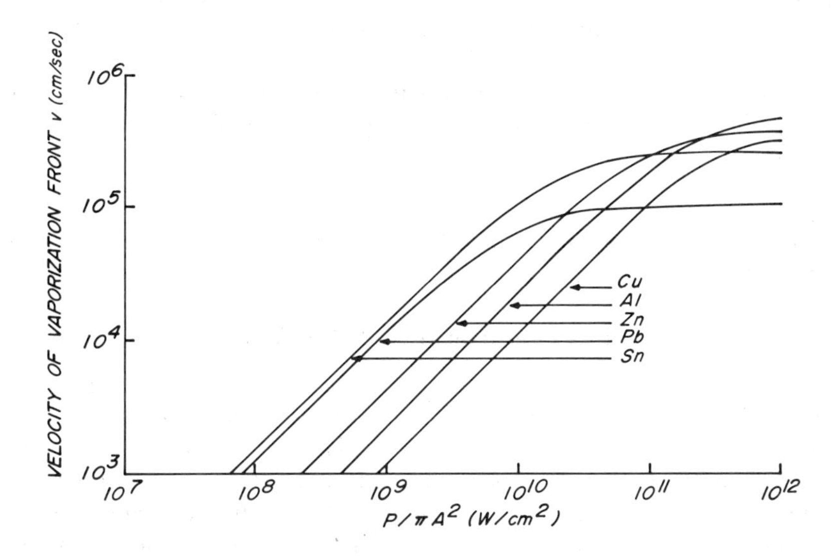

Fig. 4.23. Velocity of vaporization v of some metal surfaces under 10.6-μm radiation as a function of the incident intensity $P/\pi A^2$.

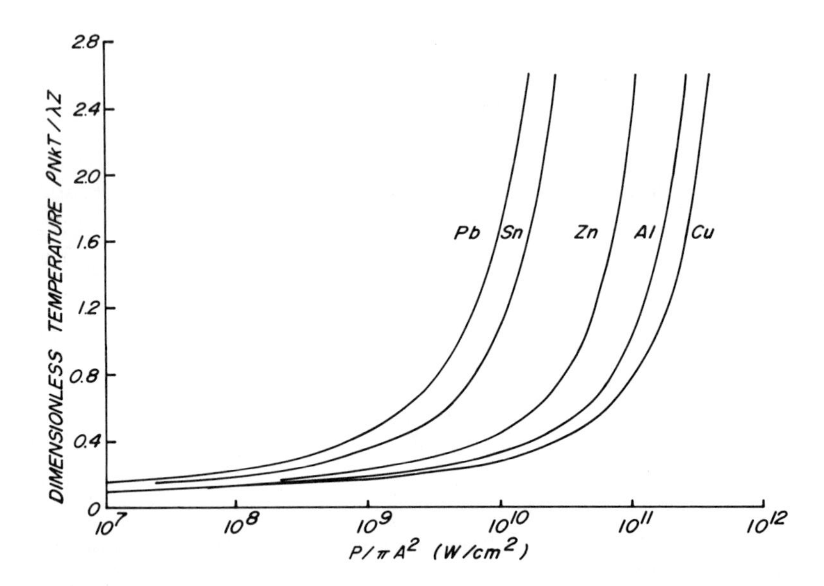

Fig. 4.24. Dimensionless temperature $\rho NkT/\lambda Z$ as a function of incident intensity of 10.6-μm radiation for some metals.

velocity of the vaporization front increases linearly with intensity everywhere except at very high intensities, where it approaches asymptotically the speed of sound in the material.

Using Eqs. (109) and (110) to predict v and knowing the duration of the applied pulse t_p, the depth of drilling can be predicted from the expression

$$d = v(t_p - t_{vap})$$

where t_{vap} is obtained from (108). For varying temporal input power, d is obtained by time integration.

4.10.4 Limitations of the Theory

In the analysis of the previous sections, apart from the assumptions stated, there are a number of points that were deliberately overlooked. No attention was given to the effect of the spatial distribution of the incident intensity on the vaporizing process. The effect of the variation of the angle of incidence of the radiation on the moving boundary was also neglected. The attempt made to take into account the temporal distribution of the pulse is usually accomplished by taking the envelope of the laser pulse. This procedure ignores temporal spiking in the applied radiation, which causes pulsations in the emission of vaporized material (Grechikhin and Min'ko, 1967). Consideration has also not been given to the case where molten material is ejected in the drilling process (Chun and Rose, 1970).

Ready (1971) has compared the depth of drilling observed with that derived on the basis of an analysis similar to that described in Section 4.10.2. Using data adapted from measurements of mass removal by Braginshii *et al.* (1967) he was able to conclude that the predictions of the simple theory describe generally the behavior observed in metals. He found, however, that discrepancies between theory and experiment suggested that reflectivity and expulsion of molten material were important. Better agreement was found when theoretical predictions were matched with data for carbon adapted from measurements by Zavitsanos (1967). This was thought to be due to the absence of molten material and the more efficient absorption by carbon.

The lack of precise knowledge of the effects discussed here and the increased complexity that they would add to the model do not warrant their inclusion. In special situations where they are of great significance empirical relations would have to be found.

4.10.5 More Exact Treatments

Although the analysis given in Sections 4.10.1–4.10.3 provides a good qualitative description of material removal rates, it is not exact in that no account is taken of the variable position of the heat source within the target as vaporization proceeds. In addition, heat is assumed to be absorbed only in an infinitesimally thin surface layer. This last approximation is not strictly valid for materials in which the absorption coefficient for laser radiation $\alpha < \infty$.

Paek and Gagliano (1972) have solved the problem of the temperature profile in an ablating solid due to a moving, uniformly distributed source (area πA^2) of constant intensity. When material is removed, the source can be thought of as varying its location with time as $z' = f(t')$. Then for a disk source in a continuous medium

$$T(r, z, t) = \int_0^a \int_0^t \frac{q(r', t')r'}{4\pi^{1/2}[K(t - t')]^{3/2}} \left[\exp\left(-\frac{(r^2 + r'^2 + [z - f(t')]^2}{4K(t - t')}\right)\right] \times I_0\left(\frac{rr'}{2K(t - t')}\right) dt'\, dr' \tag{112}$$

The method of images is used to specialize this expression for the case of a semi-infinite half-space:

$$T(r, z, t) = \int_0^a \int_0^t \frac{F(r', t')}{4\rho C_p \pi^{1/2}[K(t - t')]^{3/2}} \exp\left(-\frac{(r^2 + r'^2)}{4K(t - t')}\right) \times I_0\left(\frac{rr'}{2K(t - t')}\right) r' \left[\exp\left(-\frac{[z - f(t')]^2}{4K(t - t')}\right) + \exp\left(-\frac{[z + f(t')]^2}{4K(t - t')}\right)\right] dt'\, dr' \tag{113}$$

where $F(r', t')$ is the absorbed laser intensity $= \rho C_p q(r', t')$ W/cm^2. A similar expression was derived for a moving-disk source in a slab of finite thickness. Solution of these equations requires knowledge of $f(t')$, the position of the source at time t'. This can be obtained by measuring the depth of penetration of the hole as a function of time during the drilling process. Paek and Gagliano (1972) give several plots of $T(r, z, t)$ for points in the vicinity of holes drilled in Al_2O_3 ceramic with ruby and CO_2 radiation. The integrals have to be evaluated numerically.

In an interesting paper, Dabby and Paek (1972) examine the temperature profile inside a semi-infinite solid that is vaporizing on its free surface when the incident laser radiation partially penetrates the solid. The boundary conditions for this problem are shown in Fig. 4.25. When the temperature distribution in the solid at $t = 0$ (i.e., when vaporization begins) can be approximated by

$$T = T_v(1 + qz)e^{-qz} \tag{114}$$

then the normalized temperature θ_i valid for short times is

$$\begin{aligned}\theta_i(\tau, s) = {} & \left[1 + \frac{1}{\Delta B}\right] \operatorname{erfc}\left[\frac{s}{2\tau^{1/2}}\right] - \frac{\exp(B^2\tau)}{2\lambda B}\left[e^{-Bs} \operatorname{erfc}\left(\frac{s}{2\tau^{1/2}} - B\tau^{1/2}\right) + e^{Bs} \operatorname{erfc}\left(\frac{s}{2\tau^{1/2}} + B\tau^{1/2}\right)\right] \\ & + \frac{\exp(Q^2\tau)}{2}\left[(2Q^2\tau - Qs - 1)e^{-Qs} \operatorname{erfc}\left\{\frac{s}{2\tau^{1/2}} - Q\tau^{1/2}\right\} + (2Q^2\tau + Qs - 1)e^{Qs} \operatorname{erfc}\left\{\frac{s}{2\tau^{1/2}} + Q\tau^{1/2}\right\}\right] \\ & - \frac{e^{-Bs}}{\Delta B}[1 - \exp(B^2\tau)] - \exp(Q^2\tau - Qs)[2Q^2\tau - Qs - 1]\end{aligned} \tag{115}$$

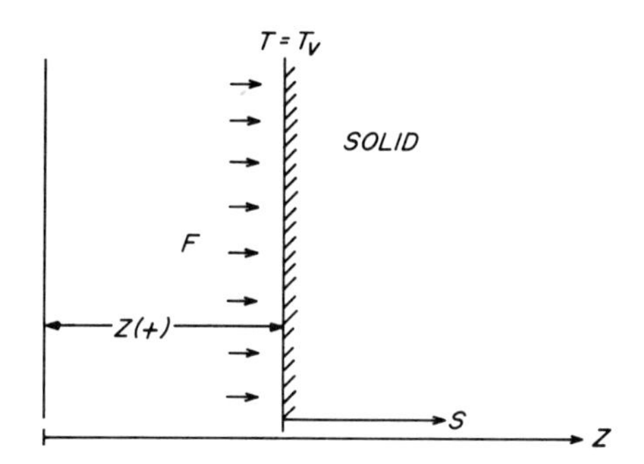

Fig. 4.25. Boundary conditions for semi-infinite solid vaporizing at receding surface $Z(t)$.

The normalized temperature θ_0 valid for large τ is

$$\theta_0(\tau, s) = \frac{1}{2}\left(1 + \frac{1}{\Delta(B - v)}\right)\left\{e^{-vs} \operatorname{erfc}\left[\frac{s}{2\tau^{1/2}} - \frac{v}{2}\tau^{1/2}\right]\right.$$

$$\left. + \operatorname{erfc}\left[\frac{s}{2\tau^{1/2}} + \frac{v}{2}\tau^{1/2}\right]\right\} - \frac{e^{B(B-v)\tau}}{2\Delta(B - v)}$$

$$\times \left\{e^{-Bs} \operatorname{erfc}\left[\frac{s}{2\tau^{1/2}} - \left(B - \frac{v}{2}\right)\tau^{1/2}\right]\right.$$

$$\left. + e^{(B-v)s} \operatorname{erfc}\left[\frac{s}{2\tau^{1/2}} + \left(B - \frac{v}{2}\right)\tau^{1/2}\right]\right\}$$

$$+ \frac{e^{Q(Q-v)\tau}}{2}\left\{\left[2Q\left(Q - \frac{v}{2}\right)\tau - Qs - 1\right]e^{-Qs}\right.$$

$$\times \operatorname{erfc}\left[\frac{s}{2\tau^{1/2}} - \left(Q - \frac{v}{2}\right)\tau^{1/2}\right]$$

$$+ \left[2Q\left(Q - \frac{v}{2}\right)\tau + Qs - 1\right]e^{(Q-v)s}$$

$$\left. \times \operatorname{erfc}\left[\frac{s}{2\tau^{1/2}} + \left(Q - \frac{v}{2}\right)\tau^{1/2}\right]\right\} - \frac{e^{-Bs}}{\Delta(B - v)}\left[1 - e^{B(B-v)\tau}\right]$$

$$- e^{Q(Q-v)\tau - Qs}\left[2Q\left(Q - \frac{v}{2}\right)\tau - Qs - 1\right] \qquad (116)$$

where

$$\theta = T/T_v, \qquad s = (FC_p/K\lambda)(z - Z), \qquad u = \rho\lambda\dot{Z}/F, \qquad \tau = F^2C_pt/\rho K\lambda^2$$

$$\Delta = C_pT_v/\lambda, \qquad B = K\alpha\lambda/FC_p, \qquad Q = Kq\lambda/FC_p$$

and units are λ (J/g), C_p (J/g-°C), F (W/cm²), ρ (g/cm³), K (W/cm-°C), α (cm⁻¹), and v is the normalized steady state velocity given by $v = 1/(1 + \lambda)$ in units of $\rho\lambda\dot{Z}/F$. Initially, the vaporization front recedes with normalized velocity

$$U_i = 1 - \exp(B^2\tau)\,\mathrm{erfc}(B\tau^{1/2}) + 2\Delta Q^3\tau\exp(Q^2\tau)\,\mathrm{erfc}(Q\tau^{1/2}) - \frac{2\Delta}{\pi^{1/2}}Q^2\tau^{1/2} \tag{117}$$

At larger τ this solution is replaced by

$$\begin{aligned} U_0 = {} & 1 - \Delta v + \frac{v}{2}\left(\Delta + \frac{1}{B - v}\right)\mathrm{erfc}\left(\frac{v\tau^{1/2}}{2}\right) \\ & - \frac{(B - v/2)}{B - v}\,e^{B(B-v)\tau}\,\mathrm{erfc}\left[\left(B - \frac{v}{2}\right)\tau^{1/2}\right] \\ & + \Delta\left[2Q\left(Q - \frac{v}{2}\right)^2\tau + \frac{v}{2}\right]e^{Q(Q-v)\tau}\,\mathrm{erfc}\left[\left(Q - \frac{v}{2}\right)\tau^{1/2}\right] \\ & - \frac{2\Delta}{\pi^{1/2}}\,Q\left(Q - \frac{v}{2}\right)\tau^{1/2}\exp\left(-\frac{v^2\tau}{4}\right) \end{aligned} \tag{118}$$

Some conclusions that can be drawn from this analysis are as follows:

(i) The vaporization front does not reach its equilibrium value v immediately. The steady state value is approached only after several time constants τ.

(ii) The temperature for $z > Z$ is not always less than T_v, the temperature at the vapor–solid interface. Under certain conditions (B small) the temperature at these points can be significantly higher than T_v.

(iii) When initial heating produces a slowly varying temperature (Q small) such that $B \gg Q$, then the initial temperature distribution may peak at a higher value than the steady state temperature. The speed of the vaporization front then reaches a maximum value $>v$ and declines to v for τ large.

(iv) Subsurface boiling at elevated temperatures will result in high pressures and explosion of the superheated material. Thus the material removal rate may be dominated by explosive evaporation under certain conditions. This effect has been observed experimentally (Ready, 1963; Klocke, 1969; Gagliano and Paek, 1974). In the experiments of Gagliano and Paek on alumina and copper excited with high-power ruby laser radiation, $B \ll 1$ for alumina, while $B \simeq 1$ for copper when $F = 2 \times 10^7$ W/cm^2. Thus alumina should show strong superheating of layers beneath the surface, while copper should not under these excitation conditions. High-speed framing camera photographs of the interaction region show that alumina ejects a cloud of particles during the interaction while copper does not. Furthermore, the amount of material ejected in the form of particles depends greatly on the laser intensity.

4.11 MOVING HEAT SOURCES

4.11.1 Cutting

In the laser cutting of thin sheets, one needs to know the temperature distribution in the sheet at points removed from the actual laser focus. We consider the geometry of a thin sheet irradiated with a beam of laser radiation incident on an area πA^2 of the sheet. The beam is uniform both in time and spatially over the circular focus. Then if the sheet lies in the xy plane and moves with velocity v in the positive x direction, the temperature $T(x, y, t)$ can be approximated for points $r \neq 0$ (Carslaw and Jaeger, 1959; Gonsalves and Duley, 1972) by

$$\exp\left(\frac{vx}{2\kappa}\right) = \frac{2\pi KlT(x, y, t)}{\epsilon PfK_0(rv/2\kappa)} \tag{119}$$

where r is the radial distance to the point under consideration, P the incident power, ϵ the emissivity at the laser wavelength, l the sheet thickness, K_0 a Bessel function of the second kind of order zero, and K and κ the thermal conductivity and thermal diffusivity, respectively. This approximation assumes that laser power absorbed over a disk of thickness l and area πA^2 can be replaced by a point source of strength ϵPf located at the origin.

With the dimensionless generalized coordinates

$$X = vx/2\kappa, \qquad Y = vy/2\kappa, \qquad R = vr/2\kappa \tag{120}$$

and with

$$C = 2\pi KlT_{\mathrm{m}}/\epsilon P$$

Eq. (119) becomes, for the location of the melting isotherm $T = T_{\mathrm{m}}$,

$$\exp(X) = C/fK_0(R) \tag{121}$$

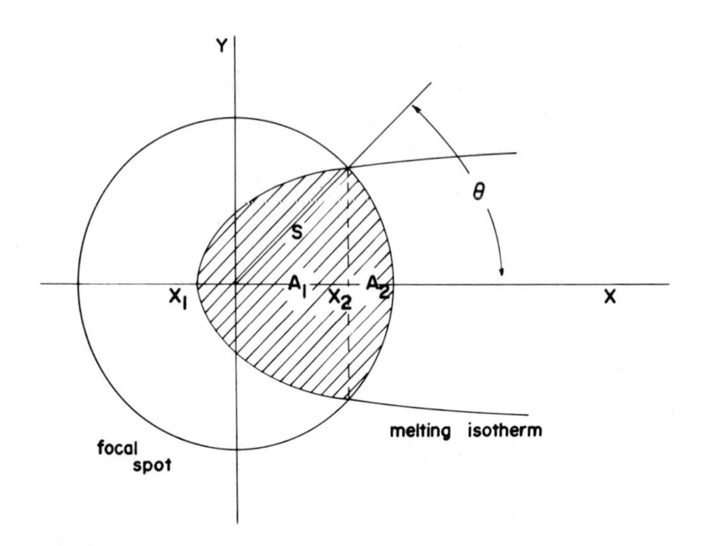

Fig. 4.26. Generalized coordinate system showing focal spot and melting isotherm for cutting speeds well below the critical value.

Since the laser is focused to a spot of radius A, in the normalized coordinate system the spot radius becomes

$$S = vA/2\kappa \tag{122}$$

and its equation is

$$X^2 + Y^2 = S^2 \tag{123}$$

Figure 4.26 shows a typical melting isotherm and the focal spot in the moving coordinate system (X,Y). All material within the melting isotherm will be removed and thus only a fraction f of the total power ϵP will contribute to the heating process.

In evaluating the fraction f, two cases must be considered: first, the situation where the maximum width of the melting isotherm occurs outside the focal spot, and second, that where it occurs inside the focal spot. In the first case, the region of the focal spot removed is the shaded region in Fig. 4.26 and has area

$$A_1 + A_2 = S^2\theta - \frac{S^2}{2}\sin 2\theta + 2\int_{X_1}^{X_2} Y\,dx \tag{124}$$

where $X_2 = \ln[C/fK_0(S)]$ and $\theta = \cos^{-1}(X_2/S)$. Substituting in the integral

$$Y = (R^2 - X^2)^{1/2} = \{R^2 - [\ln(C/fK_0(R))]^2\}^{1/2}$$

and $dX = \{K_1(R)/K_0(R)\}\, dR$ as derived from Eq. (121) we get

$$A_1 + A_2 = S^2\theta - \frac{S^2}{2}\sin 2\theta$$
$$+ 2\int_{R=|X_1|}^{S} \{R^2 - [\ln(C/fK_0(R))]^2\}^{1/2}\{K_1(R)/K_0(R)\}\, dR \tag{125}$$

The region of the focal spot that remains has area $\pi S^2 - A_1 - A_2$ and constitutes a fraction f of the total spot area given by

$$f = (\pi S^2 - A_1 - A_2)/\pi S^2 \tag{126}$$

Substituting for $A_1 + A_2$ from Eq. (125) this expression becomes

$$f = 1 - \frac{\theta}{\pi} + \frac{\sin 2\theta}{2\pi}$$
$$- \frac{2}{\pi S^2}\int_{R=|X_1|}^{S} \{R^2 - [\ln(C/fK_0(R))]^2\}^{1/2}\{K_1(R)/K_0(R)\}\, dR \tag{127}$$

In the second case shown in Fig. 4.27,

$$A_1 = 2\int_{R=|X_1|}^{R_{\text{max width}}} \{R^2 - [\ln(C/fK_0(R))]^2\}^{1/2}\{K_1(R)/K_0(R)\}\, dR$$

$$A_2 = 2Y_2(S\cos\beta - X_2), \qquad A_3 = S^2\beta - \frac{S^2}{2}\sin 2\beta \tag{128}$$

Using (126),

$$f = 1 - \frac{\beta}{\pi} - \frac{\sin 2\beta}{2\pi} - \frac{2}{\pi S^2}[Y_2\,(S\cos\beta - X_2)]$$
$$+ \int_{R=|X_1|}^{R_{\text{max width}}} \{R^2 - [\ln(C/fK_0(R))]^2\}^{1/2}\{K_1(R)/K_0(R)\}\, dR \tag{129}$$

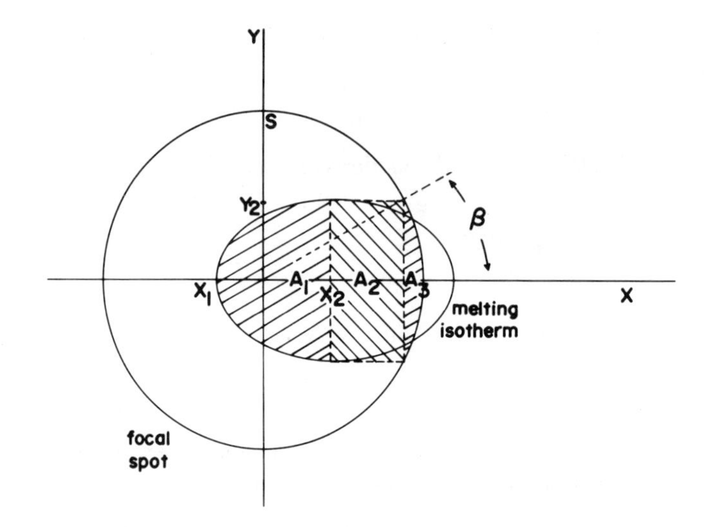

Fig. 4.27. Generalized coordinate system showing focal spot and melting isotherm for cutting speeds close to critical value.

Equations (127) and (129) have been solved numerically for f as a function of C and S (Gonsalves and Duley, 1972) and the results are plotted in Fig. 4.28. This plot can be used to predict the variation of f with v, P, and l for any material if the thermal parameters and the focal spot radius A are known. This is done by transforming S and C to the variables cutting speed v and power thickness ratio P/l by substituting appropriate values for K, κ, ϵ, T_m, and A in the relations $v = 2\kappa S/A$ and $P/l = 2\pi K T_m/\epsilon C$. Care must be taken in applying the theory. At small f values, the section of the focal spot for which the beam strikes the metal surface represents a heat source that is displaced from the origin and produces a temperature distribution that cannot be closely approximated by a point source at the origin. At very high f values the point source is a good approximation in determining the location of the melting isotherm. However, predictions made in this region might correspond to speeds exceeding the critical cutting speed, that is, speeds above which a cut is not produced. For f values lying between these two extremes, the predictions are thought to be fairly accurate.

Since the cut width corresponds to the maximum width in the melting isotherm, we use (121) to maximize Y. From (121),

$$K_0[(X^2 + Y^2)^{1/2}] = [C \exp(-X)]/f \tag{130}$$

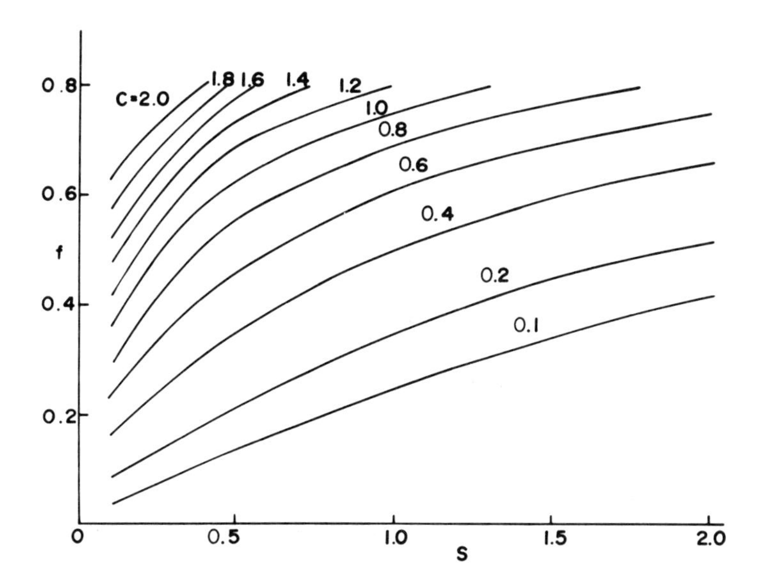

Fig. 4.28. Theoretical curves of f vs. S for various C (Gonsalves and Duley, 1972).

differentiating with respect to X we get

$$-K_1[(X^2 + Y^2)^{1/2}](X + Y\,dY/dX)(X^2 + Y^2)^{-1/2} = [-C\exp(-X)]/f \tag{131}$$

If $dY/dX = 0$, then

$$[XK_1(R)]/R = [C\exp(-X)]/f \tag{132}$$

and using

$$[XK_1(R)]/R = K_0(R) \tag{133}$$

then for maximum Y

$$X = RK_0(R)/K_1(R) \tag{134}$$

and

$$K_0(R) = C\exp[-RK_0(R)/K_1(R)]/f \tag{135}$$

Solution of this equation gives R for the cut width and hence Y, since $Y = R\sin\phi$, where $\phi = \cos^{-1}[K_0(R)/K_1(R)]$. Equation (133) has been solved numerically for various C/f and the results combined with the solution of Eqs. (125) and (127) to produce a plot of the nondimensional half-cut width Y_{max} versus S for various C (Fig. 4.29). Again predictions

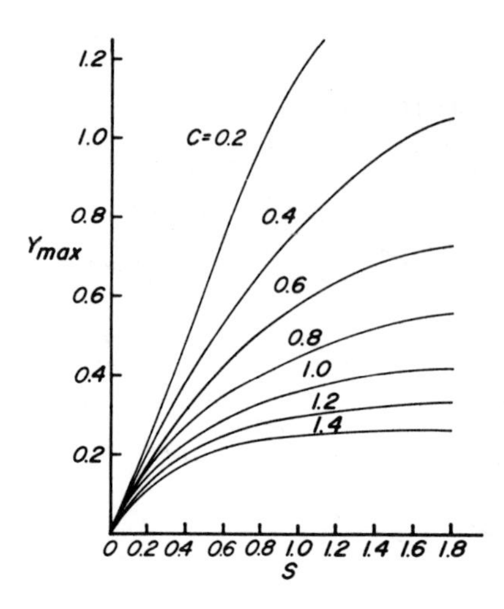

Fig. 4.29. Theoretical curves of Y_{max} vs. S for various C (Gonsalves and Duley, 1972).

made from this graph are expected to be accurate except in regions where the speed and power–thickness ratio are such that very high or very low f values are involved.

The generalized plots of Figs. 4.28 and 4.29 can now be used in determining the interrelation of cutting speed, cut width, and power requirements for metals. Assuming that a thin metal sheet is to be cut at speed v by a beam focused to a spot of radius A, then the nondimensional spot radius $S = vA/2\kappa$ can be calculated. f and C values are obtained from Fig. 4.28, where the choice of large f ensures high efficiency in utilization of the applied energy. The power required is then determined by the equation $P = 2\pi\kappa l T_m/\epsilon C$ using the appropriate thermal values for that material, and the cut width calculated using $W = 4\kappa Y_{max}/v$, where the value of Y_{max} is obtained from Fig. 4.29 for the required S and C. The predictions of Figs. 4.28 and 4.29 are expected to be valid for $l < (2\kappa A/v)^{1/2}$, where $(2\kappa A/v)^{1/2}$ is the characteristic distance heat has penetrated into the sheet in the time it has moved one focal diameter.

Siekman (1968) has developed a theoretical description of thermal processes in the CO_2 laser machining of thin metal films on a thick insulating substrate. The heat transfer to the film is assumed to be via the substrate, an approximation that is justified in view of the low emissivities of most insulators at 10.6 μm. Thus, when a hole in the thin film has been opened up (by momentarily increasing the laser power or by introducing a defect in the surface), the subsequent steady state absorption of laser power will occur mainly in the area of the substrate just behind the evaporating metal surface (Fig. 4.30). When the substrate is considered to be a semi-infinite sheet, the temperature at the point (r, x) is (Rosenthal, 1946)

$$T(r, x) = \frac{q}{2\pi K r} \exp\left[-\frac{vr}{2\kappa} - \frac{vx}{2\kappa}\right] \tag{136}$$

where $q = f'P$ and the sheet moves with velocity v in the positive x direction. $r = (x^2 + y^2 + z^2)^{1/2}$ and f' is the fraction of the total power absorbed by the substrate. The thermal constants are those of the substrate.

Equation (136) can be written

$$\theta(R, X) = (1/R) \exp(-R - X) \tag{137}$$

where X, Y, and Z are as defined previously and $R = (X^2 + Y^2 + Z^2)^{1/2}$. The normalized temperature is

$$\theta(R, X) = (4\pi K\kappa/qv) T(r, x) \tag{138}$$

The theoretical cut width (in the metal film) can now be obtained by assuming that material is removed for all $\theta > \theta_1$. On the limiting isotherm, we have

$$\partial Y/\partial X \,|_{\theta=\theta_1} = 0$$

which gives $R_1 + X_1 = -X_1/R_1$, and X_1 will be negative since the maximum cut width lies in the $-x$ direction. One can then show that for high velocities

$$Y_1^2 \simeq 0.736/\theta_1 \tag{139}$$

and the cut width

$$W \simeq 0.968 (\kappa/KT_1)^{1/2} (f'P/v)^{1/2} \tag{140}$$

Siekman (1968) shows that the critical temperature T_1 can be found ap-

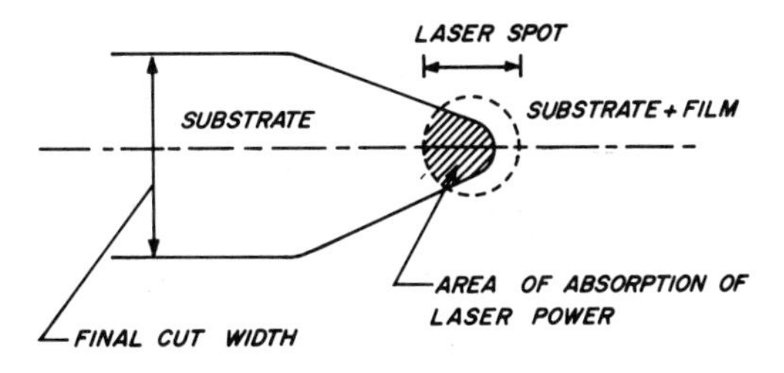

Fig. 4.30. Area of absorption of laser power on an insulating substrate coated with a thin metal film.

proximately from

$$8.54KBvD/fP \simeq A \exp(-B/T_1) \tag{141}$$

where A and B are evaporation constants, and D is the film thickness in g/cm^2.

Extension of these calculations to a system in which the coating film is also absorbing have been reported by Siekman (1969).

4.11.2 Welding

In welding metals with high-power cw CO_2 lasers, material is removed completely from a long roughly elliptical cylinder and incident radiation is able to penetrate deeply into the material. This effect, which is known as "keyholing," permits welds to be obtained whose depth is much larger than that expected simply on the basis of heat transfer theory. The geometry of the melt region is shown schematically in Fig. 4.31. Heat transfer at the surface of the keyhole forms an egg-shaped melt region whose flat end lies ahead of the laser beam. The width and depth of the melted zone depend on laser power and the speed at which the weld is produced. Swift-Hook and Gick (1973) have calculated this dependence using a moving

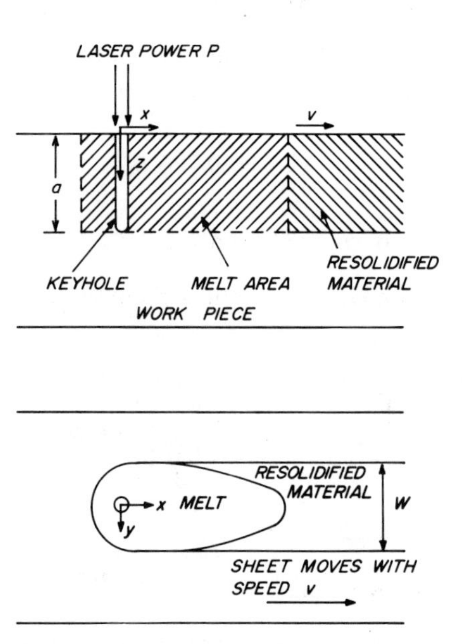

Fig. 4.31. Geometry for penetration welding of a semi-infinite sheet.

line source model (Carslaw and Jaeger, 1959). Isotherms can be obtained from the equation

$$\theta = \frac{q}{2\pi}[\exp(Ur\cos\phi)]K_0(Ur) \tag{142}$$

where $q = P/a$, $\theta = KT$, $x = r\cos\phi$, $U = v/2\kappa$, and a is the penetration depth. Writing the power per unit depth $M = P/a\theta$, this equation becomes

$$M = [2\pi/K_0(Ur)]\exp(-Ur\cos\phi) \tag{143}$$

It can be shown that at the point where the melt has its greatest width the following condition is satisfied (putting $T = T_m$):

$$\frac{\partial M/\partial\phi}{\partial M/\partial r} = \frac{\partial y/\partial\phi}{\partial y/\partial r}$$

so that

$$\cos\phi = -K_0(Ur)/K_0'(Ur) \tag{144}$$

The normalized maximum melt width*

$$Y_{max} = vW/\kappa = 2UW = 4Ur[1 - K_0^2(Ur)/K_0'^2(Ur)]^{1/2} \tag{145}$$

Substituting $\cos\phi$ in Eq. (143) one gets

$$M = \frac{2\pi}{K_0(Ur)}\exp\left(\frac{UrK_0(Ur)}{K_0'(Ur)}\right) \tag{146}$$

The relation between absorbed power P and the melt width W can be found by eliminating Ur in Eqs. (145) and (146). Swift-Hook and Gick (1973) discuss two limiting cases when this can be done analytically.

In the high-speed limit (Ur large), the Bessel functions can be expanded to give

$$M \simeq 8.26(Ur)^{1/2} \quad \text{and} \quad Y_{max} \simeq 4(Ur)^{1/2}$$

so that

$$Y_{max} \simeq 0.484M \quad (Ur\ \text{large}) \tag{147}$$

When the speed is low (Ur small),

$$M \simeq \frac{2\pi}{\ln(2e^{-\gamma}/Ur)} \quad \text{and} \quad Y_{max} \simeq 4Ur$$

* Note that this value of Y_{max} differs by a factor of 2 from that used in Section 4.11.1.

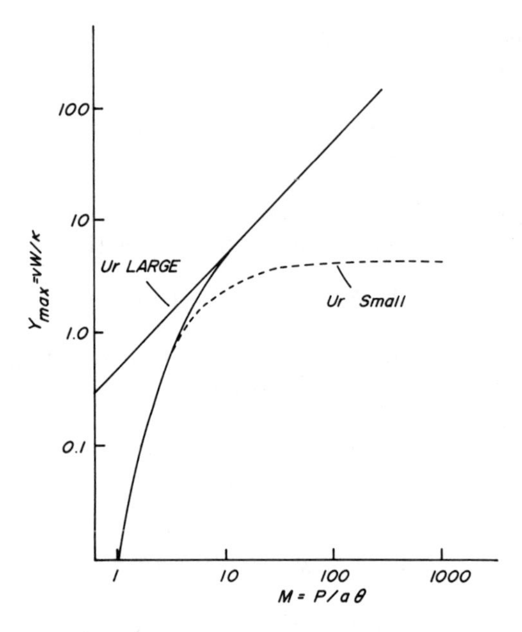

Fig. 4.32. Relation of maximum width of weld W to absorbed laser power P and penetration depth a.

so that

$$Y_{\max} \simeq \exp(1.50 - 2\pi/M) \qquad (Ur \text{ small}) \tag{148}$$

where $\gamma = 0.577\ldots$ is Euler's constant. Figure 4.32 shows a plot of $Y_{\max}$ versus M constructed from these two limiting solutions with an interpolation in the intervening region where neither solution is strictly valid (Swift-Hook and Gick, 1973).

Consider the problem of penetration welding of type 304 stainless steel to depth $a = 1$ cm and width $W = 0.5$ cm at the rate of 1 cm/sec. Then using $\kappa = 0.049$ cm²/sec, $Y_{\max} = vW/\kappa = 10.2$. The graph then gives $M = 21 = P/a\theta = P/1 \times 3.6 \times 10^2$, where the average value for θ given by Swift-Hook and Gick has been used. The power required would be $\simeq$7.6 kW assuming 100% efficiency of energy transfer to the workpiece.

4.12 THE VALIDITY OF CLASSICAL HEAT TRANSFER THEORY

It is surprising that there have been few examinations of the limitations of conventional heat transfer theory in the context of the rapid heating rates possible with high-power lasers. Even for the relatively low incident laser intensity of 10^6 W/cm^2, the surface of a sheet exposed to this flux will rise to a temperature of several thousand degrees in 10^{-6} sec. In this time, layers even 10^{-3} cm deeper within the material have not yet experienced significant heating. Thus, $dT/dt \simeq 10^9$ deg/sec and $dT/dx \simeq 10^6$ deg/cm. At higher values of laser flux, these derivatives will be many orders of magnitude greater. It would be remarkable if classical heat conduction theory still held rigorously under such extreme conditions.

Harrington (1967) has discussed some of the possible limitations of heat conduction theory when a material is heated rapidly with an intense radiative flux. Classically, Q, the heat transferred through unit area on a slab of thickness Δz when the temperature difference between the faces of the slab is ΔT, is

$$Q = -K\,\Delta T/\Delta z \tag{149}$$

One then lets $\Delta z \to 0$ so that

$$Q = -K\,dT/dz \tag{150}$$

Harrington points out that although one requires $\Delta z \to 0$ mathematically, physical considerations determined by the heat transfer mechanism in metals limits the minimum value for Δz to 10Λ, where Λ is the mean free path for electrons. Λ is typically 100–500 Å and is also a measure of the distance over which radiant energy is absorbed by a metal. Hence absorption of incident radiation is some 10 times smaller than the minimum distance Δz for which Eq. (150) will be valid. Consequently, the temperature at the surface would not seem to be exactly predictable from classical heat conduction theory.

Consider two isothermal planes, one at temperature T_1 and the other at T_2. Then classically

$$K[dT/dz\,|_1 - dT/dz\,|_2]\Delta t = \rho c\,\Delta z\,\Delta T \tag{151}$$

Then the term in the brackets can be written

$$T_1' - T_2' = T_2''\,\Delta z + T_2'''(\Delta z/2!)^2 + T_2''''(\Delta z/3!)^3 + \cdots$$

Classically one neglects T''' and all higher order derivatives. This requires

$$T_2'' \gg T_2'''(\Delta z/2!) \tag{152}$$

Harrington's conclusion on consideration of the heating of a semi-infinite medium by absorption of flux at its surface according to the expression $F(z) = F_0 e^{-\alpha z}$ is that the temperature distribution within the first few electron mean free paths (typically 100 Å) of the surface cannot be specified by the classical theory [Eq. (28)] for short times. However, a straightforward application of the requirement (152) to the case of heating with a surface source, which normally yields the temperature distribution

$$T(z,t) = \frac{2\epsilon F_0}{K} (\kappa t)^{1/2} \operatorname{ierfc}\left[\frac{z}{2(\kappa t)^{1/2}}\right] \tag{153}$$

places the following restriction on the region for which this solution is valid:

$$z\,\Delta z/2(\kappa t) \ll 1$$

Taking $\Delta z = 10\text{Å} \simeq 10^{-5}$ cm, this becomes

$$0.5 \times 10^{-5} z/\kappa t \ll 1$$

When $\kappa = 0.5$ cm^2/sec, $z \ll 10^{-1}$ cm at $t = 10^{-6}$ sec and $z \ll 10^2$ cm when $t = 10^{-3}$ sec. Hence Eq. (153) would seem to be valid for all regions of interest for most values of t. Only when $t \to 10^{-12}$ sec, does this requirement place some constraints on the solution of Eq. (153).

Chapter 5

Drilling

5.1 INTRODUCTION

This chapter outlines some measurements that have been made on drilling metals and nonmetals with various types of pulsed and cw lasers. Depending on the laser intensity the incident beam may interact in a variety of ways with a solid target. Section 5.2 summarizes the various effects that can occur as the incident laser intensity is increased. Examples of actual drilling operations using lasers are outlined in Sections 5.3 and 5.4, and a comparison of the results obtained with the predictions of heat transfer theory are given where possible. Section 5.5 discusses some applications of lasers in the drilling of holes in thin metal sheets.

5.2 INTERACTION MECHANISMS

The means by which intense optical radiation is coupled to solid surfaces and subsequently dissipated is a subject still under active investigation. At low levels of irradiation ($<10^5$ W/cm^2) there would seem to be little justification on the basis of present knowledge to suppose that the interaction is anything other than "classical." In this case, one assumes that the incident radiation is coupled via a time- and temperature-dependent reflectivity $R(\lambda, T, t) = 1 - \epsilon(\lambda, T, t)$ into an effective intensity which produces heating in the material. This radiation will be absorbed in a surface layer whose thickness is $\simeq \alpha^{-1}$, where α is the absorption coefficient at the laser wavelength. Matter ejected from the target may attenuate the incident beam either by means of absorption or by scattering, but this effect will be small because of the low evaporation rates attainable with fluxes of this magnitude. Heat absorbed at the surface will cause a temperature rise in the material but the magnitude and extent of this rise will depend on the thermal constants of the material together with the ratio of the pulse length to the thermal time constant. When this ratio is small, little heat will be conducted away from the focal area during the pulse. When this ratio is greater than one, a higher temperature will be reached in the focal area, but utilization of absorbed intensity will be inefficient as much of this heat will be conducted away from the interaction region.

If the melting temperature is not reached, the zone of interaction may be distinguishable from the bulk material only by structural changes or by an increase in hardness. When melting is produced, a fusion front will propagate into the material. However, the maximum extension of this front into the material will be limited in the case of metals by the large fraction of the absorbed power that is needed just to balance conduction losses. Intensities $\lesssim 10^5$ W/cm^2 are usually not able to give rise to significant vaporization in metals (see, for example, Table 4.5 taking $A = 10^{-2}$ cm). When vaporization does occur it will be at a temperature less than or approximately equal to the normal boiling temperature of the metal. Insulators can be drilled with intensities $\lesssim 10^5$ W/cm^2 since $\epsilon \simeq 1$ generally and K and κ are smaller than for metals, and holes may be drilled in thin metallic sheets when the pulse length is larger than the thermal time constant of the sheet.

Intensities in the range $10^5 \leq F \leq 10^7$ W/cm^2 are easily produced by conventional solid state lasers and by pulsed TEA and kilowatt cw CO_2 lasers. Much work has been reported on interaction mechanisms in this intensity range and a variety of useful thermal effects can be produced. Focused radiation from the laser will be partially attenuated before reaching the surface due to material ejected during the beginning of a pulse. This material may consist of neutral atoms and molecules, ions and electrons, and small particles of liquid. Absorption and scattering will be the primary attenuation mechanisms. Laser-supported combustion waves have been reported to shield an irradiated surface completely from incident 10.6-μm radiation (Stegman *et al.*, 1973) at an intensity of $1\text{–}2 \times 10^6$ W/cm^2. The target will be exposed to a periodic flux of incident radiation as the attenuating material alternately forms, blocks the beam, and then dissipates. Locke *et al.* (1972) have shown that this cloud of attenuating material that forms above a metal under irradiation with a high-power cw CO_2 laser can be removed by a transverse gas jet of some inert gas. Some discussion on the "tailoring" of laser pulses to minimize the effects of scattering and absorption by the plume has been given by Herziger *et al.* (1973). For optimum drilling rates, the surface should be irradiated with a series of pulses such that the separation between pulses is greater than the time required for the dissipation of the plume.

Radiation passed by the plume will be absorbed in a layer of thickness α^{-1} cm on the surface of the target after suffering some attenuation due to the nonzero reflectivity of the gas–solid or gas–liquid interface. Since the reflectivity will depend on the temperature and the geometry of the surface in the interaction zone, this quantity will hardly be independent of time during irradiation. However, experimental measurements of the dynamic reflectivity of metals (Bonch-Bruevich *et al.*, 1968b) show that significant reflectivity changes are produced only for fluxes greater than 10^6 W/cm^2. When $F \gtrsim 10^7$ W/cm^2, the reflectivity of metals has been observed to decrease drastically (Basov *et al.*, 1969; Chun and Rose, 1970). At low levels of the incident flux, the reflectivity has actually been observed to increase slightly (Bonch-Bruevich *et al.*, 1968b; Muzii *et al.*, 1973) possibly due to the evaporation of a thin surface oxide layer. Reflectivity changes in laser-irradiated germanium with intensities in this range have been shown to be due to optically generated carriers (Bonch-Bruevich *et al.*, 1968a; Birnbaum and Stocker, 1968) and to the onset of surface damge (Muzii *et al.*, 1973). The former effect can result in an increase in reflectivity when the intensity exceeds a threshold value.

Continued irradiation of a sample with $10^5 \lesssim F \lesssim 10^7$ W/cm^2 will result in a temperature rise to the melting point, at which time a fusion front will then propagate into the material. When the surface temperature rises toward the boiling temperature an evaporation front begins to move into the material, reducing the thickness of the liquid layer. Nevertheless, even when rapid evaporation is occurring, the evaporating surface will be preceded by a thin liquid layer whose thickness has been estimated by Rykalin and Uglov (1971). Boiling is enhanced when this layer encounters imperfections in the target material. This may result in the ejection of droplets of molten material. As the hole generated by the evaporation front deepens, incident radiation will be more effectively trapped and the surface of the hole will be coated with a liquid layer. The interaction between escaping vapor and this layer may result in a "flushing" mechanism, whereby liquid is swept out of the hole. Thus material removal rates can exceed those predicted from a consideration of one-dimensional evaporation driven by the absorbed laser flux. Evaporation will occur at a temperature that may be greater than the normal boiling temperature of the material. In addition, this temperature will depend on F and therefore, under excitation with pulsed lasers, on the time t.

A number of measurements have been made of the mass removed and specific impulse imparted to an evaporating target for intensities in this range generated by pulsed ruby and Nd lasers (Afanas'ev *et al.*, 1969; Batanov *et al.*, 1970). For metals, P_r/E, the specific impulse, and $\Delta m/E$, the specific mass removed, both rapidly increase with F in this intensity range. (P_r is the recoil momentum, E the pulse energy, and Δm the mass removed.)

As incident laser intensity rises above 10^7 W/cm^2 a host of new interaction effects are observed. A full discussion of these effects is beyond the scope of this book. However, reviews on this subject are available (Ready, 1971; Caruso, 1971; Mallozzi *et al.*, 1973). A few comments on these effects in the context of laser processing of materials will be given.

Prokhorov *et al.* (1973) have predicted that when a critical incident intensity in the range $10^7 \lesssim F_{md} \lesssim 10^8$ W/cm^2 is exceeded, a transparency wave begins to propagate into the target. Passage of this wave converts a liquid metal into a liquid dielectric. This effect occurs only as the temperature of the vaporization front approaches the critical temperature T_{cr}. The final temperature T_{md} reached on conversion of a thin surface layer from a metal to a dielectric is always $< T_{cr}$. Furthermore, because of the transparency of this layer, the temperature does not exceed T_{md} and a further increase in F above F_{md} will not raise T. Near the transition temperature there will be a sharp drop in the reflectivity of the surface. Such abrupt changes in reflectivity have been observed experimentally (Bonch-Bruevich *et al.*, 1968b; Basov *et al.*, 1969; Chun and Rose, 1970). Prokhorov *et al.* (1973) attribute this effect to the onset of the metal–dielectric transition. They further predict that the evaporation rate should be independent of F for $F \gtrsim F_{md}$ since an increase in $F > F_{md}$ only increases the speed of the transparency front. This may limit the depth of craters produced by high-intensity pulses. Experimental observations on the variation of P_r/E and $\Delta m/E$ at high intensities show that both these quantities maximize for bismuth and lead to values of $F \simeq F_{md}$. The subsequent decrease in these quantities that is observed for $F > F_{md}$ (Batanov *et al.*, 1970) is compatible with the existence of a dielectric surface layer.

The effect of superheating and subsurface explosions on the ejection of material from some metals as well as alumina has been discussed by

Gagliano and Paek (1974). It was shown that excitation conditions that give small values of B [see Eq. (4.116)] yield strong erosion of the target through the explosive ejection of material. This evaporation regime typically occurs for metals when $F \simeq 10^8$ W/cm^2.

5.3 METALS

There have been a number of studies of the relation between hole depth, entrance diameter and shape, and the thermophysical parameters of materials using lasers (Deming *et al.*, 1969; Akimov and Mirkin, 1969; Klocke, 1969; Chun and Rose, 1970; Ready, 1971; Suminov and Kuzin, 1972). Table 5.1 gives some details of holes drilled in metals with a ruby laser (Moorhead, 1971). It has been generally found that when the laser pulse energy is kept constant, the largest hole depths are produced for low-melting-point materials. This correlation can be most clearly seen in the report of Akimov and Mirkin (1969), where hole depths and diameters were examined in 20 elemental solids under standard irradiation conditions with a ruby laser. Hole depths of 1–1.5 mm were observed in samples of gallium, indium, and bismuth, all of which have melting temperatures less than 500°C. The smallest hole depths occurred in irradiating molybdenum,

Table 5.1

Data on Holes Drilled in Some Metals with a Ruby Laser[a]

Material	Thickness ($\times 10^{-3}$ in.)	Pulse length (msec)	Energy (J)	Hole diameter entrance ($\times 10^{-3}$ in.)	Hole diameter exit ($\times 10^{-3}$ in.)
PE Magnesium	62	1.8	2.1	14	8
	62	2.0	3.3	16	12
Molybdenum	20	2.0	3.3	10	8
	20	2.25	4.9	10	8
	20	2.35	5.9	10	10
Copper	32	2.25	4.9	8	—
304 Stainless steel	36	2.35	5.9	20	10
Ti–6%Al–4%V	96	2.35	5.9	16	6
	96	2.4	7.0	18	6
Tungsten	20	2.0	3.3	8	6
	20	2.1	4.0	8	8
	20	2.35	5.9	10	12

[a] After Moorhead (1971).

tantalum, and tungsten, whose melting temperatures are in the 2500–3500°C range. Klocke (1969) found similar results but noted that, in addition, holes drilled in low-melting-point materials tended to have larger cross-sectional areas than did those drilled in more refractory metals.

Material is removed on laser drilling a metal by a variety of processes. Vaporization is most important for short pulse lengths and high peak powers. For longer pulses of lower power, material may be removed primarily in liquid form by a flushing mechanism. The measurements of Chun and Rose (1970) show that the mass of material removed increases slowly with the duration of the laser pulse for the first 100 μsec or so. Subsequently, the amount of material removed increases almost linearly with the duration of the pulse. These experiments were performed with a constant average power. As the amount of material removed increases with pulse length, the fraction of this material ejected in liquid form also increases. All the materials studied (Al, Cu, Mo, and Ni) were observed to eject mass mainly in liquid form for pulse durations greater than about 100 μsec. Figure 5.1 shows the mass removal rate, and the rate of removal of material in the form of vapor, as a function of pulse length. These curves are based on measurements on Mo and Ni. It can be seen that the vaporization rate actually diminishes with time after 50 μsec. Suminov and Kuzin

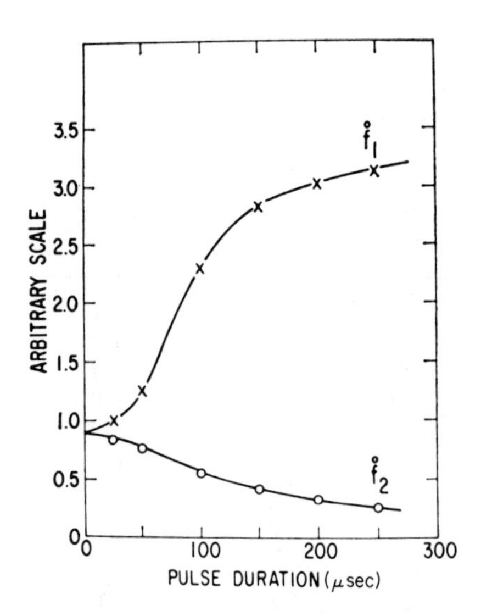

Fig. 5.1. Total mass removal rate ($\dot{f}_1$) and rate of removal of mass as vapor ($\dot{f}_2$) as a function of time for variable pulse duration. $f_1 = M(t)$, $f_2 = M(t)[1 - f_L(t)]$. These data were obtained for Mo and Ni (from Chun and Rose, 1970).

(1972) have examined the dependence of mass removal in the form of liquid and vapor on melting temperature for several metals. Particles of liquid ejected by subsurface explosions have been shown to shield the surface partially from incident laser radiation (Zhiryakov *et al.*, 1971). These particles may exhibit a complex time-dependent motion on leaving the target. Some are blown completely away from the interaction region, while others can remain suspended for some time above the focal area before returning to the workpiece. Suspended particles can absorb and scatter incident laser light.

The light absorbed by the particles may cause them to heat rapidly and evaporate part of their mass. The impulse due to this evaporation propels the particle back toward the target. The excellent photographs of Klocke (1969) show that beads of molten material are redeposited on the target outside the hole. Zhiryakov *et al.* (1971) report that particles are ejected at speeds in the range $1\text{–}5 \times 10^3$ cm/sec.

The energy dependence of hole depth and entrance diameter (Klocke, 1969; Suminov and Kuzin, 1972) shows that both increase rapidly with increasing energy at low energies. Subsequently both increase more slowly, but even at high incident energies there appears to be little tendency for the curves to flatten out.

Similar results have been reported by Gagliano *et al.* (1969). As the pulse energy increases, the plasma generated above the workpiece will become more and more opaque to the incident laser radiation. There is thus little apparent advantage to increasing the pulse energy indefinitely in an attempt to drill deeper holes. Repetitive pulsing with pulses of lower energy can just as effectively drill holes with large aspect ratios with a much more efficient use of laser energy. Furthermore, drilling with a superposition of pulses usually yields holes whose sides have less taper than those of holes drilled with one pulse of higher energy. Gagliano *et al.* (1969) report an interesting exception to this rule. Complete penetration of 2.4-mm 70:30 brass sheet was accomplished with only one pulse of a ruby laser, yielding an intensity of 10^7 W/cm^2 on the surface of the brass. The pulse length was 5 msec and the pulse energy 75 J. High penetration was attributed to the rapid evaporation of the zinc component of the brass. With high-intensity irradiation, pockets of zinc-enriched alloy were superheated well above the normal boiling point of zinc. This resulted in the creation of enormous pressures and consequently in the explosive removal of material.

In pure metals, residual impurities and gases may act as localized centers to promote boiling, which ejects material at a higher rate than expected from a consideration of the thermal parameters of the material and the incident laser flux. A study of this effect has been reported by Brekhovskikh *et al.* (1970). Several types of copper stock were subjected to a pulse from a neodymium glass laser at an intensity of 10^6–10^7 W/cm^2. At low incident intensities, cathodic copper showed only a fused zone with individual fine craters. Porous copper showed a hole under the same conditions. At higher powers, craters were formed in all materials, but these were always deeper in the porous copper samples than in those of cathodic or ordinary stock copper. In addition, the holes drilled in porous copper had irregular profiles. A calculation of the maximum one-dimensional evaporation rate and the maximum depth of the hole that could be produced with the laser used showed that evaporation alone could not account for the observed depth in porous samples. It was suggested that both chemical and physical defects in porous copper can act as nucleation centers that promote vigorous boiling of the liquid phase. This would enhance the material removal rate.

Rykalin and Uglov (1971) have examined the role of rapid evaporation at inclusions in the surface layer of an irradiated metal. Even when vaporization of the bulk material dominates the interaction, a thin liquid layer precedes the vaporization front. The thickness of this layer will vary as the flux changes. For incident intensities in the range $\gtrsim 10^6$ W/cm^2, the liquid layer thickness can vary from several microns (large F) to several hundred microns (small F). As the liquid layer encounters inclusions of nonmetallic particles, clumps of impurities, and gas bubbles on moving into the metal, these centers can act as nuclei for the growth of bubbles in the melt. Rykalin and Uglov (1971) estimate the radius and lifetime of these bubbles in molten copper as a function of incident intensity. The radius may be several hundred microns for $F \simeq 10^6$ W/cm^2, reducing to several microns for $F \simeq 10^8$ W/cm^2. The maximum size of liquid droplets ejected due to this process should therefore decrease as F increases. Experimental verification of this process is made difficult by the fact that the calculated relation of bubble size to incident flux is appropriate only when a crater has not yet formed in the material. When a crater has formed, droplets are ejected primarily from the sides of the crater.

It should be noted at this point that the impurity-dominated evaporation processes discussed above are not the same as those investigated by Ready (1965) and Dabby and Paek (1972). Subsurface explosions due to finite penetration of laser radiation into the material and the creation of a superheated layer ahead of the vaporization front will occur even in the absence of impurity centers and will enhance the material removal rate.

The shape of holes drilled in uranium with multiple pulses from a CO_2 laser has been investigated by Spitz (1969). It was found that the volume of the material removed by the laser could be fitted by the expression

$$V = V_0 [1 - \exp(-\beta S)]$$

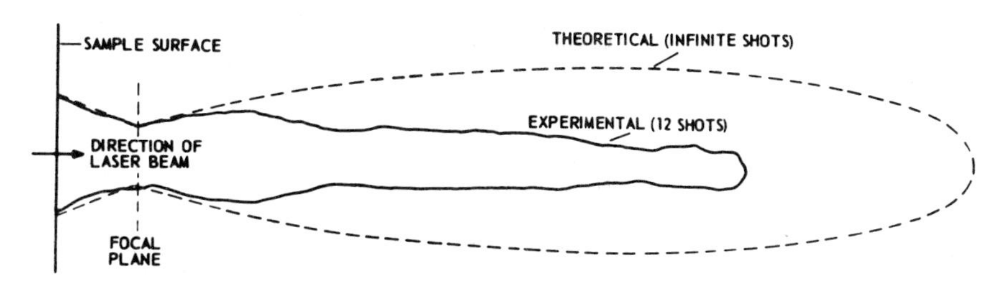

Fig. 5.2. Comparison of experimental and theoretical results for a sample of uranium (Spitz, 1969).

where V_0 is the limiting volume removed by an infinite number of shots, S the number of shots, and β a constant. Each "shot" consisted of a 1-sec burst of 245 pulses with each pulse lasting for 1 μsec. When the laser output was focused just below the surface of the uranium sheet, the holes produced had the shape shown schematically in Fig. 5.2. The constriction at the laser end of the hole corresponded in position to that of the focal plane of the lens used. A theoretical hole profile calculated for an infinite number of shots is also shown in Fig. 5.2. It can be seen that the theoretical prediction of hole shape is excellent close to the focal plane. Spitz calculated the depth and radius (r and z in cylindrical coordinates centered on the optical axis) of points at which the incident laser intensity was maintained at a constant value. This intensity was then identified with the critical intensity for the production of significant evaporation. The surface over which the intensity is maintained at the critical value then defines the limiting boundaries of the hole for an infinite exposure of the target to laser pulses. Although this method neglects the change in intensity at a point on the hole surface due to the slope of the sides and reflection and channeling of incident radiation, which increase the intensity at the end of the hole, reasonable agreement with the experimental results was obtained. The good agreement between theory and experiment is particularly interesting in view of the fact that the theory requires no input of thermodynamic parameters of the workpiece. These data would, however, be required for a calculation of the critical intensity. Empirical values of the critical intensity were approximately 10^8 W/cm^2.

Spitz examined three samples of uranium with different hardnesses. The depth of penetration and the volume of material removed for a given number of shots were found to be smaller, the harder the material. Penetration depths were typically 1 mm for 10 shots of 1-sec duration and a peak power per pulse of about 10^7 W/cm^2.

The initial stages of laser damage to metals have been followed by electron and optical microscopy (Vogel and Backlund, 1965). The central melting zone was found to be surrounded by a concentric ring containing craterlike formations. The maximum diameter of these craters was 10 μm and topographically they fell into two types. The first type (called *ejection craters*) were characterized by a central peak. The other types (called *surface craters*) were similar to impact craters without a central peak. This type was found clustered around surface scratches and other defects. Surprisingly, craters were formed on the surface behind a shield that effectively blocked part of the incident beam. As the intensity increased, radial grooves were observed, which terminated in a droplet of target material.

Other studies of this effect have been reported by Bastow and Bowden (1968), Bastow (1969), and more recently by Siegrist *et al.* (1973). Bastow also reports two types of microcrater and associates one with the pure metal and the other with impurities, but there seems to be some disagreement between different groups as to the conditions that give rise to the various kinds of microcrater. Bastow finds that the craters formed on the surface of very pure metals tend to line up in rows. This was attributed to the formation of unipolar arcs in the surface plasma. Siegrist *et al.* (1973) found that the interaction of 150-nsec TEA CO_2 laser pulses with peak power $\simeq$2 MW with either metallic or insulating surface produced a periodic structure of resolidified material. The "wavelength" of this structure was that of the laser (10.6 μm).

5.4 NONMETALS

Fine holes, particularly those with a large aspect ratio (the ratio of hole depth to entrance hole diameter), are difficult to drill in many insulating materials using conventional machine tool technology. The aspect ratio of holes drilled in materials like high-temperature-fired alumina, for example, rarely can exceed 4:1. Holes may, of course, be drilled prior to firing, but then the precision of hole location and the tolerance in hole diameter are lost during the firing process. Lasers on the other hand have produced holes in ceramics with aspect ratios of 25:1 (Cohen, 1967). Such large aspect ratios are due in part to the channeling effect of laser radiation to the end of a partially drilled hole. This has the effect of maintaining the incident intensity at a high value at the end of the hole even at distances much greater than the depth of focus of the optics used to converge the beam. Refocusing the beam to points deeper inside the target between laser pulses may enhance this effect.

Small-diameter holes are best drilled with lasers whose wavelengths are in the visible or ultraviolet, since the wavelength of the light used limits the theoretical spot size on focusing. Infrared lasers are, however, useful in drilling glasses and some ceramic materials that are partially transparent to visible light. In this case, the limiting spot size is approximately 10 μm in diameter. It should be remembered, however, that diameters this small are obtained only on focusing the output from a laser operating in the fundamental mode with distortionless optics.

Historically, one of the first industrial applications of high-power pulsed lasers was in the drilling of fine holes in diamonds for the fabrication of diamond dies (Epperson *et al.*, 1966). This required creation of a hole that tapered to 0.46 mm in diameter.

Laser drilling of holes in alumina ceramic has been treated theoretically by Paek and Gagliano (1972) and experimentally by Longfellow (1971) and Nakada and Giles (1971). Holes drilled in slabs and in the bulk material are slightly tapered, with the exit hole in slabs having a smaller diameter than that of the entrance hole. Both holes are usually surrounded by a small annular ring of debris and melt material from the hole. X-ray diffraction studies of the structure of this material show it to be a mixture of crystalline α and γ Al_2O_3 (Nakada and Giles, 1971). The hole is coated internally with a thin layer of resolidified alumina, which shows a grain structure quite different from that of the bulk material. Nakada and Giles found no evidence for radial cracks propagating from the hole. Stresses exist, however (Paek and Gagliano, 1972), and may produce cracks when holes are drilled close to an edge. Cracks were most apparent when holes were drilled by the superposition of several pulses. This was attributed to the incomplete stress removal in the finite interval between pulses. Holes drilled close together with one laser pulse per hole showed no evidence of crack formation in the region between them. Since the maximum stress that can be supported by the alumina used in these experiments without fracture is somewhat less than 28 kg/mm^2, thermal stresses generated during drilling must be significantly smaller than this value. The theoretical calculations of Paek and Gagliano (1972) indicate that the maximum stress does not exceed 25 kg/mm^2 when drilling occurs with a ruby laser at an intensity of 3.2×10^7 W/cm^2.

Paek and Gagliano found that the depth of holes drilled in alumina ceramic with a ruby laser could be fitted to the expression

$$d = 0.53t^{0.85} \qquad (1)$$

where d is measured in units of 10^{-2} cm and t is time in msec. Since the derivative of d with respect to t gives the instantaneous speed of the vaporization front, it is apparent that this speed is not independent of time. This is to be expected since $d = \int_0^t v(t)\,dt$, where $v(t)$ is the speed of the vaporization front and

$$v(t) = F(t)/(\lambda + \rho c T_v)$$

for one-dimensional vaporization. Heating with a ruby laser operating in the free-running mode will subject the target to a large number of short high-peak power pulses, $F(t)$, during 1 to 2 msec. The vaporization speed will therefore vary rapidly over a time scale of microseconds. d, which integrates over these rapid fluctuations, is thus unlikely to be directly related to t. What is remarkable is that the exponent of t in Eq. (1) differs only slightly from unity despite the fact that the vaporization is not one dimensional and $F(t)$ is not constant. Paek and Gagliano used $v(t)$ determined experimentally from Eq. (1) to find the speed of a moving heat source, which was then used as input to the theory of Section 4.5.2 to calculate the temperature distribution in the irradiated solid. The resulting temperature distribution was used to estimate the time-dependent shape of the hole. Good agreement was found between theoretical and experimental hole shapes.

Two advantages of laser drilling of ceramics are that holes can be accurately positioned and that patterns of holes can be preprogrammed automatically. A study of these two factors has been reported by Longfellow (1971). Using a cw CO_2 laser with a programmable shutter and an alumina workpiece in an X–Y numerically controlled table, 0.125–0.3-mm diameter holes were drilled with a positional accuracy of better than 0.01% over a distance of 12.7 cm. Material removal was aided by the addition of a gas jet concentric with the laser beam and a vacuum chamber behind the sheet. Debris ejected during drilling was forced away from the hole by the combined action of the gas jet and suction from the vacuum chamber. Good quality tapered holes were produced in 0.7-mm-thick alumina.

In drilling thick slabs of alumina with a pulsed laser, refocusing between pulses has been shown (Cohen and Epperson, 1968; Gagliano *et al.*, 1969) to have a deleterious effect on hole shape. Fifteen shots from a ruby laser each with an energy of 3.1 J and a duration of 0.5 msec produced a hole with an aspect ratio of about 8:1 and roughly cylindrical cross section when the pulses were focused on the surface of the material. Refocusing between each shot to move the focal plane farther into the material generated a highly tapered hole of approximately the same aspect ratio. It would seem that refocusing appears to enhance the "light-pipe" or channeling effect of incident radiation reflected off the walls of the hole. The profiles of holes with refocusing are quite similar to those observed in fused quartz drilled with a cw CO_2 laser (see below).

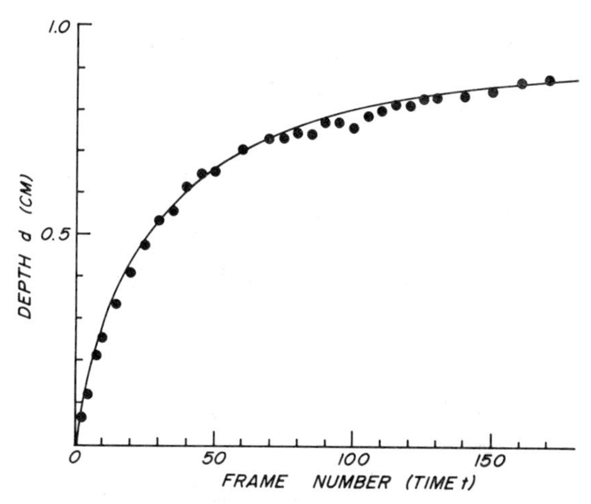

Fig. 5.3. Depth d of a hole drilled in fused quartz vs. time t. The incident intensity was 0.6×10^4 W/cm². The time evolution of the hole depth and profile was followed photographically. The interval between frames is 0.056 sec.

Drilling of fused quartz sheet with a cw CO_2 laser has been reported by Duley and Gonsalves (1972) and Duley and Young (1973). Quartz is well suited to working with the CO_2 laser since it absorbs strongly in the vicinity of 10 μm. A large absorption coefficient together with relatively low thermal diffusivity and thermal conductivity means that significant thermal effects can be produced with low laser power. As the melting range of quartz is relatively small, careful control over laser power and focusing must be exercised if welding is desired instead of vaporization.

The depth d of a hole drilled in quartz with a cw CO_2 laser intensity of 0.6×10^4 W/cm² as a function of time is shown in Fig. 5.3. The depth first increases rapidly with time and then increases less quickly. It has been found that the slope of the initial part of this curve is proportional to laser intensity (Duley and Gonsalves, 1972). This suggests that the initial rapid rise is due to the propagation of a vaporization front into the material since

$$v = \partial d/\partial t = F/(\lambda + \rho c T_v) \tag{2}$$

describes the rate of recession of a vaporizing surface [Eq. (4.101)]. A linear relation between $\partial d/\partial t$ and F is expected only when the absorbed intensity is small, so that $T_v \simeq T_b$ the normal boiling point of quartz (Section 4.10.3). Chang, D. B., *et al.* (1970) have discussed the problem of vaporizing quartz with a high-power cw CO_2 laser. They give the following expressions for the vapor pressure of quartz:

$$p\ (T > 2270°\mathrm{K}) = \exp(21.9)\ \exp(-40{,}600/T)\, T^{0.73} \tag{3}$$

$$p\ (T < 2270°\mathrm{K}) = \exp(30.6)\ \exp(-42{,}900/T)\, T^{-0.27} \tag{4}$$

where p is in units of N/m² and T is in °K. The evaporation rate β will be

$$\beta = [\bar{m}/2kT]^{1/2}p \tag{5}$$

where β is in units of kg/m²/sec and $\bar{m}$ is the average mass of an evaporated molecule. β is directly related to v, and hence one can show

$$F\ (T > 2270°\text{K}) = 5.6 \times 10^{-14}(1 + 2.26 \times 10^{-4}T_v)T^{0.23} \times \exp(-40{,}600/T)\ \text{W/m}^2 \tag{6}$$

and

$$v = (7.66 \times 10^{-11}\ F)/(1 + 2.26 \times 10^{-4}\ T_v)\ \text{m/sec} \tag{7}$$

where $T = T_v + 273$. The numerical factors are obtained by using the following values for fused quartz:

$\rho = 2.2 \times 10^3$ kg/m³, $c = 1.34 \times 10^3$ J/kg°C, $\lambda = 1.31 \times 10^{10}$ J/m³

In fitting the experimental results, one first plots F versus T and then obtains the *actual* vaporization temperature from this plot using the known value for F. This temperature is then used in Eq. (7) to derive v, the initial slope of the d versus t plot. For short times, the total depth of the hole can be obtained from $\int_0^t d(t)\ dt$. A theoretical plot of v versus F using this result is shown in Fig. 5.4. It can be seen that the temperature changes only slightly over the range of laser intensity $0 < F < 10^8$ W/m² making this plot linear. At higher laser intensities this plot would no longer be linear.

The d versus t curve shown in Fig. 5.3 was obtained with $F = 0.6 \times 10^4$ W/cm². Figure 5.4 predicts that the initial slope of this curve should be $v \simeq 0.3$ cm/sec. This should be compared with the slope $v \simeq 0.25$ cm/sec from Fig. 5.3.

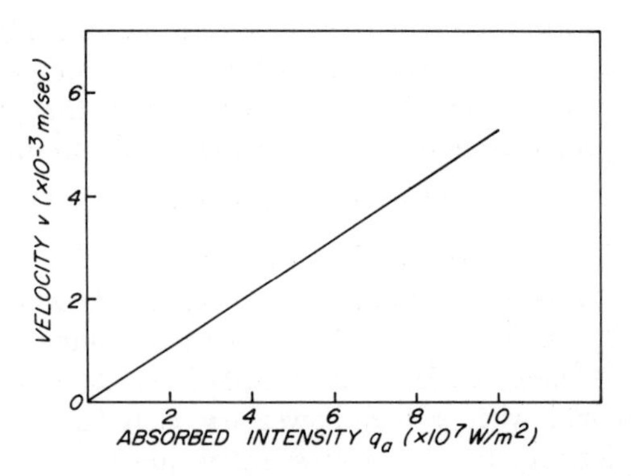

Fig. 5.4. Theoretical plot of v as a function of F, the absorbed intensity, for fused quartz calculated from Eqs. (6) and (7).

As shown in Section 4.10.3, the problem of evaporation under a constant flux can be solved in a general way. We take the vapor pressure

$$p = \alpha \exp(A) \exp(-\zeta/T) \qquad (8)$$

where A and ζ are evaporation constants for a particular material, and $\alpha = 1.013 \times 10^5$ N/m² for p in N/m². Then as above,

$$v = (\eta/\zeta^{1/2})[\zeta/T]^{1/2} \exp(-\zeta/T) \qquad (9)$$

where

$$\eta = (\alpha/\rho)[\bar{m}/2k]^{1/2} \exp(A) \text{ m}(°\text{K})^{1/2}/\text{sec} \qquad (10)$$

Table 5.2 gives values of A, $\bar{m}$, η, and ζ for a variety of refractory compounds from which these equations can be reduced to numerical form. Figure 5.5 shows a generalized plot of $\ln[v/\eta]$ against ζ/T for various ζ.

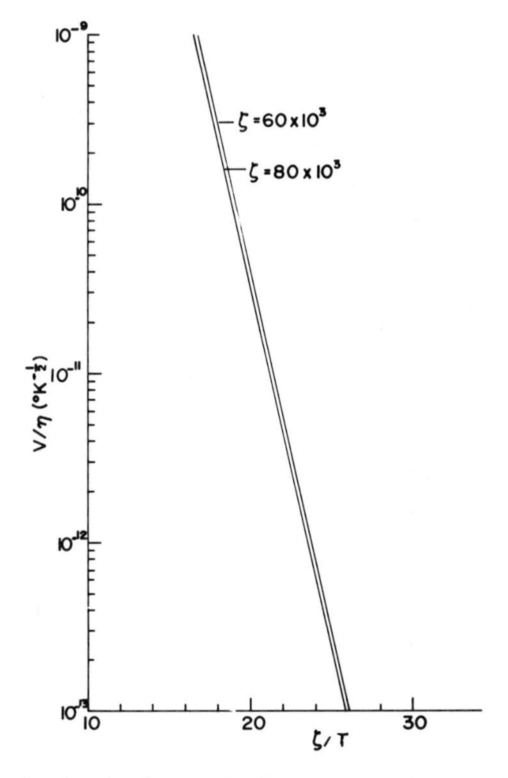

Fig. 5.5. Plot of reduced velocity v/η of vaporization front against reduced temperature ζ/T.

Table 5.2

Evaporation and Thermodynamic Constants (Handbook Values) for Several Refractory Oxides

Oxide	A	m^a (amu)	η (m°K$^{1/2}$/sec)	ζ (×10^{-4} °K)	λ (×10^{-10} J/m^3)	c (×10^{-3} J/kg°C)
MgO	18.3	30	1.05×10^8	6.0	4.41	1.34
CaO	18.1	47	1.17×10^8	6.45	3.14	1.00
Al_2O_3	18.9	27.5	1.69×10^8	7.35	2.34	1.46
ZrO_2	20.6	76	1.01×10^9	8.56	3.42	0.60
TiO_2	21.6	60	3.43×10^9	6.91	3.00	0.92
ThO_2	21.9	250	4.02×10^9	8.66	2.56	0.42
SiO_2	19.4	40	5.9×10^8	5.9	1.83	1.34

[a] Estimated from vapor composition at $\simeq$2500°K given by Kulikov (1967).

Note that this plot is linear for most ζ/T of interest and that, in addition, the running parameter ζ on these curves has little effect in determining ζ/T for particular v/η. For a given v this plot enables T, the temperature at which vaporization occurs, to be obtained. The requisite laser intensity can then be found from

$$F = v[\lambda + \rho c(T\text{-}273)] \text{ W/m}^2 \tag{11}$$

As an example, suppose one wants to drill MgO sheet at the rate $v = 1$ cm/sec. Then $v/\eta = 1.05 \times 10^{-10}$ °K$^{-1/2}$ and from Fig. 5.5, $\zeta/T = 19$ or $T = 6 \times 10^4/19 = 3160$°K. Then the laser intensity required would be 5.8×10^4 W/cm^2 ($\rho = 3.6 \times 10^3$ kg/m^3).

Although the initial slope of the $d(t)$ curve can be well understood in terms of the propagation of a vaporization front into the material, as d becomes larger other effects become important. Some of these have been discussed by Duley and Young (1973). As the hole deepens, the incident intensity along the optical axis is diminishing because of the finite depth of focus of the condensing optics. At the same time, as the angle of the sides of the hole increases, more and more incident radiation is channeled down to the end of the hole by multiple reflections. The measured reflection coefficient for fused quartz at room temperature and at a wavelength of 10.6 μm as a function of incidence angle is shown in Fig. 5.6 (Young, 1973)

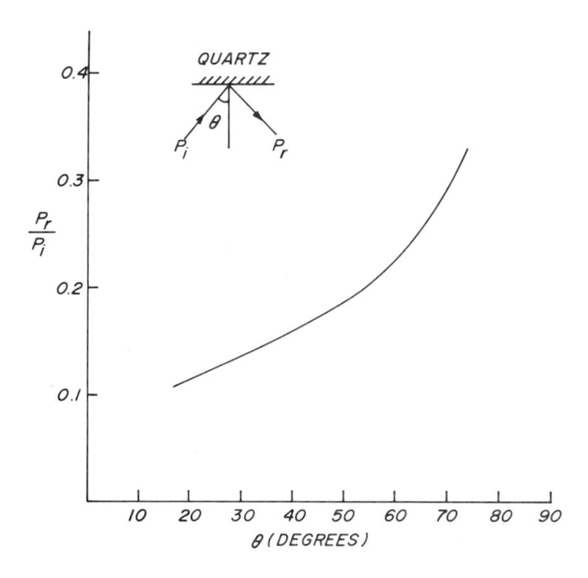

Fig. 5.6. Measured reflectivity at 10.6 μm of fused quartz as a function of angle of incidence.

and can be high for large angles of incidence. It seems likely that the angle of the side of the hole at any point adjusts itself (by vaporization) so that the absorbed intensity at that point is just sufficient to maintain a particular critical temperature at which vaporization is negligible.

The time evolution of the shape of holes drilled with cw CO_2 laser radiation in fused quartz is shown in Fig. 5.7 (Duley and Young, 1973). It was found that the propagation of the hole into the bulk material is highly irregular after the initial rapid increase in depth shown in Fig. 5.3. The tip of the hole often moves at an angle with respect to the optical axis of the system and may execute a helical motion on moving into the sheet. This peculiar behavior is attributed to the effect of channeling of incident radiation down to the end of the hole. At long times, further increases in depth appear to occur in a pulsating manner (Fig. 5.7b). The complexities exhibited in Fig. 5.7 provide a good illustration that while simple models can be evolved to explain the basic mechanisms of laser drilling, much more sophisticated treatments are required to account for the details of such processes.

Metal oxide molecular absorption coefficients at the 10.6-μm CO_2 laser line have been calculated by Chang *et al.* (1970) for SiO and by Boni and Su (1973) for SiO, FeO, AlO, and TiO with a view to predicting the opacity of vapor ejected from solids under heating with CO_2 laser radiation.

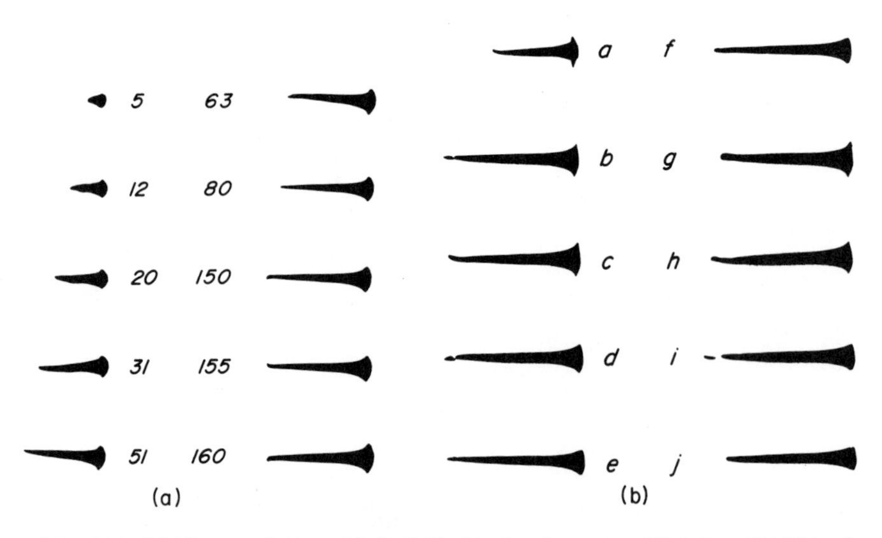

Fig. 5.7. (a) Time evolution of hole drilled in fused quartz with 0.6×10^4 W/cm². Frame numbers are shown. The camera speed was 18 frames/sec. (b) A selection of holes drilled in fused quartz with an incident intensity of $\simeq 10^4$ W/cm². Time increases from (a) → (j).

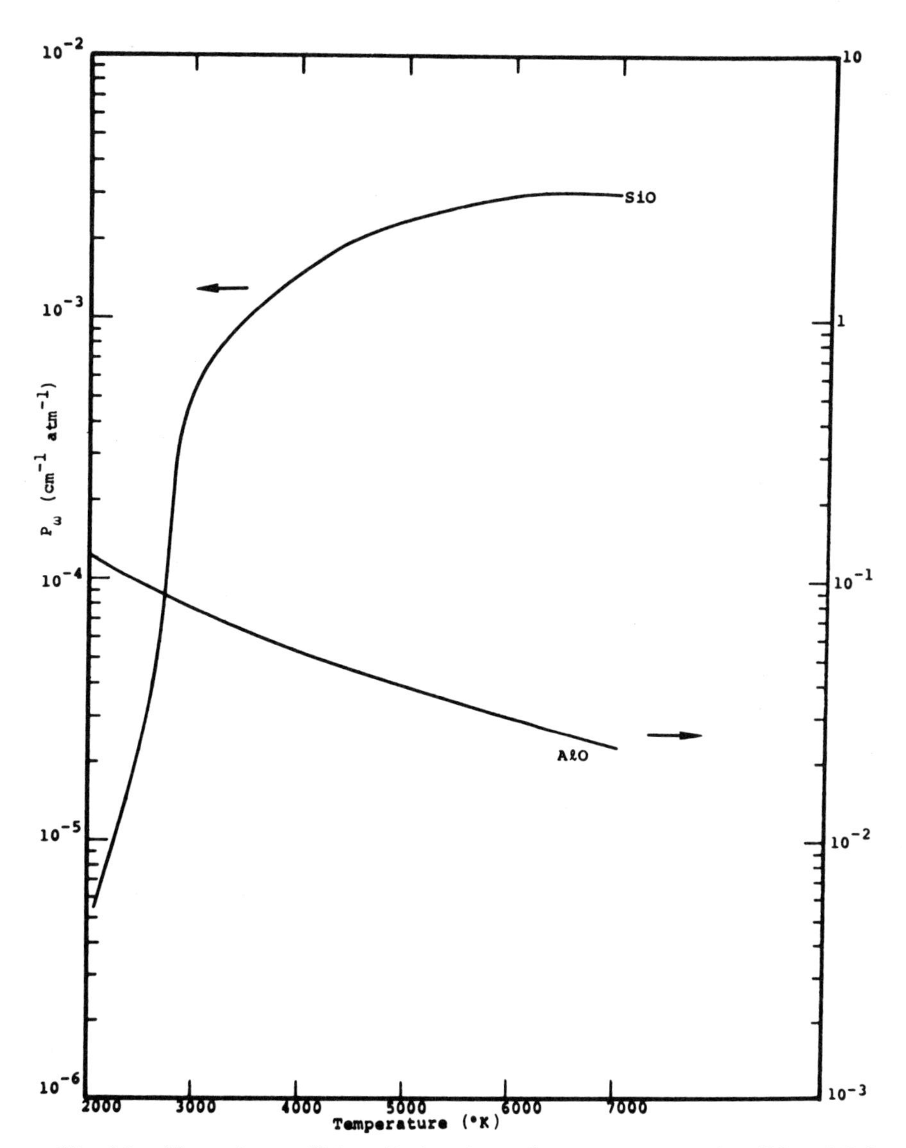

Fig. 5.8. Absorption coefficient P_ω (cm^{-1}-atm^{-1}) vs. temperature for AlO and SiO at 938.67 cm^{-1} (from Boni and Su, 1973).

Broadening of individual vibrational–rotational lines due to interactions between gas phase molecules and due to thermal motion make such calculation of temperature-dependent absorption coefficients extremely difficult. Boni and Su (1973) adopt a somewhat simplified model in which the spectral absorption coefficient is approximated by the ratio of the local value of the integrated intensity of a rotational line divided by the local spacing between two rotational lines. This model is most exact when the width of the vibrational–rotational lines is comparable to the separation between them. Because the broadening of these levels due to collisions with like molecules or with foreign molecules increases greatly at high pressures, the approximate method of Boni and Su is most reliable at high pressures ($\geq$10 atm). Reduction of these data to provide predictions of the opacity of vapor evaporating from solids that produce these molecules requires a knowledge of the chemical equilibrium existing over the solid at the temperature of interest. Figure 5.8 shows the spectral absorption coefficient P_ω (cm^{-1}-atm^{-1}) for AlO and SiO as a function of temperature. To estimate the opacity at 938.67 cm^{-1} due to these molecules *alone*, the partial coefficient k_i is then

$$k_i = P_\omega p_i \text{ cm}^{-1}$$

Boni and Su conclude that the calculations of Chang *et al.* (1970) will not provide a good estimate of the opacity of the vapor emanating from fused quartz.

5.5 THIN FILMS

Since the conduction of heat in thin films can often be considered one dimensional and simple analytic expressions are available (Section 4.7) to describe the time-dependent temperature, experimental studies on the laser penetration of thin films offer a good opportunity to compare theory with experiment. Although the capability of producing small diameter ($\lesssim$several microns) holes in thin metallic or insulating sheets is of intrinsic interest, a more immediate application would seem to lie in the area of the development of optical memories employing laser "writing" (Carlson *et al.*, 1966; Harris *et al.*, 1970; Cohen *et al.*, 1968; Amodei and Mezrick, 1969; Maydan, 1971; Sard and Maydan, 1971). In this process, a focused laser beam is used to create a minute hole in a thin metallic film on a substrate. The "bit" thus created is read by scanning the film and detecting changes in reflection or transmission of light.

Aboel Fotoh and von Gutfeld (1972) have produced micron-sized holes in very thin (150 Å) aluminum sheets coated on Mylar substrates. Holes were drilled using the 5145 Å line of an argon laser at power levels in the range 240–550 mW and pulse lengths of 0.07, 0.20, and 2 μsec. Above the threshold for drilling (240 mW), the resulting holes were observed to have irregular edges. Near threshold the holes were more regular, but all showed a lip of resolidified material. The minimum hole diameter was approximately 1 μm. A theoretical analysis of the results was performed using the model of Section 4.7.3, which assumes that the intensity distribution on the target is Gaussian and that the temperature in the thin film is independent of depth. However, there is some doubt that such a calculation will be valid since no account was taken of the finite penetration of laser radiation into the film. Since the films studied were only 150 Å thick while the absorption coefficient for light of the laser wavelength was given as 6.93×10^5/cm ($\alpha^{-1} = 144$ Å) the surface source model used would not seem to be appropriate.

Laser light incident on a thin metallic film through a transparent substrate has been shown to result in extensive crystallographic damage to the substrate for incident fluxes well below the usual damage threshold (Masumura and Achter, 1970). This effect was attributed to the momentary confinement of a plasma created at the metal–substrate interface. Low-intensity cw CO_2 laser radiation incident on thin gold films coated on quartz has been shown to increase the reflectance of the gold surface in the infrared by several percent. The visible transmittance of films treated with CO_2 laser radiation at intensity levels of 20–1.2×10^3 W/cm^2 also increased by several percent (Poulsen, 1972). This effect was attributed to face heating of the gold, which melted smaller particles into a smooth layer of larger particles.

The removal of a portion of a thin film on a substrate has been the subject of many investigations. Applications of this process occur in the trimming of thin-film resistors (Unger and Cohen, 1968) and capacitors (Gagliano *et al.*, 1969) and in the generation of capacitors and patterns on thin films coated on a substrate (Cohen *et al.*, 1968). Only a few details of these processes of relevance to the question of material removal with lasers will be discussed here.

As expected from heat transfer considerations, care must be taken in selecting the energy and duration of laser pulses for the selective evaporation of thin films without damaging the substrate. Cohen and Epperson (1968) report on the evaporation of a 1200 Å thick tantalum film coated on a glazed alumina substrate with both Q-switched and free-running ruby lasers. When the energy in both pulses was the same, the Q-switched pulse of 50-nsec duration produced total evaporation of the metal film in the vicinity of the laser focus with little damage to the substrate, while the free-running mode of operation, generating a 0.3-msec pulse, yielded cracking of the metal film around the hole. Paek and Kestenbaum (1973) define an "accommodation" coefficient

$$\eta = 1 - Q_s/Q = 1/(1 + [2\beta/(\pi\sigma)^{1/2}]\sqrt{\tau}) \tag{12}$$

which is a measure of the heat conducted to the substrate, Q_s, compared to that delivered to the system, Q. The assumptions used in arriving at this expression have been given in Section 4.8. It is strictly valid only for laser pulses of duration $\lesssim 1$ μsec, when a metallic film of thickness $\simeq 1000$ Å is coated on an insulating substrate. The parameters are

$$\beta = K_2/K_1, \qquad \sigma = \kappa_2/\kappa_1, \qquad \tau = \kappa_1 t/l^2 \tag{13}$$

where 1 and 2 refer to film and substrate, respectively, and t can be taken as the pulse length. This expression shows that heat conduction to the substrate will be most important for pulse durations such that $2\beta\sqrt{\tau}/(\pi\sigma)^{1/2} \gtrsim 1$. Thus, laser power will be most efficiently used when the pulse length is kept less than this value. Equation (12) tends to overestimate η for pulse lengths in which radial conduction of heat is important.

Gagliano *et al.* (1969) have shown that the energy required to remove a small volume of a metallic film on a substrate can be approximately calculated from the heat content of the material at its normal vaporization temperature. They give an example of a calculation of the energy required to evaporate a 10^{-3}-cm diameter hole in a gold film of 0.5×10^{-4}-cm thickness. The heat content of gold at its normal boiling point (3264°K) is $\Delta H = 2360$ J/g. Since the volume to be removed is 39.27×10^{-12} cm^3 and the density of gold is 19.3 g/cm^3, 1.8×10^{-6} J would be required. This should be increased by a factor of about 60 to allow for the high reflectance of gold in the visible region of the spectrum. The laser would then have to generate 120×10^{-6} J in a time comparable to the thermal diffusion time for such a layer. A Nd:YAG laser yielding 150 μJ/pulse with a pulse length of 300 nsec ($\simeq 10^2$ times the thermal diffusion time) was able to produce the desired evaporation.

More exact fits to available experimental data and predictions for other systems are available from the theory developed by Paek and Kestenbaum (1973). The theory has been briefly outlined in Section 4.8. It was applied to the experimental results of Maydan (1971) on the drilling of thin (1000 Å) bismuth films on Mylar substrates. The second-order correction to the temperature in the film is found to be of importance only when the pulse length exceeds 5 μsec for a Gaussian spot size of 10 μm. For gold on the same substrate, however, $\epsilon\theta_{12}$ is comparable to θ_{11} for pulse lengths longer than $\simeq 0.5$ μsec. Good agreement between theory and experiment was obtained using the first term in the series expansion for θ_1 for all pulse lengths ≤ 5 μsec used in the drilling of bismuth–Mylar composite slabs. In fitting these data it was assumed that $T_1 = T_v$, the vaporization temperature of bismuth. The theoretical threshold intensity was then compared with measured thresholds.

Table 5.3

Threshold Laser Intensity $F_m/(1 - R)$ and Absorbed Intensities F_m for Drilling of Holes in 0.1-μm Thick Metal Films on Pyrex and $\lambda = 1.06\ \mu$m[a]

Material	F_m (W/cm²)	$F_m/(1 - R)$ (W/cm²)
Tantalum	1.7×10^6	4.5×10^6
Chromium	1.5×10^6	3.9×10^6
Manganese	1.2×10^6	2.6×10^6
Silver	5.4×10^5	1.1×10^7
Aluminum	5.4×10^5	6.8×10^6
Lead	1.7×10^5	4.9×10^5

[a] After Nakayama *et al.* (1973).

When the laser pulse length is such that lateral heat conduction in the film can be neglected* the diameter of the hole produced can be predicted from

$$r_m^2 = d^2 \ln[F_0/F_m] \tag{14}$$

where d is the parameter describing the extent of the Gaussian beam distribution on the target, F_m a critical or threshold intensity for material removal, and r_m the radius of the resulting hole. Nakayama and Kashiwabara (1972) and Nakayama *et al.* (1973) report a series of measurements on the diameter of holes drilled in a variety of metal films on Pyrex substrates with pulses from a Q-switched Nd–YAG laser. Individual pulses were of 350-nsec duration, which means that some lateral conduction of heat must have occurred since d was 21 μm. However, the experimental data were shown to fit Eq. (14) quite well. Some values of F_m and $F_m/(1 - R)$, where R is the reflectivity of the metal at $\lambda = 1.06\ \mu$m, are given in Table 5.3. These values are those given by Nakayama *et al.* (1973) for drilling films of 0.1-μm thickness coated on Pyrex.

A rim of resolidified material was noted around the periphery of these holes but the volume of the rim decreased with increasing hole diameter. Sard and Maydan (1971) report a comprehensive study of the structure of holes machined in thin bismuth films or bismuth/germanium layered films coated on Mylar. The films were 300–600 Å thick and machining was accomplished by means of He–Ne or argon lasers. The structure in the vicinity of laser-drilled holes was examined by both scanning and trans-

* An approximate criterion would be t_p = length of pulse $\lesssim A^2/\kappa$, where A is the radius of the beam ($A = d$ for a Gaussian beam distribution),

mission electron microscopy. In all cases, a rim of material was observed adjacent to the holes. This rim was well defined when the films were drilled with 30-nsec pulses but became irregular when the pulse length was increased to 300 nsec. Large, well-defined rims were observed with 1-μsec pulses. All holes were several microns in diameter.

Laser intensities just below threshold were shown to melt the film in the area of the focus but no hole was produced. At threshold, a small hole formed within this melted area. This hole could be as small as 1 μm for a focal spot diameter of about 3.5 μm. The hole subsequently grows by a combination of surface tension and vaporization effects. With laser intensities well above threshold the majority of the material within the hole is apparently removed by vaporization and the ejection of small particles of liquid. Some molten material is, however, pulled back to the edge of the hole, forming a rim.

A parametric study of machining micron-sized holes in bismuth films on Mylar (Maydan, 1971) showed that the area of the machined spot increased linearly with incident laser intensity. The energy flux (J/cm^2) required to machine holes of constant diameter also increased linearly with film thickness.

Maydan (1971), Harris *et al.* (1970), and Carlson *et al.* (1966) have reported on the recording of video information on thin films coated on substrates using the technique of selective evaporation of small holes with argon and He–Ne lasers. The writing speed is about 10^6 holes/sec (Maydan, 1971) and 8–10 shades of grey can be produced by modulating the laser intensity to vary hole size. Holograms have been prepared by laser evaporation of a thin bismuth film on a glass substrate (Amodei and Mezrick, 1969) and Curie point writing has been used to generate magnetic holograms utilizing a similar technique (Mezrick, 1969, 1970). Thermostrictive recording on Permalloy films has been reported by Kump and Chang (1966). Here no hole is drilled, but recording is accomplished by producing a local stress with a low-power laser beam. This stress causes a switching of magnetization over a small volume of the film.

Further discussion of curie point writing can be found in the articles by Mayer (1958); Tchernev and Lewicki (1968), Chen *et al.* (1968), and Fan and Greiner (1968). Low-temperature recording is reported by Treves *et al.* (1969) and Silverman (1972). Ashkin and Dziedzic (1972) have discussed the interaction of a laser beam with magnetic domains, and thermomagnetic recording in thin garnet layers has been reported by Krumme *et al.* (1972).

Experiments on the drilling of thin metal sheets with CO_2 lasers have been reported by Asmus and Baker (1969) and Gonsalves and Duley (1971). In both studies cw lasers were used with a mechanical switch used for obtaining pulses of variable duration. Asmus and Baker measured the temperature on the irradiated surface of the sheet with a high-speed infrared pyrometer and that on the back surface of the sheet directly behind the focal spot with a thermocouple. Temperature versus time at the front surface for various incident intensities and 0.010-in. stainless steel is shown in Fig. 5.9. These curves are similar to those predicted from the cylindrical source model of Section 4.7.2 for low values of $P/\pi A^2$. As the incident intensity rises, the initial shape of the $T(t)$ curve remains as predicted from the above model until a critical temperature is reached above which the temperature rises abruptly. This rapid rise was attributed to a rapid increase in absorption of laser power due to high-temperature oxidation of the metal surface. When this process is allowed to continue, a hole quickly forms in the area of the laser focus. The oxidation proceeds on both sides of the sheet and material appears to be removed simultaneously from both sides. When heating occurred in vacuum, the nonlinear temperature rise was not observed.

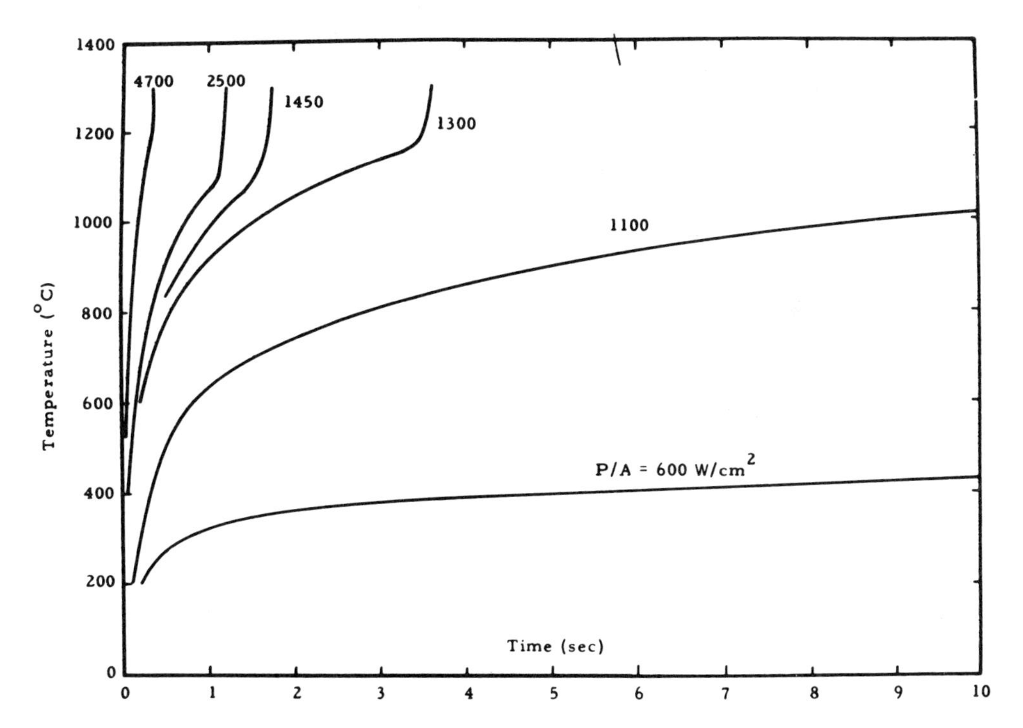

Fig. 5.9. Temperature rise profiles for 0.010-in. stainless steel for various laser power densities (Asmus and Baker, 1969).

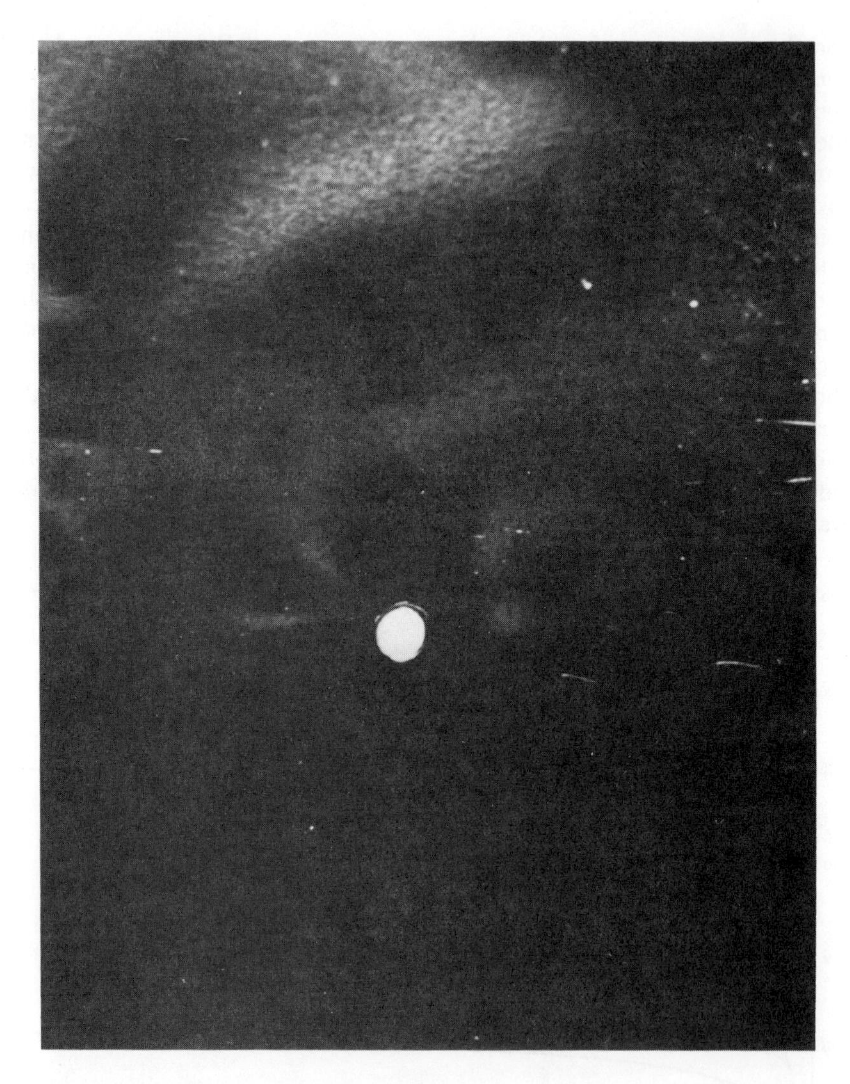

Fig. 5.10. Hole produced in 0.001-in. thickness stainless steel when drilled in vacuum.

The quality of the holes produced depended greatly on the intensity at which drilling occurred. Low-power drilling was accompanied by an extensive heat-affected region adjacent to the hole boundary and some of the melt was deposited on the surface of the sheet. Drilling occurs in a few milliseconds at high incident intensities and little heat is transferred laterally into the sheet. The result is a clean hole with well-defined edges and no evidence of a residual melt region. Similar differences are seen between holes drilled in air and in vacuum. Even at low intensities holes drilled in vacuum are much more uniform than those drilled in air (Figs. 5.10 and 5.11).

Figure 5.12 shows a plot of the power required to drill stainless steel sheets of various thickness as a function of the time taken for the hole to be drilled. It can be seen that there is a critical power below which the time for drilling increases drastically. If a critical temperature must be reached before the hole develops, then the theory of Section 4.7.2 predicts that a plot of $\ln t_m$ versus $4\pi Kl/P_m\epsilon$ should be linear, where t_m is the time to reach

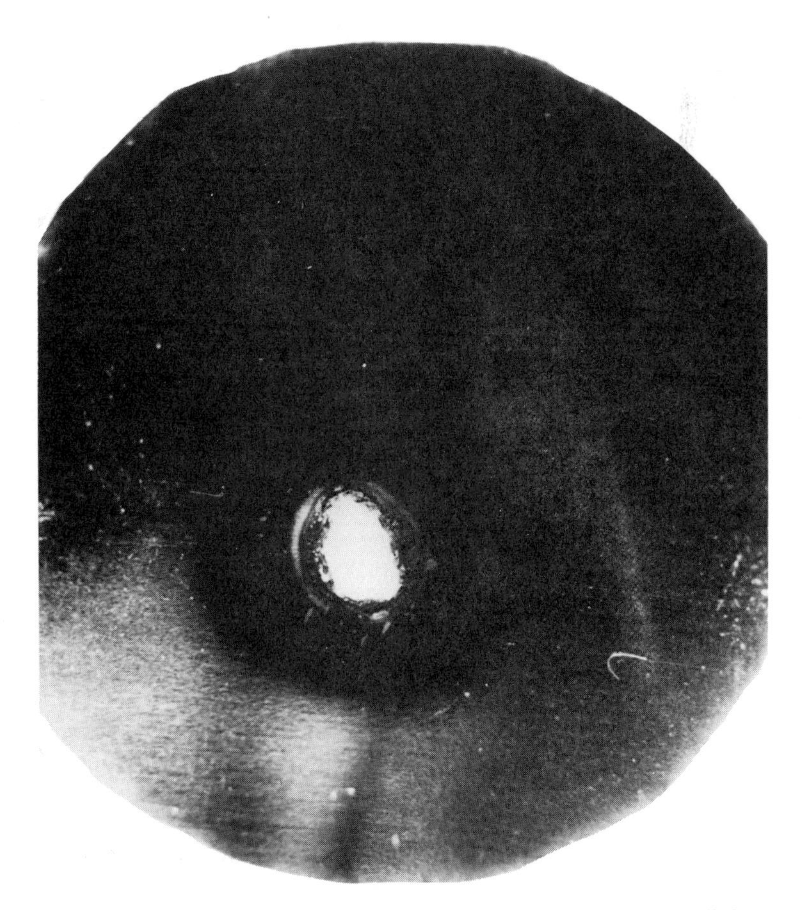

Fig. 5.11. Hole produced in 0.001-in. thickness stainless steel when drilled in air.

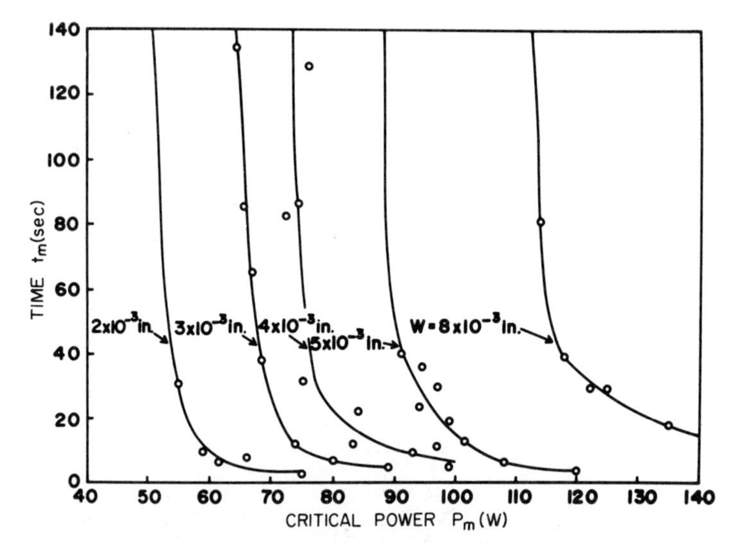

Fig. 5.12. P_m vs. t_m for several thicknesses of type 302 stainless steel in air. A for these curves is 0.04 cm.

the critical temperature T_m and P_m is the incident laser power. Furthermore, a plot of l versus P_m for t_m constant should yield a straight line whose slope is proportional to ϵ, the emissivity of stainless steel at $\lambda = 10.6\ \mu m$ and $T = T_m$. l versus P_m is plotted in Fig. 5.13 from the data given in Fig. 5.12. It is evident that this graph is indeed linear but that it has an intercept at $P_m = P_c$ for $l = 0$. P_c is identified with the incident power required to balance convection losses due to the fact that the samples were heated in air. From the graph, and using $\kappa = 0.05\ cm^2/sec$ with $A = 0.04$ cm, the constant $4\pi KT_m/\epsilon = 3.7 \times 10^4$ W/cm. This implies that $\epsilon(T_m) \simeq 0.12$ when T_m is taken to be 1100°C and $K \simeq 0.30$ W/cm/°C. The emissivity of type 302 stainless steel in vacuum at temperatures in this range is $\simeq$0.05. This indicates that laser heating in air is accompanied by a significant increase in absorption of incident radiation at high temperatures. Some 90% of the incident flux is apparently still reflected even when heating occurs in air. This illustrates one limitation of theoretical predictions of laser heating effects. In the absence of experimental data on the appropriate value of ϵ, estimates of laser power required to drill holes in thin sheets may be incorrect by an order of magnitude. Only when heating occurs in vacuum is the value of ϵ fairly accurately predictable.

Figure 5.14 shows the experimental data plotted in terms of the reduced variables θ and τ using the previously determined value for $4\pi KT_m/\epsilon$.

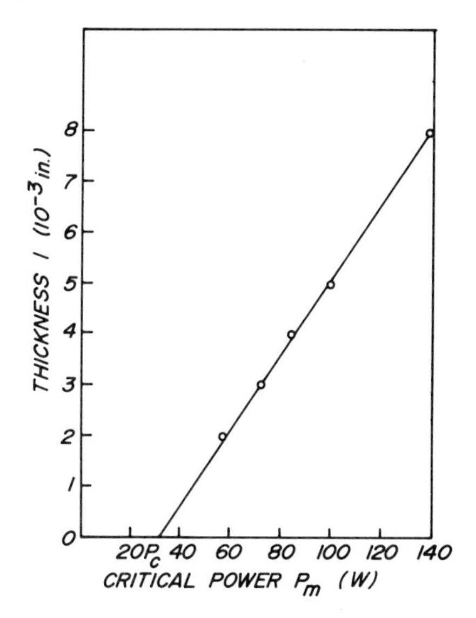

Fig. 5.13. l vs. P_m for Fig. 5.12 with t_m = 15 sec.

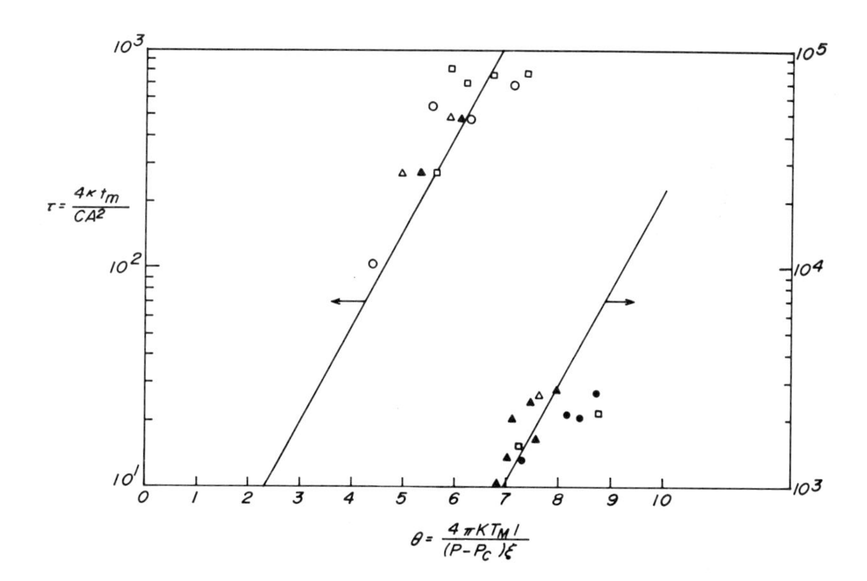

Fig. 5.14. Data obtained on the drilling of thin stainless steel sheet with the cw CO_2 laser plotted in terms of the variables θ and τ. ○, 2 × 10^{-3} in.; △, 3 × 10^{-3} in.; □, 4 × 10^{-3} in.; ▲, 5 × 10^{-3} in.; ●, 8 × 10^{-3} in.; A = 0.04 cm; κ = 0.05 cm^2/sec; $4\pi KT_m/\zeta$ = 3.7 × 10^4 W/cm.

Although the data show some scatter, it is evident that the theory provides a reasonable match to the experimental points and can provide an approximate estimate of either P_m or t_m in particular situations of interest in the drilling of thin sheets with a cw CO_2 laser.

As the power and incident intensity increase, the time to reach the drilling temperature will decrease. However, both the cylindrical source model and the Gaussian source model are valid only for times such that the sheet can be considered thermally thin, i.e., for $t_m \gtrsim l^2/\kappa$. This is $\simeq 5 \times 10^{-4}$ and 1.2×10^{-2} sec, respectively, for 5×10^{-3} and 25×10^{-3} cm thick sheets of stainless steel. Thus for drilling thin sheets with pulsed lasers where the pulse length is usually 1 msec or less, both of these models are no longer valid. In fact, when the pulse length is less than the thermal time constant of a thin sheet, the sheet can be thought of as infinitely thick. Assuming that the time to reach the vaporization temperature is much shorter than the pulse length, the time t_m to penetrate a thin sheet with a laser pulse is approximately given by the solution to the following equation:

$$l = \int_0^{t_m} v(t)\, dt \tag{15}$$

where

$$v(t) = F(t)/(\lambda + \rho c T_v) \tag{16}$$

Since T_v does not depend on $F(t)$ for laser intensities $F \lesssim 10^8$ W/cm² at a wavelength of 10.6 μm, the time to drill can be obtained from

$$E(t_m) = l(\lambda + \rho c T_v) \tag{17}$$

where $E(t_m)$ is the energy delivered to the sheet in the time it takes to drill. The pulse from a TEA CO_2 laser can often be approximated by

$$F(t) = a_1 \exp(-b_1 t) + a_2 \exp(-b_2 t) \tag{18}$$

and in this case t_m is obtained as the solution to the expression

$$\frac{a_1}{b_1}[1 - \exp(-b_1 t_m)] + \frac{a_2}{b_2}[1 - \exp(-b_2 t_m)] = l(\lambda + \rho c T_v) \tag{19}$$

Similar expressions can be derived for other laser pulse shapes. This analysis omits any consideration of rapid evaporation due to the melting–flushing mechanism.

As the incident intensity increases, T_v will start to depend on the value of the flux and prediction of t_m becomes more difficult. At high intensities, shielding of the target by material ejected during the initial part of the pulse will cause t_m to approach a constant value independent of $F(t)$. This effect has been studied experimentally by Andreev *et al.* (1972) using a neodynium laser oscillating at $\lambda = 1.06\ \mu m$. Saturation of t_m occurred at intensities $F \gtrsim 10^8\ W/cm^2$ for a 0.8-μm aluminum film.

The remote opening of thin-walled metal tubes containing hazardous materials by puncturing with pulses from a high-power ruby laser has been reported by Horrocks and Studier (1965).

Chapter 6

Welding and Machining

6.1 INTRODUCTION

The past ten years have seen many applications develop for high-power lasers in the areas of micromachining, microwelding, welding, and scribing. While it is unlikely that the laser will replace conventional machine tools in routine metal-working operations, many specialized applications exist. Several of these will be discussed in this chapter and particular emphasis will be placed on those processing operations that involve or potentially involve the CO_2 laser.

6.2 MICROWELDING

By 1965, a variety of laser systems had already been developed for the production of microwelds in the fabrication of electronic circuit boards, inside vacuum tubes, and in other specialized applications where conventional welding technology was unable to provide reliable joining. Early studies had shown the feasibility of laser welding in the research laboratory and this was rapidly translated into industry-wide acceptance of lasers as another very valuable welding tool. Today lasers are routinely used in a variety of microwelding applications.

The localized heating obtained with laser sources was soon realized to be an important advantage. Anderson and Jackson (1965b) report an interesting comparison between heating effects produced with a conventional arc source and those occurring with a pulsed laser. Their result is shown in Fig. 6.1. The laser pulse with an intensity of 1.9×10^5 W/cm² and a duration of 2×10^{-4} sec produces melting to a depth of 0.001 in. with a heat-affected region (T = 500°C) limited to $\simeq$0.005 in. The arc source would produce melting to the same depth in 0.0246 sec but the heat-affected zone would be $\simeq$0.03 in. thick. Furthermore, the laser source is more efficient since it requires only 37.8 J/cm² to produce melting to the required depth, while the arc source must deliver 246 J/cm² to the workpiece. Localized heating makes the laser ideal for welding of circuit elements on printed-circuit boards where high average temperatures even in small volumes surrounding the weld region cannot be tolerated.

Some microweld configurations encountered in practical systems are shown in Fig. 6.2. The welds shown at the bottom of this figure are similar to those required for welding integrated circuits to circuit boards. The

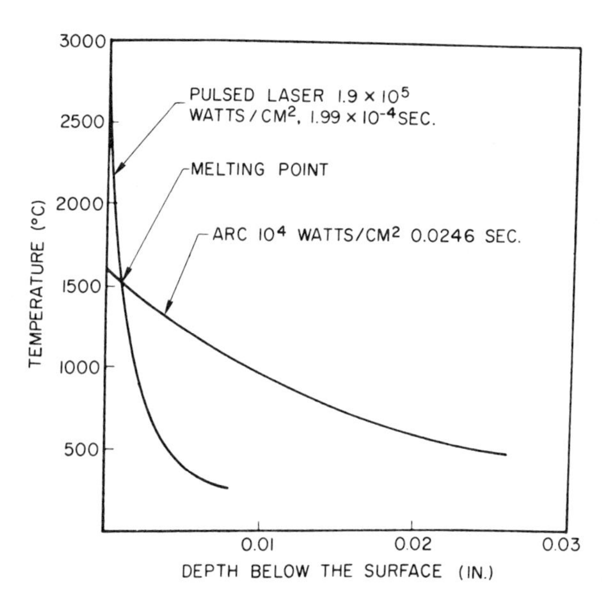

Fig. 6.1. Maximum temperature reached as a function of depth in iron for heating with a laser pulse and the pulse from a conventional arc source (from Anderson and Jackson, 1965b).

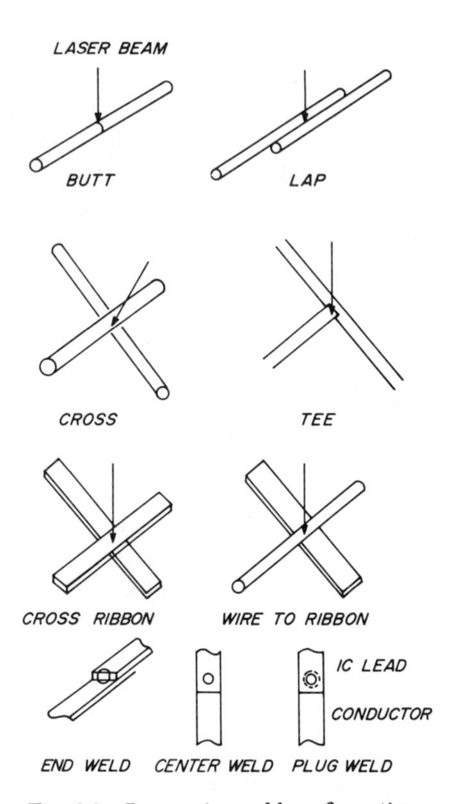

Fig. 6.2. Laser microweld configurations.

plug weld is formed by having the diameter of the laser beam somewhat larger than that of a hole in the integrated circuit lead so that laser energy is absorbed around the periphery of this hole and on the conductor lead below. To produce an end weld, the laser is directed so as to impinge on the edge of the integrated circuit lead. Part of the incident energy is then absorbed by the lower conductor. Center welds, which are more difficult to produce, rely on the propagation of a melt region completely through one conductor to fuse with the conductor beneath. All the configurations shown in Fig. 6.2 have been welded with lasers.

Pfluger and Maas (1965) have discussed the problems associated with making wire–wire and wire–ribbon welds. Care must be taken in making cross-wire welds to ensure that both wires are heated during the laser pulse. Pfluger and Maas (1965) experienced some difficulty in welding thin wires using this configuration due to a tendency for either incomplete penetration of the weld through the top wire or complete penetration followed by severing. This problem was overcome by Anderson and Jackson (1965b) by directing the laser beam at an angle to the joint so that both wires were heated simultaneously. They show a nice example of a cross weld produced between 0.005-in. diameter tungsten and 0.020-in. nickel wires.

Either parallel or antiparallel lap wire–wire welds are relatively easy to produce by focusing the laser spot between the two wires. This heats both wires simultaneously and promotes an even flow of molten material into the adjoining void. The tensile shear strength of laser welds in 0.020-in. nickel wire in the antiparallel configuration varied from 25 to 73% of that of the wire itself (Pfluger and Maas, 1965). More than one weld in the same region (but without overlapping) significantly increased the shear strength.

Wire to ribbon cross welds are most easily made by penetration through the ribbon to melt the wire, although careful control over the energy and pulse duration permits welds to be made from the wire side. Once again it is advantageous to have the laser beam hit the joint at an angle, so that both wire and ribbon are heated simultaneously. Cross ribbon welds are similar to lap welds in thin sheets and can be made under conditions that give good melt penetration from the upper to the lower sheet.

Application of laser-formed wire–wire welds to the generation of a plated-wire magnetic memory device has been described by Cohen *et al.* (1969). The individual wires were 0.005-in. diameter beryllium copper plated with 1.5 μm of copper and 0.6 μm of permalloy. Pairs of wires were located only 0.025 in. apart, so careful control over the welding process had to be maintained so that short circuits did not occur. Most welds were performed on pairs of wires presented to each other at an angle of 60°. Either the ends of the wires of a pair could be touching or contact could be made slightly back of the ends so that an abbreviated cross was formed. For a given pulse duration in the range 2–5 msec, the strength of the resulting welds depended quite strongly on the energy in the laser pulse. The 60° welds were about 50% as strong as the wire itself. The heat-affected region under optimized welding conditions was characterized by a length equal to twice the weld nugget diameter down each of the wires. The feasibility of producing such welds rapidly using a suitable jig was demonstrated. Since it was desirable to have all pairs of wires coplanar after welding, pairs were mechanically forced together by the jig such that welding tended to bring both wires of a pair into the same plane.

Laser welds have been produced between a wide variety of dissimilar metals. Miller and Nunnikhoven (1965) working at the AiResearch Manufacturing Co. have described successful welds between a B-1113 steel feed through and type 321 stainless steel casing in a thermistor enclosure.

Garashchuk and Molchan (1969) have reported a metallographic analysis of laser welds between nickel and copper, nickel and titanium, and copper and titanium. The weld zone in the copper–nickel weld showed macroscopic regions of both copper and nickel inside a melt consisting of copper–nickel solution. These inclusions were the result of the short pulse duration, which prevented equilibrium from being reached in the melt. The fusion region in the nickel–titanium weld showed a finely dispersed structure and an intermetallic phase was present at the boundary of the melt. An alloy between copper and titanium was formed when these two metals were welded. This was interspersed with particles of copper.

Tantalum-molybdenum welds showed the presence of a tantalum–molybdenum alloy along the fusion line (Garashchuk *et al.*, 1969). These welds were of high quality. The same group also studied laser welds in nickel–tungsten combinations. Again, the welds were of good quality with no embrittlement of the tungsten, although tongues of tungsten penetrated into the nickel. Laser welding of brass, mild steel, and stainless steel to copper has been reported by Baranov *et al.* (1968).

Although this list of materials welded with lasers is not by any means complete, it does serve to indicate that a wide variety of different types of weld are possible. Some general rules for the production of successful laser welds have been listed by Anderson and Jackson (1965b):

(1) The location of the laser spot on the weldment should be within 20% of the characteristic dimension.

(2) The distance between the laser and the workpiece should be within 2% of the focal length of the lens.

(3) Reactive materials require shielding. When welding titanium, zircaloy, and other oxygen-sensitive materials, argon shielding is necessary.

(4) Symmetrical heat input is preferred. When welding two wires together, it is better to put heat into both wires rather than put all of it into one.

(5) Small weldments require short-focal-length lens (or mirror) systems. It is (usually) not possible to put the workpiece at a large distance from the welding head.

Fine wires may often be laser welded together or to terminals without the need for removing insulation from the wires. At the high intensities produced by the laser, the insulation appears to be rapidly evaporated or degraded thermally, leaving no detectable residue. Studies have been reported on welding polyurethane (Anderson and Jackson, 1965a) and enamel-coated conductors (Lebedev and Granitsa, 1972). The strength of lap welds of coated wires 0.1–0.2 mm in diameter were found to be 70–90%

that of the wires (Lebedev and Granitsa, 1972). Intimate contact between the two pieces to be welded is not always necessary for the production of a sound weld since under proper conditions the molten metal will fill a small gap resulting in fusion of both materials. A quantitative study of the strength of laser spot welds in sheets made with a gap between the sheets (Velichko *et al.*, 1972a) shows that gaps of 0.1 mm before welding do not seem to affect the subsequent strength of the bond. In this case, however, the laser power and pulse duration must be tailored to produce optimum melt penetration.

Some specialized laser welds have been discussed by Miller and Nunnikhoven (1965) and Miller (1966). One involved the welding of a bearing assembly made of type 321 stainless steel to a massive type 440C stainless steel bearing housing. Gas tungsten arc welding, resistance spot welding, and electron beam welding had previously been used without satisfactory results. A circumferential weld was made with a ruby laser by overlapping individual spot welds. There was no significant heat transfer to the ball race area using this technique and the final assembled piece met all design requirements. Welding measurements on Rene 41, columbium D-36, and

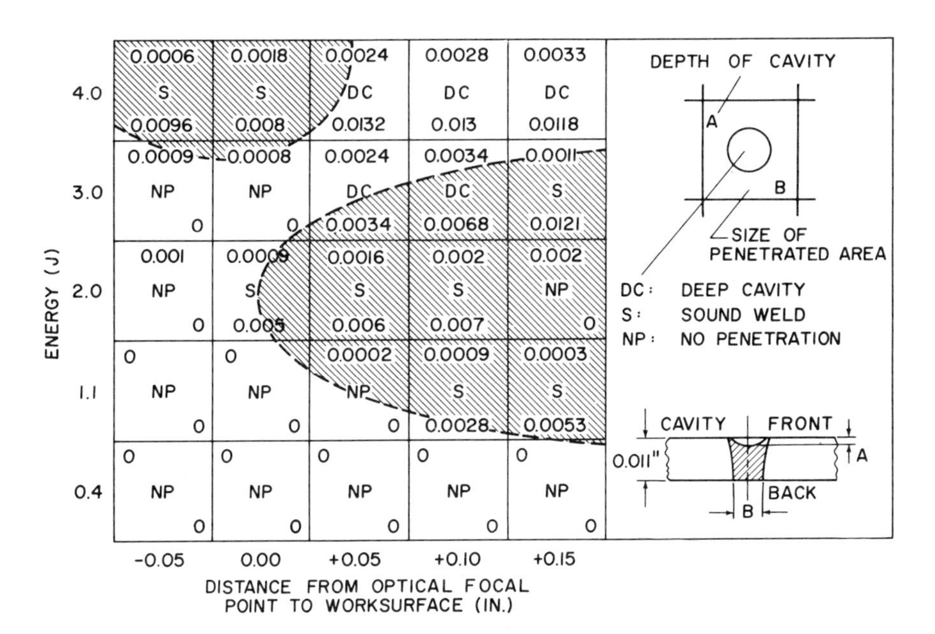

Fig. 6.3. Weldability test results with 0.011-in.-thick 18% Ni maraging steel sheet; the cross-hatched areas indicate the conditions for sound welding (from Schmidt *et al.*, 1965).

molybdenum TZM materials have been reported by Earvolino and Kennedy (1966). The slow process of overlapping welds produced by individual laser pulses has now largely been replaced by continuous welding using cw CO_2 and YAG lasers of higher power. Some data on welding thin sheets with a pulsed CO_2 laser are, however, reported in Table 6.1.

Although numerical predictions can be made concerning the feasibility of laser welding in particular instances, it is often simpler and more reliable to perform a series of experiments with one or more lasers to determine the conditions under which welds can be produced. An approach that could be taken in such a feasibility study has been discussed by Schmidt *et al.* (1965). The weldability of type 302 stainless steel and of 18% Ni maraging steel was carefully examined under a variety of test conditions that involved changing the sheet thickness, the incident laser spot size, and the energy in the light pulse. A typical result for 0.011-in.-thick 18% Ni maraging steel sheet is shown in Fig. 6.3. Optimum penetration is obtained for a laser energy of 4 J and slight defocusing of the light spot on the workpiece.

Figure 6.4a shows how the laser beam may be directed to a remote location to effect a weld. This configuration was used by Moorhead (1971) to

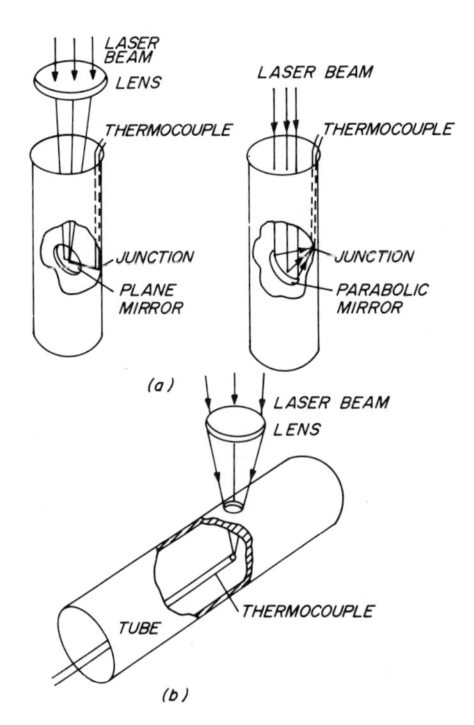

Fig. 6.4. Laser welding of thermocouples to the inside of tubes (after Moorhead, 1971).

Table 6.1

Conditions for Edge Lap Welds with a Pulsed CO_2 Laser[a]

Material	Power (W)	Pulse width (sec)	Repetition rate (sec/pulse)	Speed (IPM)	Material ultimate strength (lb/in.)	Peel strength (% of ultimate)
0.0045-in. Phosphor bronze A	95	0.30	0.35	5	49,000	65
0.004-in. 304 Stainless	95	0.0002	0.001	3	86,000	45
	95	0.22	0.28	6.5		
0.004-in. Silver 752	95	0.065	0.075	3	55,000	19
0.004-in. Monel	95	0.07	0.2	3	66,000	23
0.004-in. Cupronickel	95	0.30	0.35	3	75,000	12

[a] After Conti (1969).

Table 6.2

Thermocouples Welded with a Ruby Laser to Some Metals[a]

Base metal	Thickness ($\times 10^{-3}$ in.)	Thermocouple	Diameter ($\times 10^{-3}$ in.)	Pulse length (msec)	Energy (J)
Molybdenum	62	Pt vs. Pt–10% Rh	10	4.0	3.2
	62	W vs. W–26% Re	10	4.35	4.2
Tantalum	0.5	Pt vs. Pt–10% Rh	3	2.75	0.03
	62	W vs. W–26% Re	20	5.2	6.5
304 Stainless steel	20	Pt vs. Pt–10% Rh	3	3.0	0.04
Zircaloy-4	—	Chromel-P vs. Alumel	13	2.75	0.78
Niobium	1	Pt vs. Pt–10% Rh	3	3.50	0.06
Tungsten (arc cast)	125	Pt vs. Pt–10% Rh	10	4.50	4.6

[a] After Moorhead (1971).

weld thermocouples to the inside wall of a tube. Alternatively, the laser beam may be directed at the thermocouple through a small hole drilled in the tube (Fig. 6.4b). The hole is resealed by laser welding a small plug into the hole after the thermocouple is attached. Some data reported by Moorhead (1971) on the welding of thermocouples to various metals with a ruby laser are given in Table 6.2.

6.3 PENETRATION WELDING

The limitations of current welding technology together with the availability of very high-power cw CO_2 lasers have stimulated much interest in deep penetration welding using these devices. The conventional method using electron beams requires not only a vacuum system but frequent replacement of the electron gun. On the other hand, it would be expected that laser welding could be performed at atmospheric pressure and would provide more flexibility in terms of the geometry of welds that could be produced because of the ease with which the laser beam could be directed to remote points on the workpiece. A series of studies (Banas, 1971; Locke, 1972; Locke *et al.*, 1972; Baardsen *et al.*, 1973; Locke and Hella, 1974; Hoag *et al.*, 1974; Ball and Banas, 1974) have examined the parameters with cw CO_2 lasers and have noted the similarity of the welding process to that obtained with high-power electron beams. In both cases, radiation trapping by formation of a keyhole permits the workpiece to absorb most of the incident laser radiation. Heat is then transferred from the surface of this keyhole to the bulk material. Power levels in the most recent of these studies have been in the 4–20 kW range.

Figure 6.5 shows a plot of penetration depth versus power for the Avco CO_2 laser welding type 304 stainless steel (Locke and Hella, 1974). It can be seen that penetration increases almost linearly with incident power in the high-power regime. The correlation of penetration depth with welding speed is shown in Fig. 6.6 together with a curve obtained with electron beam welding. The penetration in the laser weld is consistently less than that possible with an electron beam, but the difference between the two penetration depths diminishes as the welding speed increases. This is somewhat surprising, since as pointed out by Baardsen *et al.* (1973) the time to form a void or "keyhole" may become comparable to the illumination time for a particular area on the surface of the workpiece as the welding speed increases. When this occurs, the average power dissipated in the sheet is expected to drop because the keyhole is no longer a completely effective trap for the incident laser radiation. For an electron beam, the absorptivity of the material is independent of the shape and extent of the

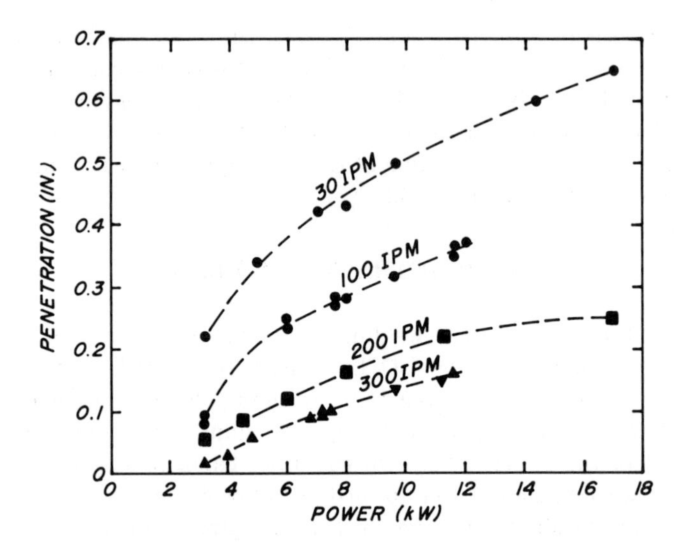

Fig. 6.5. Relation between penetration depth vs. laser power for welding with the AVCO CO_2 laser (from Locke and Hella, 1974).

keyhole and hence the total power dissipated in the workpiece will be less strongly dependent on the welding speed. At very low welding speeds, the penetration depth of laser welds becomes significantly less than that attainable with the electron beam. This has been attributed (Locke *et al.*, 1972) to the formation of a plasma cloud, which attenuates the incident beam.

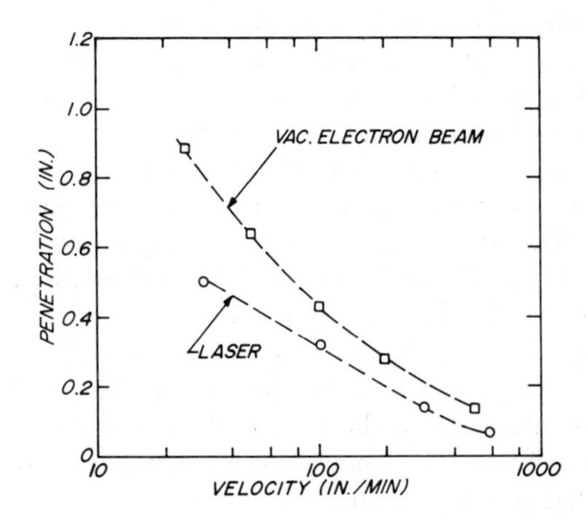

Fig. 6.6. Weld penetration vs. weld speed for type 304 stainless steel welded with a 10-kW CO_2 laser (from Locke and Hella, 1974).

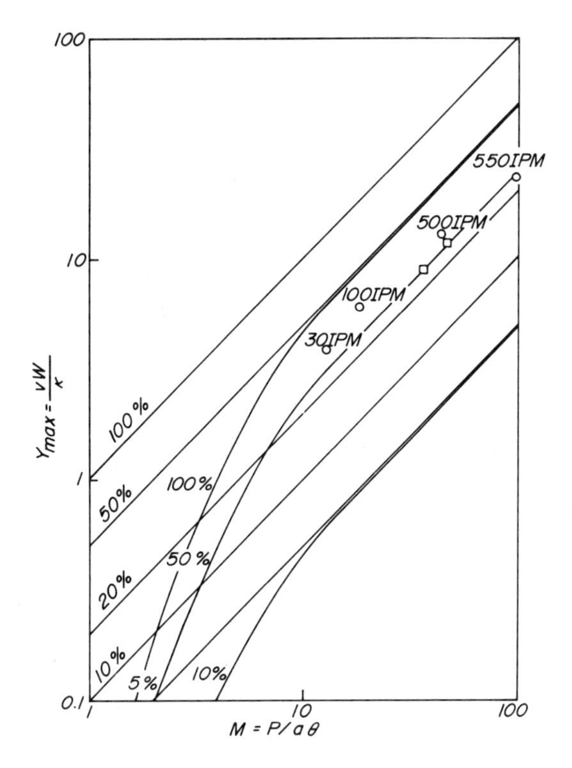

Fig. 6.7. Power per unit depth $M = P/a\theta$ vs. normalized maximum melt width $Y_{max} = vW/\kappa$ (see Section 4.11.2) for penetration welding with the CO_2 laser. Experimental points corresponding to observed relations for 8 (○) and 20 (□) kW lasers are shown.

Figure 6.7 shows the available experimental results in the context of the theory described in Section 4.11.2. Also plotted on this graph are straight lines that denote the melting ratio (Swift-Hook and Gick, 1973)

$$q = HvaW/P \tag{1}$$

where H is the heat content of the metal at the melting temperature, and q the ratio of the power required to melt the volume of metal in the fusion zone to the total laser power. The curves in Fig. 6.7 are the solution to Eqs. (4.147) and (4.148), assuming various efficiencies of power transfer to the workpiece. Since $Y_{max} = 0.484M$ when Ur is very large, the limiting melting ratio (for thick sheets) is 48%. Swift-Hook and Gick (1973) point out that q has often been mistaken for welding efficiency. The efficiency is, in fact, measured by the ratio of the power transferred in the form of heat

Table 6.3

Data on Penetration Welding with cw CO_2 Lasers

Material	Power (kW)	Thickness (mm)	Width (mm)	Rate (cm/sec)	Remarks	Reference
321 Stainless steel	0.25	0.125	0.45	3.8	Full penetration butt welds in slabs; edge, lap-fillet, and corner welds also reported	Webster (1970)
		0.250	0.70	1.48		
		0.417	0.75	0.47		
302 Stainless steel	0.25	0.125	0.50	2.11		
		0.203	0.50	1.27		
		0.250	1.00	0.42		
17-7 PH	0.25	0.125	0.45	4.7		
Inconel	0.25	0.100	0.25	6.35		
		0.250	0.45	1.69		
Nickel	0.25	0.125	0.45	1.48		
Monel	0.25	0.250	0.62	0.64		
Titanium	0.25	0.125	0.37	5.90		
		0.250	0.55	2.11		

1010 Sheet steel	3.9	0.94	—	6.4–5.1	Fillet weld	Banas (1971)
302 Stainless steel	3.5	12.7	—	2.1	Butt weld	
304 Stainless steel	17	6	1.2	8.4	Butt weld	Locke and Hella (1974)
		12.5	2	2.08		
		17	4	1.0		
		16.5		1.26		
	11.5	3.8		12.6		
		5.6		8.4		
		8.9		4.2		
	9.5	12.3		1.26		
	8	8.9	2.3	1.26	Butt weld	Locke *et al.* (1972)
	20	20.3	3.3	2.11		
		12.7	2.3	4.2		
Low carbon steel	4.3	6.4		3.6	Butt weld, other types of weld reported	Baardsen *et al.* (1973)
		3.3		7.2		
		1.5		11.0		
X8 Cr Ni 18 8	1.2	0.5		5	10-mm diameter tube, wall 5 mm thick	Ruffler and Gürs (1972)

to the workpiece to the total incident laser power and can approach 100%, as can be seen from the figure. The total efficiency of the system must, however, include the efficiency with which electrical power taken by the power supplies is converted to laser output power. Thus, even when the power transfer to the workpiece is 100% effective, the overall efficiency of the system may only be 20%.

Good penetration and the efficient use of incident laser power necessitates the incorporation of a gas jet "assist" (Locke *et al.*, 1972). Best results are obtained for a gas jet of helium or argon directed through the laser beam parallel to the workpiece surface. This produces a combination of good penetration and weld smoothness. Directing the gas jet toward the surface yields greater penetration but also tends to blow off the head of the weld. At high powers without a gas jet assist, a stationary plasma is formed in the path of the incident beam remote from the surface of the workpiece. This plasma is maintained by a combination of evaporation from the workpiece and absorption of laser energy in the resulting cloud of material. The resulting plasma is nearly opaque to 10.6-μm radiation with the result that only a small fraction of the incident beam actually reaches the target. The flux of an inert gas through this cloud of material apparently prevents the density of evaporated species from building up to the point where the cloud has high opacity at the laser wavelength.

Locke and Hella (1974) have investigated the effect of focusing on the depth of penetration for constant power and welding speed. For focusing to a point within the workpiece, the weld is cone-shaped and the penetra-

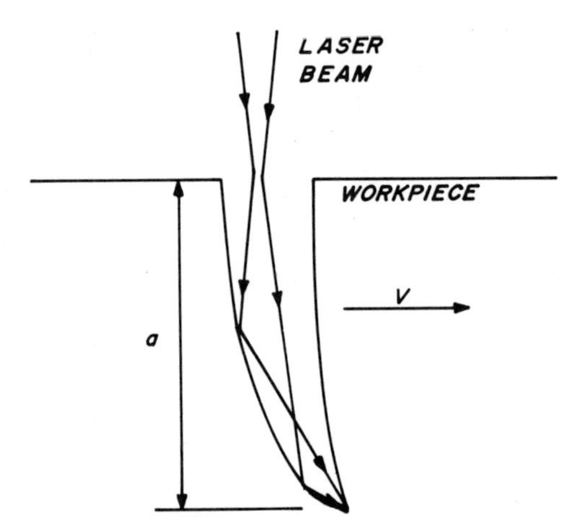

Fig. 6.8. Shape of "keyhole" during laser welding of quartz (after Siekman and Morijn, 1968).

Table 6.4

Comparison of Hardness Data on Laser and Electron Beam Welds in Type AMS 5525 Material[a]

Point	DPH hardness (kg/mm^2)	
	Laser weld	Electron beam weld
1	179	176
2	179	182
3	179	179
4	182 (within weld)	176
5	182 (within weld)	193 (within weld)
6	182 (within weld)	199 (within weld)
7	179 (within weld)	193 (within weld)
8	176 (within weld)	193 (within weld)
9	179 (within weld)	193 (within weld)
10	179 (within weld)	193 (within weld)
11	176 (within weld)	196 (within weld)
12	196 (within weld)	193 (within weld)
13	176 (within weld)	193 (within weld)
14	179 (within weld)	193 (within weld)
15	182	182
16	179	176
17	176	176
18	176	—

[a] From Alwang *et al.* (1969).

tion is less than that obtained for focusing closer to the target surface. The highest penetration and best uniformity of the weld is obtained for focusing to a point just inside the sheet surface. As expected, focusing with $f/18$ optics was less critical than with a $f/6$ system, although the penetration for a given laser power was smaller. A summary of currently available data on deep penetration welding with CO_2 lasers is given in Table 6.3.

An interesting experiment on the mechanism of deep-penetration welding with a cw CO_2 laser has been reported by Siekman and Morijn (1968). This experiment was performed on transparent fused quartz so that the development of the weld in time could be directly followed photographically. The laser was seen first to drill a hole in the quartz, which was then translated through the material. However, the profile of the hole was found to vary as the welding speed increased. A schematic representation of this profile at high speeds is shown in Fig. 6.8. The tip of the hole is seen to bend around toward the direction in which the workpiece is translated. This process is caused by the reflection of laser light from the leading edge of the hole. Material evaporated at this surface is effectively trapped by the cooler trailing edge. Thus, material is transported across the laser beam from the hot leading edge to the cooler trailing edge, without significant ejection of material back out toward the beam. For welding speeds in the range 10–45 mm/min, the depth of penetration was found to be linearly related to welding speed. As expected, the penetration was least for the highest welding speeds.

Samples of AMS 5525 and AMS 5544 material butt welded with a 200-W CO_2 laser have been subjected to detailed hardness measurements across the weld region by Alwang *et al.* (1969). A comparison was also made with electron beam welds produced in the same materials. Table 6.4 lists the hardness at various points in the region of the welds. It is evident that the electron beam weld has a more uniform hardness than that observed in the laser weld. This may be due in part to the nonuniformity of intensity within the laser focus.

6.4 CUTTING METALS

Gonsalves and Duley (1972) have reported a study of the cutting of thin metal sheets with a cw CO_2 laser. The purpose of this study was to ascertain the extent to which a theoretical model could be developed to describe the interrelation of the cutting parameters.

Figure 6.9 shows a series of cuts produced with a laser intensity of 1.1×10^4 W/cm^2 in 0.003-in. stainless steel sheet (Gonsalves, 1973). The cuts were produced at different speeds under constant focusing conditions. It can be seen that the cut width and heat-affected zone both decrease as the cutting speed is increased. Furthermore, the edges of the cut become sharper as the speed increases. A critical speed exists, however, above which molten material is incompletely removed from the cut and islands of resolidified material remain after the laser beam has passed. In the limit, as the speed increased still further, only a line of damage is visible in the interaction region.

Figures 6.10 and 6.11 show some of the relations between cutting parameters obtained in this study. The parameters are

P total laser power
A radius of circular focal spot
v cutting speed
v_{max} maximum cutting speed
D sheet thickness
f fraction of laser power used in heating
W cut width

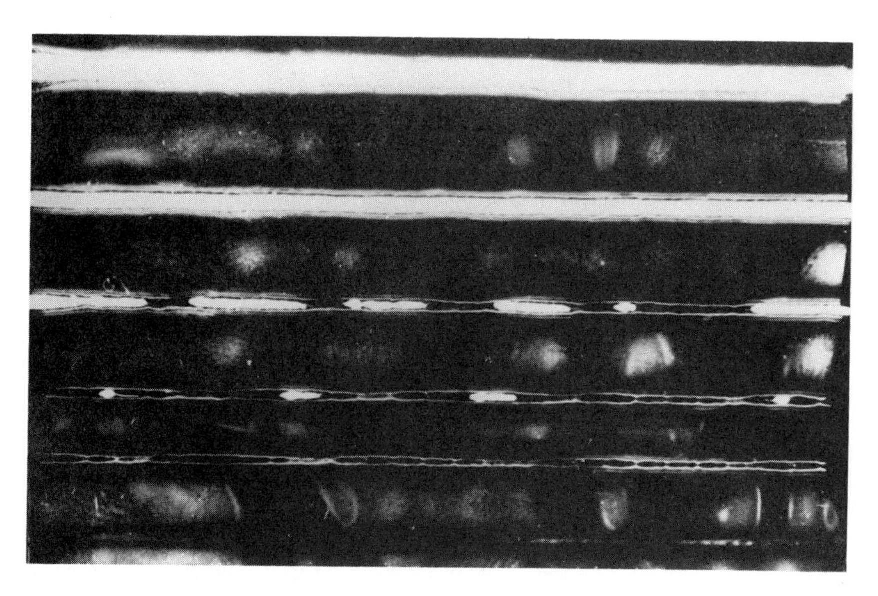

Fig. 6.9. A sequence of cuts produced in 0.003-in.-thick stainless steel sheet at increasing speeds with $P = 195$ W. A line of damage is observed for speeds in excess of the critical cutting speed, while large cut widths are observed for low-speed cutting.

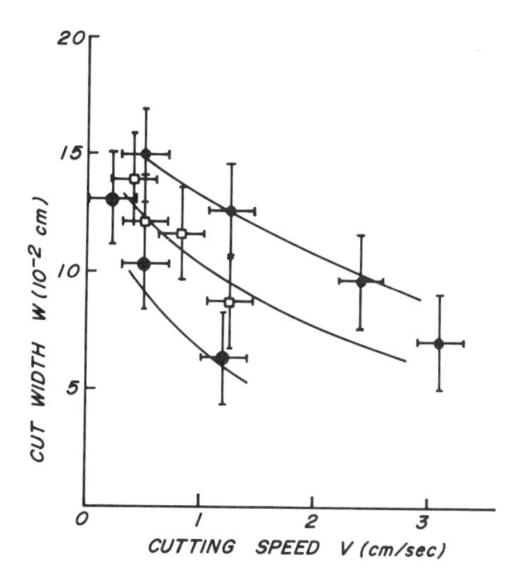

Fig. 6.10. Experimental data and theoretical curves of W vs. v for various powers with $D = 2 \times 10^{-3}$ in. and $A = 7.5 \times 10^{-2}$ cm. •, $P = 185$ W; □, $P = 113$ W; ●, $P = 65$ W.

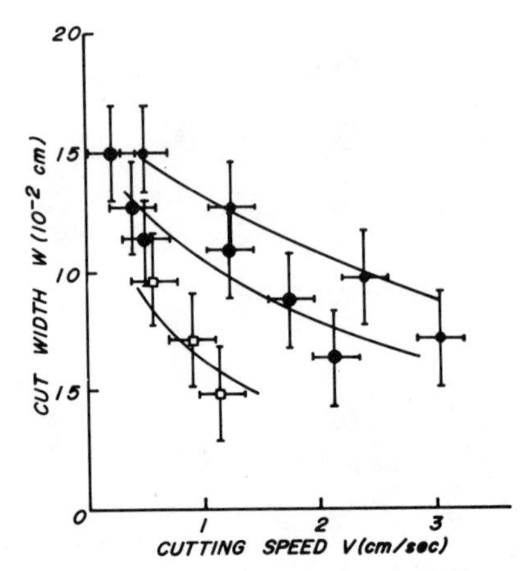

Fig. 6.11. Experimental data and theoretical curves of W vs. v for various thicknesses with P = 185 W and A = 7.5 × 10^{-2} cm. •, D = 2 × 10^{-3} in.; ●, D = 3 × 10^{-3} in.; □, D = 6 × 10^{-3} in.

Figures 6.10 and 6.11 show that W decreases rapidly with v until a critical cutting speed v_{max} is reached, which is seen (Fig. 6.12) to increase almost linearly with laser power for a sheet of constant thickness. Comparison of figures indicates that curves with different P and D values but with the same P/D ratio are coincident. Such behavior is predicted from the theoretical considerations of Section 4.11.1, where the thermal response of a thin sheet is seen to depend on the P/D ratio.

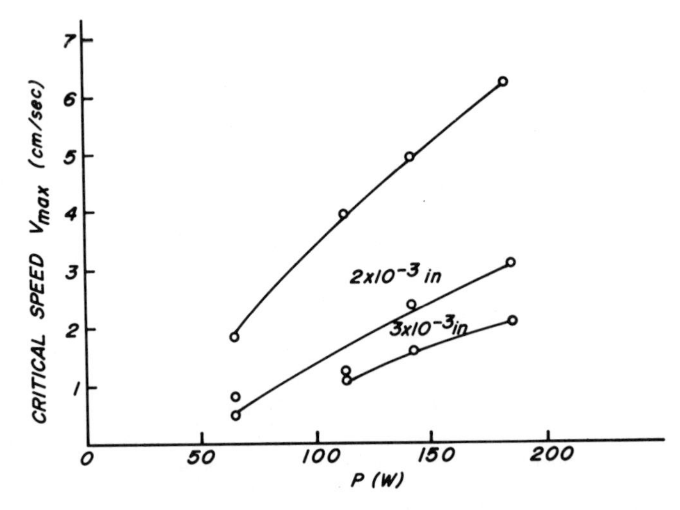

Fig. 6.12. Plot of critical cutting speed vs. power for various thicknesses with A = 7.5 × 10^{-2} cm, D = 10^{-3} in.

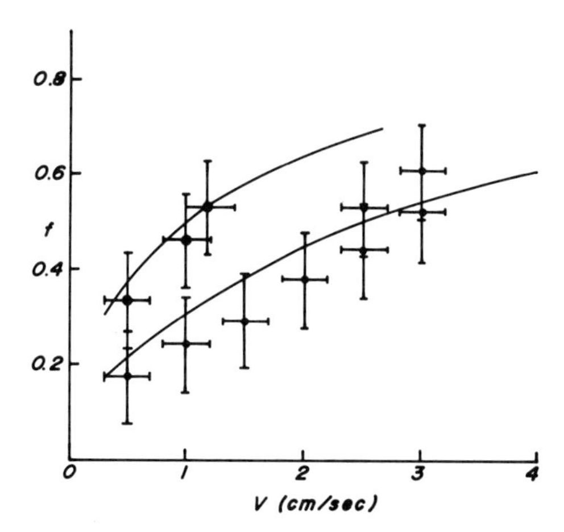

Fig. 6.13. Experimental data and theoretical curves of f vs. v for various P/D values with $A = 5 \times 10^{-2}$ cm. •, $P = 185$ W, $D = 2 \times 10^{-3}$ in.; ●, $P = 142$ W, $D = 3 \times 10^{-3}$ in.

Figure 6.13 shows that the fraction of the laser power actually used in the cutting process increases with v until v_{max} is reached. At low cutting speeds, however, f may often be less than 0.5. The shape of these curves is as predicted from the calculations given in Section 4.11.1.

Solid lines plotted on these figures represent the fit of the data to the point source model of Section 4.11.1 using appropriate values for the thermal constants and emissivity of stainless steel (Gonsalves and Duley, 1972).

Siekman (1968) has found that CO_2 laser machining of a thin metal film on an insulating substrate yields a cut cross section similar to that shown in Fig. 6.14. From Eq. (4.140) one expects

$$W^2 \propto P/v \tag{2}$$

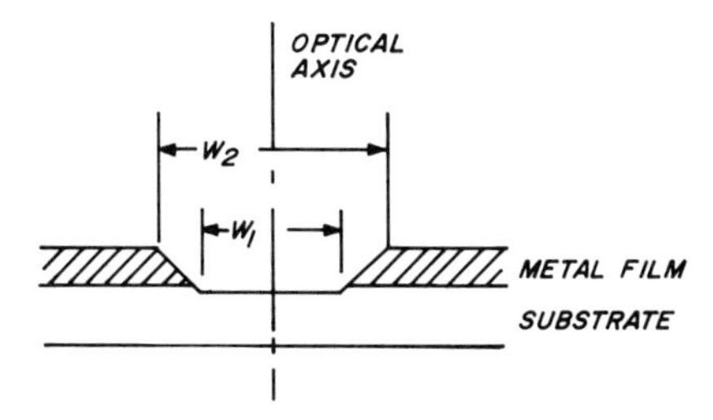

Fig. 6.14. Shape of groove on machining thin metal film on an insulating substrate (Siekman, 1968).

Table 6.5

Cutting Rates for Metal Sheets Using Gas Jet Assist

Metal	Power	Thickness	Rate	Gas	Reference
2219 Aluminum alloy	3.8 kW	0.25 in.	12 IPM	CO_2	Banas (1971)
Mild steel	320 kW	0.64 mm	18 cm/min	O_2	Harry and Luman (1971)
Stainless steel	350 W	0.30 mm	432 cm/min	O_2	Harry and Luman (1971)
	350 W	3.25 mm	22.9 cm/min	O_2	Harry and Luman (1971)
Nimonic (75)	225 W	0.79 mm	40.6 cm/min	O_2	Harry and Luman (1971)
Titanium	240 W	0.17 mm	610 cm/min	O_2	Harry and Luman (1971)
Titanium alloy (Ta 115)	225 W	0.91 mm	482 cm/min	O_2	Harry and Luman (1971)
Stainless steel	225 W	0.25 mm	350 cm/min	O_2	Harry and Luman (1971)
	225 W	0.5 mm	210 cm/min	O_2	Harry and Luman (1971)
	225 W	0.7 mm	80 cm/min	O_2	Harry and Luman (1971)
	225 W	1.2 mm	50 cm/min	O_2	Harry and Luman (1971)
	225 W	1.6 mm	45 cm/min	O_2	Harry and Luman (1971)
Steel	1.2 kW	5 mm	60 cm/min	O_2	Ruffler and Gürs (1972)
6061 Aluminum	10 kW	0.5 in.	40 IPM	He	Locke and Hella (1974)
Inconel 718	11 kW	0.5 in.	50 IPM	He	Locke and Hella (1974)
Titanium	10 kW	1 in.	200 IPM	O_2	Locke and Hella (1974)

Table 6.5 (Continued)

Metal	Power	Thickness	Rate	Gas	Reference
302 Stainless steel	185 W	10^{-3} in.	360 IPM	None	Gonsalves and Duley (1972)
	185 W	2×10^{-3} in.	180 IPM	None	Gonsalves and Duley (1972)
	185 W	3×10^{-3} in.	120 IPM	None	Gonsalves and Duley (1972)
	200 W	3×10^{-3} in.	240 IPM	O_2	Duley and Gonsalves (1974)
	200 W	4×10^{-3} in.	180 IPM	O_2	Duley and Gonsalves (1974)
	200 W	8 in.	120 IPM	O_2	Duley and Gonsalves (1974)
	200 W	12 in.	90 IPM	O_2	Duley and Gonsalves (1974)
Steel	300 W (100 Hz)	0.10 in.	40 IPM	O_2	Barber and Linn (1967)
Aluminum	15 kW	0.5 in.	90 IPM	None	Locke *et al.* (1972)
Carbon steel	15 kW	0.25 in.	90 IPM	None	Locke *et al.* (1972)
304 Stainless steel	20 kW	0.187 in.	50 IPM	None	Locke *et al.* (1972)

This dependence was verified experimentally for aluminum and gold films on soft glass, pyrex, and fused silica substrates. Cutting speeds were of the order of 250 cm/min with laser powers $\lesssim$30 W cw focused to a spot of approximately Gaussian distribution with diameter $\simeq 1.5 \times 10^{-2}$ cm. Both W_1 and W_2 were found to exhibit the P, v dependence given by Eq. (2).

Similar results were obtained in machining carbon films on pyrex and ceramic substrates (Siekman, 1969). De Jong and Knapen (1969) report the helixing of carbon film resistors using similar equipment to that described by Siekman.

Sullivan and Houldcroft (1967) were the first to suggest that addition of a gas jet assist could aid in cutting, welding, and drilling with cw lasers.

The effects of a gas jet seem to be at least twofold: First, it assists in the removal of material from the focal area and reduces the amount of material ejected back toward the laser. This helps to prevent a cloud of attenuating material from building up in front of the workpiece. By removing material from the focal area it ensures a cleaner cut. Second, it can either promote or inhibit reactions that may occur due to heating in air. Inert gas assists may be used when cutting flammable materials, while oxygen gas jet assist has been shown to enhance the burning of metals in air and hence to increase the maximum attainable cutting rate with a given laser power (Babenko and Tychinskii, 1973; Adams, 1968; Duley and Gonsalves, 1974). A high flow of gas inhibits heat flow in the material away from the interaction region by cooling the target and thus minimizes the heat-affected region. This helps prevent charring in cutting flammable materials.

Studies of gas jet assisted cutting with the cw CO_2 laser have also been reported by Lunau and Paine (1969), Lunau *et al.* (1969), Higuchi *et al.* (1971), Harry and Lunau (1972), Tandler (1971), Scott and Stovell (1968), Ruffler and Gürs (1972), and Locke and Hella (1974). We will consider the results of these experiments next (Table 6.5).

Figure 6.15a shows a gas jet nozzle that has been effectively used in the author's laboratory. The inner aperture must be larger than the focal spot on the target to prevent absorption of laser radiation by the nozzle. This design is not optimized since it is advantageous to have the gas flow exactly

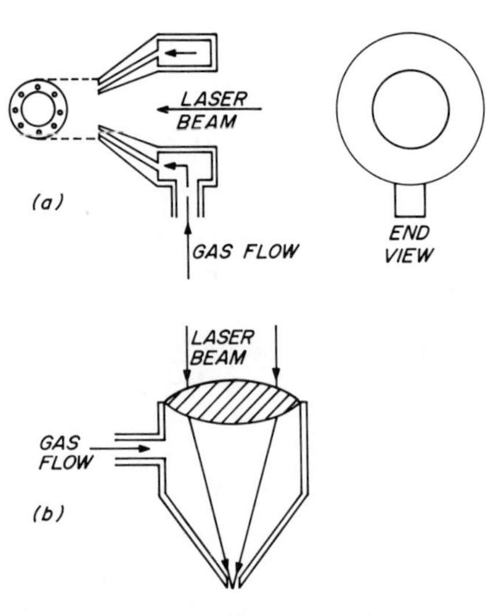

Fig. 6.15. Gas jet nozzles.

coincident with the optical axis. One alternate design that overcomes this problem is shown in Fig. 6.15b. In this case, however, either a lens or window must be provided, since the gas pressure within the nozzle is often several atmospheres. Optimum cutting seems to be obtained when the gas jet orifice is placed closer than one diameter from the workpiece. A summary of observed cutting rates is given in Table 6.5.

Some results on the cutting of thin metal sheets with a 300-W cw CO_2 laser using an oxygen gas jet assist are shown in Figs. 6.16–6.20 (Duley and Gonsalves, 1974). In these curves $v_{critical}$ (v_c) refers to the maximum speed of the workpiece at which a continuous and defect-free cut is produced. For speeds slightly in excess of v_c the cut is discontinuous with islands of melted metal filling the gap at intervals along the cut. Usually the minimum cut width is obtained at v_c. Figure 6.16 shows a plot of v_c versus G, the oxygen flow rate, for constant laser power and focusing to a circular spot of radius $A = 5 \times 10^{-2}$ cm. The sheet thickness was varied from 0.003 to 0.012 in. Maximum cutting speeds are seen to be essentially independent of the oxygen flow rate over a wide range of Q. The variation of v_c with Q using different laser intensities (obtained by changing P while keeping A constant) but with $l = 3 \times 10^{-3}$ in. is shown in Fig. 6.17. The shape of all of these curves is similar but a greater percentage increase in v_c occurs with gas flow at low incident laser intensities. The widths of the cuts produced in 3×10^{-3}-in. thick sheet with $P = 200$ W at various critical speeds are shown in Fig. 6.18. The curve drawn through these points is shifted to higher W and v when an oxygen gas jet assist is used compared to the result obtained when $Q = 0$. Figure 6.19 shows that oxygen assist actually decreases the fraction f of the incident power used in the heating process. A theoretical curve calculated from the theory of Section 4.11.1 is shown for comparison.

Quantitative data on gas-assisted cutting of thicker metals has been reported by Babenko and Tychinskii (1973). Figure 6.21 shows some of their results. An order of magnitude improvement in cutting speed is seen to occur with the gas jet at high oxygen flow rates. However, it is unclear from the report of Babenko and Tychinskii whether v refers to v_c or to some lower speed.

One of the advantages of gas jet-assisted CO_2 laser cutting of metals would seem to be that thick slabs of metal can be cut at high speeds. Locke and Hella (1974) report that this is particularly true for cutting oxidizable metals such as steels and titanium with the aid of an oxygen gas jet. An example is given in their article of the cutting of 1-in.-thick titanium slab at a rate of 200 in./min.

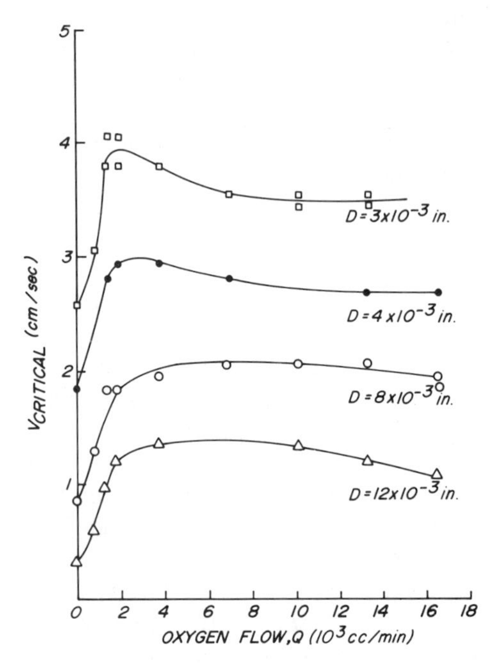

Fig. 6.16. Variation of critical cutting speed with oxygen flow for constant incident intensity and various sheet thicknesses. $P = 200$ W, $A = 5 \times 10^{-2}$ cm.

Some advantages and disadvantages of gas jet assisted laser cutting of metals can be summarized as follows:

(1) Oxidizable metals can be cut at high rates using an oxygen gas jet assist.
(2) Cut widths are usually smaller than those attainable with conventional thermal cutting methods.
(3) The edges of the cuts are square and a planar surface is produced.
(4) The heat-affected zone can usually be kept small but may be different from one side of the slab to the other.
(5) It is difficult to cut metals with a high melting point, high reflectivity at 10.6 μm, and/or large thermal conductivity with the cw CO_2 lasers presently available.
(6) The oxygen gas jet is most effective only for highly oxidizable metals.

Although the heat transfer situation in cutting metals with the addition of a reactive gas jet is very complex, the main features of this transfer can

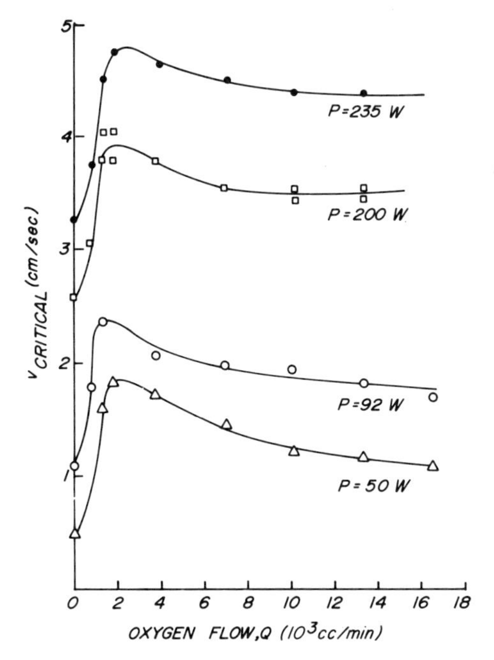

Fig. 6.17. Variation of critical cutting speed with oxygen flow for different incident intensities. $D = 3 \times 10^{-3}$ in., $A = 5 \times 10^{-2}$ cm.

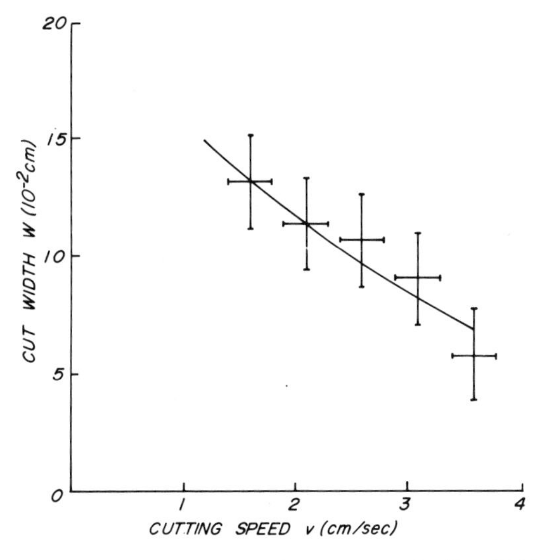

Fig. 6.18. Relation between cut width and cutting speed. $P = 200$ W, $A = 5 \times 10^{-2}$ cm, $D = 3 \times 10^{-3}$ in.

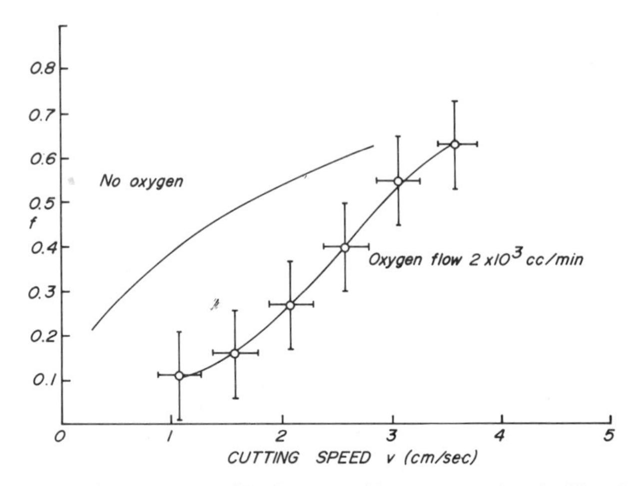

Fig. 6.19. The relation between the fraction of laser power absorbed by the workpiece as a function of cutting speed. $P = 200$ W, $A = 5 \times 10^{-2}$ cm, $D = 3 \times 10^{-3}$ in.

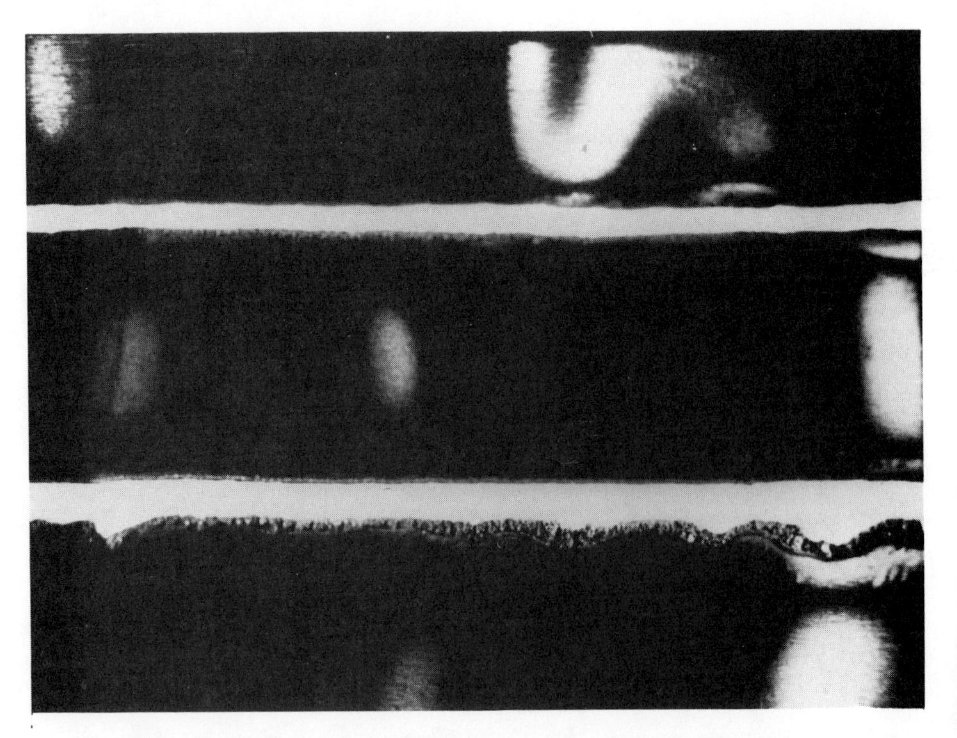

Fig. 6.20. Cuts produced in 0.003-in.-thick stainless steel sheet with the gas jet and $P = 200$ W, at speeds well below and close to the critical cutting speed.

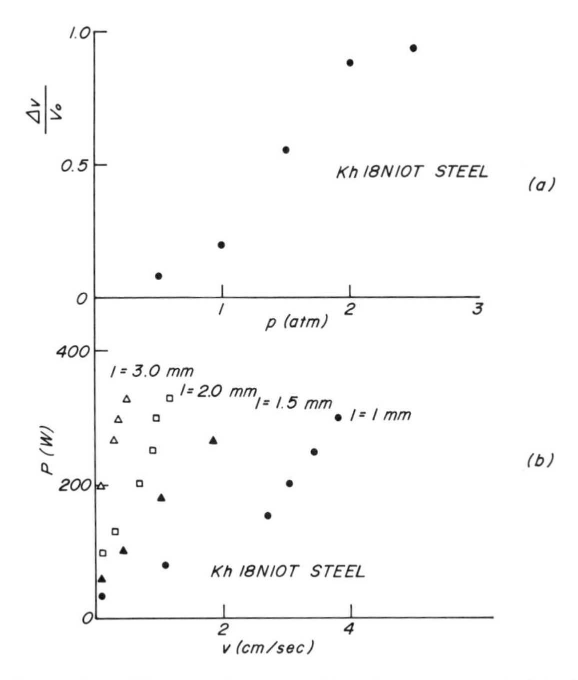

Fig. 6.21. (a) Change in cutting speed as a function of gas pressure in jet. (b) Relation between incident laser power and cutting speed for steel sheets of various thicknesses (Babenko and Tychinskii, 1973).

be described by a modification of the moving point source theory described in Section 4.11.1 (Babenko and Tychinskii, 1973; Duley and Gonsalves, 1974). As before, the temperature distribution in a sheet moving with speed v past a point source at the origin can be expressed as

$$T(r, t) = \frac{\epsilon Pf}{2\pi Kl} \exp\left(\frac{vx}{2\kappa}\right) K_0\left(\frac{rv}{2\kappa}\right) \tag{3}$$

in the absence of additional sources of heat transfer to the sheet through the point source. With a reactive gas jet, two additional heating/cooling terms must be included. These are P_1, the power transferred due to the heat of chemical reactions, and P_2, the power dissipated due to the cooling effect of the jet. In the point source approximation, both of these terms may be assumed to be incorporated in the strength of the source. Then, in terms of normalized variables, one obtains

$$C_0 + C_1 - C_2 = e^{-X} K_0^{-1}(R) \tag{4}$$

where

$$C_0 = \epsilon Pf/2\pi KlT_0, \qquad C_1 = P_1/2\pi KlT_0, \qquad C_2 = P_2/2\pi KlT_0$$

$$X = vx/2\kappa, \qquad R = vr/2\kappa$$

and T_0 is the temperature at which oxidation occurs. The term C_1 can be written

$$C_1 = (2/\pi)(q/cT_0)Y \tag{5}$$

where c is the specific heat (J/g) and q the net heat liberated (J/g) due to reactions in the cutting zone. Calling $q/cT_0 = \psi$, Eq. (4) becomes

$$C_0 - C_2 = e^{-X}K_0^{-1}(R) - (2/\pi)\psi Y \tag{6}$$

The cut width can be found by differentiating this expression with respect to X (Section 4.11.1). Then

$$C_0 - C_2 = K_0^{-1}(R_m)\exp\left[-\frac{R_m K_0(R_m)}{K_1(R_m)}\right] - \frac{2}{\pi}\psi Y_{max} \tag{7}$$

where R_m is the value of R for $Y = Y_{max}$. Since $Y = R \sin\phi$, while $\phi = \cos^{-1}[K_0(R)/K_1(R)]$,

$$Y_{max} = R_m\left[1 - \left(\frac{K_0(R_m)}{K_1(R_m)}\right)^2\right]^{1/2} \tag{8}$$

If we now put $f = 1$ and therefore assume that all power absorbed from the laser beam is converted into heat in the target (the solution will therefore be strictly valid only for thick sheets) then a plot of $C_0 - C_2$ versus Y_{max} has the form shown in Fig. 6.22 for various values of the parameter ψ. These curves show that stable cutting can be obtained as long as $\psi < 1.9$, since it is only in this case that $\partial(C_0 - C_2)/\partial Y_{max} > 0$, i.e., an increase in power leads to an increase in Y_{max}. $C_0 - C_2$ negative means either that the cut is proceeding on chemical energy alone or that C_2 is inordinately large. Curves are plotted for ψ negative since the removal of material from the reaction zone may actually yield an energy loss. For example, in the limit of strong evaporation when no reaction heat is retained by the target, $\psi \simeq q_{evap}/cT_{evap} \simeq -10$ for most metals. If liquid is formed and the latent heat is removed, then $\psi \simeq q_{melt}/cT_{melt} \simeq -0.4$. On the other hand, the known heats of reaction of O_2 with Fe limit the maximum positive value that ψ can assume to $\simeq$5.3. Thus one expects that a value of $-0.4 < \psi < 5.3$ would be appropriate for laser cutting of steel. The curves shown in Fig. 6.22 are valid for v in the range $0.1 < v < 10$ cm/sec. The upper limit is determined by the requirement that the cut width be greater than the diameter of the focal spot, while the lower limit is determined by heat transfer from the sheet (Babenko and Tychinskii, 1973).

Unfortunately, there are few quantitative cutting data that can be used as a test of these calculations. One point obtained from the experiments of Gonsalves (1973) is shown; however, more data are needed before it can be said whether or not the simple theory adequately describes the cutting kinetics with a gas jet assist. This theory should also describe the rate at which welding can be performed in slabs since ψ then can be thought of as the heat loss due to the latent heat of fusion required for the weld. Some points obtained from welding data (Babenko and Tychinskii, 1973; Webster, 1970) are also plotted in Fig. 6.22. The data of Webster have been normalized to the thermal constants of stainless steel as in the article by Swift-Hook and Gick (1973). Swift-Hook and Gick's energy transfer coefficients have been used to estimate the absorbed laser power. It can be seen that the experimental data follow the trend of the theoretical curves quite well. Webster's measurements seem to lie along the line with $\psi = 0$, while those of Babenko and Tychinskii fall on the line with $\psi \doteq -0.4$.

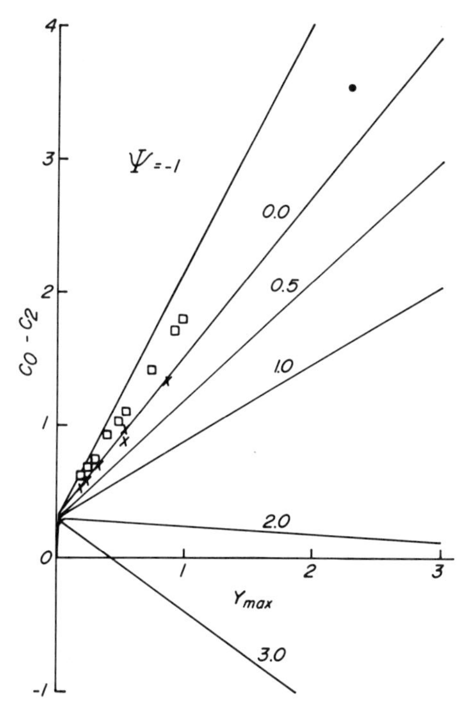

Fig. 6.22. $C_0 - C_2$ vs. Y_{max} from Eq. (7) for cutting with a gas jet assist. ×, Webster (1970); ●, Gonsalves (1973); □, Babenko and Tychinskii (1973).

Figure 6.17 shows that v_c first increases rapidly as Q increases, reaches a maximum, and then declines to a value that is almost independent of Q. This suggests that low Q promotes an exothermic reaction whose energy is partially transferred to the workpiece. As Q increases, cooling may become effective, resulting in lower v_c. P_1 is given approximately by

$$P_1 = \alpha W l \lambda v \tag{9}$$

where λ is an average heat of the reactions (J/cm^3), W the cut width, and α the fraction of this power transferred to the workpiece. P_2 can be expressed as

$$P_2 = \beta N k (T - T_g) \tag{10}$$

where N is the number of gas molecules striking the target/sec, k Boltzmann's constant, T the target temperature (°K), T_g the gas temperature (°K), and β the fraction of the incident gas flow that actually strikes the target. It is of interest to examine the relative magnitudes of P_1, P_2, and ϵPf in an actual cutting situation. We will take the example of 7.5×10^{-3}-cm-thick stainless steel cut with a power of 200 W. Figure 6.18 shows that for the maximum cutting speed $v = 4$ cm/sec, $W \simeq 5 \times 10^{-2}$ cm. Taking $\lambda = 4 \times 10^4$ J/cm^3 as representative of the heat generated by combustion,

$$P_1 \simeq \alpha \times 60 \text{ W} \tag{11}$$

The gas flow $Q \simeq 2 \times 10^3$ cm^3/min and with $(T - T_g) \simeq 1000$°K,

$$P_2 \simeq \beta \times 12 \text{ W} \tag{12}$$

The laser power absorbed is

$$P\epsilon f \simeq 28 \text{ W}$$

taking $\epsilon = 0.2$ and $f \simeq 0.7$ from Fig. 6.19. When one now considers that the gas jet will rapidly remove heated material from the interaction region so that α is likely to be considerably <1 while complete combustion is also unlikely so that the numerical factor in Eq. (11) is probably less than 60 W, it is evident that $P_1 < P\epsilon f$. Similarly, since $\beta < 1$, $P_2 < P\epsilon f$ also. This rather surprising fact suggests that little additional heat is either transferred to the workpiece or removed from it when thin sheets are cut with the aid of a gas jet assist. Instead, the main effect of the reactive gas jet is to lower the temperature at which material may be removed. This implies that for the same incident power P and focusing conditions, $F(Q) < f(0)$ and $Y_{max}(Q) > Y_{max}(0)$. This can be seen to correspond with the results shown in Fig. 6.19.

The initial rapid rise in v_c versus Q then most likely denotes a mode of operation in which the removal of material through oxidation is limited by the amount of O_2 gas available. When Q increases, however, oxidation can occur at lower temperatures and W increases while f decreases. Eventually f becomes small enough to limit severely the amount of incident laser power absorbed by the workpiece. The cutting rate then will decrease with a further increase in Q.

Babenko and Tychinskii (1973) report a modification of the moving point source model in which the heat source has a Gaussian distribution,

$$F(r) = (\epsilon P/\pi d^2) \exp[-r^2/d^2] \tag{13}$$

Then

$$C_0 - C_2 = \frac{2}{-\mathrm{Ei}(-U^2/4)} - \frac{2}{\pi} \phi U \tag{14}$$

where

$$U = vd/2\kappa, \qquad \phi = y_{\max}\psi/d$$

and Ei is the exponential integral (see Section 4.7.2).

6.5 CUTTING NONMETALS

The cw CO_2 laser has been shown to be a suitable and versatile tool in the cutting of a wide variety of nonmetallic materials. It is safe to say that almost any material can be cut rapidly and cleanly under proper conditions with the CO_2 laser. However, whether the CO_2 laser offers an economically feasible alternative to conventional cutting methods depends in detail on the application. Some examples to illustrate the range of materials cut with the CO_2 laser are given in Table 6.6.

Some of the factors that have made CO_2 lasers attractive in certain cutting applications are summarized as follows:

(1) Depth of penetration, kerf width, and cutting speed can be controlled by changing the laser power and focusing as well as the type and flow of a gas assist.

(2) Cuts are usually of good quality under optimized cutting conditions.

(3) The cutting tool can be transferred optically from one point on the workpiece to another and can describe complex geometrical patterns.

(4) Cutting complex contours can easily be preprogrammed.

(5) The beam cuts equally well in all directions, unlike a saw blade or a diamond wheel, which have definite cutting directions.

(6) Cutting can be stopped or started almost instantaneously.

(7) The beam can be directed to a remote location that may be difficult to reach with conventional tools. It can also be passed through windows into special environments.

Table 6.6

Cutting Rates for Nonmetals Using the cw CO_2 Laser

Material	Power	Thickness	Rate	Gas	Reference
Corrugated	3.5 kW	0.18 in.	350 ft/min	None	Banas (1971)
Borsical tape	3.9 kW	9×10^{-3} in.	100 ft/min	None	Banas (1971)
Asbestos (compressed)	180 W	6.4 mm	76.2 cm/min	Air	Harry and Lunau (1972)
Asbestos (cement)	335 W	6.4 mm	2.5 cm/min	Air	Harry and Lunau (1972)
Confectionary	250 W	27 mm	100 cm/min	Air	Harry and Lunau (1972)
	260 W	6 mm	150 cm/min	Air	Harry and Lunau (1972)
Glass (soda lime)	350 W	2 mm	75 cm/min	Air	Harry and Lunau (1972)
Paper (matt)	60 W	0.33 mm	2880 cm/min	Air	Harry and Lunau (1972)
Paper (gloss)	60 W	0.33 mm	4000 cm/min	Air	Harry and Lunau (1972)
Plastic (acrylic)	300 W	3.1 mm	183 cm/min	Air	Harry and Lunau (1972)
Plastic (PVC)	300 W	3.2 mm	360 cm/min	Air	Harry and Lunau (1972)
Plastic (expanded polystyrene)	300 W	20 mm	10 cm/min	Air	Harry and Lunau (1972)
Nylon	180 W	—	360 cm/min	Air	Harry and Lunau (1972)
Vinyl (36 stack)	330 W	—	2.5 cm/min	Air	Harry and Lunau (1972)
Leather	225 W	3 mm	305 cm/min	Air	Harry and Lunau (1972)
Wood (oak)	300 W	16 mm	27.9 cm/min	Air	Harry and Lunau (1972)
Wood (deal)	200 W	50 mm	12.5 cm/min	Air	Harry and Lunau (1972)
Wood (hardboard)	300 W	3.8 mm	91 cm/min	Air	Harry and Lunau (1972)
Wood (plywood)	350 W	4.8 mm	530 cm/min	Air	Harry and Lunau (1972)
	225 W	5 mm	110 cm/min	Air	Harry and Lunau (1972)
	225 W	6.5 mm	65 cm/min	Air	Harry and Lunau (1972)
	225 W	15.5 mm	30 cm/min	Air	Harry and Lunau (1972)
	225 W	19 mm	28 cm/min	Air	Harry and Lunau (1972)

Table 6.6 (Continued)

Material	Power	Thickness	Rate	Gas	Reference
Plastic (perspex)	90 W	10 mm	33 cm/min	Air	Lunau *et al.* (1969)
	200 W	20 mm	20 cm/min	Air	Lunau *et al.* (1969)
	180 W	30 mm	11 cm/min	Air	Lunau *et al.* (1969)
Boron epoxy composite	15 kW	0.32 in.	65 in./min	Air	Locke *et al.* (1972)
Fiberglass epoxy composite	20 kW	0.5 in.	180 in./min	Air	Locke *et al.* (1972)
Wood (plywood)	8 kW	1 in.	60 in./min	Air	Locke *et al.* (1972)
Plastic (plexiglass)	8 kW	1 in.	60 in./min	Air	Locke *et al.* (1972)
Glass	20 kW	0.375 in.	60 in./min	Air	Locke *et al.* (1972)
Concrete	8 kW	1.5 in.	2 in./min	Air	Locke *et al.* (1972)
Alumina	40 W	0.635 mm	60 in./min	Air	Conti (1969)

(8) There is no contamination of the workpiece by contact with the cutting tool.

(9) Since some materials absorb or dissipate CO_2 laser radiation more effectively than others, selective cutting or machining of one component in a composite may be accomplished.

(10) The tool does not exert a force on the specimen during cutting. Thermal stresses may, however, develop.

These and similar factors will decide whether or not the CO_2 laser is an attractive alternative to current material removal technology for a given process or application.

There have been few detailed descriptions of cutting applications in this area reported in the literature. Studies as reported are usually quantitative only in the sense that cutting rates are related to incident laser power. Laser mode structure, beam diameter, and focusing optics used all affect the reproducibility of results and make a comparison between the work of different groups difficult. In many cases the design of a gas jet and the rate at which gas is flowed onto the workpiece will determine whether or not good quality cuts are produced. This information is rarely reported in the literature.

Before we examine some cutting applications of the cw CO_2 laser in more detail, it is of interest to discuss the results of Babenko and Tychinskii (1973), which provide some general quantitative estimates of material removal rates for a wide variety of nonmetallic materials. The rate at which material is removed from a rectangular channel of width W and depth l when cutting proceeds at speed v is

$$\text{mass removal rate} = \rho W l v \text{ g/sec} \tag{15}$$

where ρ is the density of the material. If, on the average, λ kJ/g are required for this process then the power needed will be

$$P = \rho \lambda W l v \text{ kW} \tag{16}$$

λ is tabulated for some materials of interest in Table 6.7. As expected, low-density materials generally have smaller λ than those materials with high density. As an example of an estimate of the power required for a particular application, consider the cutting of 5-mm-thick plywood at the rate of 120 cm/min. We will assume that the kerf width will be about 1 mm. Then for $\rho \simeq 0.5$ g/cm^3,

$$P = 0.5 \times 5.4 \times 0.1 \times 0.5 \times 2 = 270 \text{ W}$$

Table 6.6 shows that Harry and Lunau (1972) have produced cuts in ply-

Table 6.7

Specific Cutting Energies for Some Nonmetallic Materials Using a CO_2 Laser[a]

Material	Specific cutting energy λ (kJ/g)
Pine	0.9
Oak	5.4
Plywood	5.4
Cardboard	0.8
Rigid PVC	1.8
Plexiglass	2.0
Rubber (oil resistant)	2.5
Rubber (vacuum)	2.1
Asbestos cement	28
Asbestos sheet	20
Glass ceramic (opaque)	25
Ceramic	30
Silicate glass	31
Silica glass	45

[a] From Babenko and Tychinskii (1973).

wood of this thickness at the rate of 110 cm/min for a laser power of 225 W. In view of the uncertainties both in the determination of λ in Table 6.7 and in the kerf width W (which was not given by Harry and Lunau), the theoretical prediction of P is remarkably accurate.

Locke *et al.* (1972) report on the cutting of 0.95-cm-thick glass at the rate of 2.54 cm/sec with a laser power $P = 20$ kW. Taking $\rho = 2.4$ g/cm^3, $W = 0.1$ cm, and $\lambda = 31$ kJ/g the estimated power required would be $\simeq$18 kW. Once again there is good agreement.

Individual Materials

Wood. The cutting rate for plywood sheet has been found to be almost linearly related to incident laser power under constant focusing and gas flow conditions (Harry and Lunau, 1972). Cuts are of good quality with, however, some tendency for charring to occur on the side of the sheet not subjected to the gas assist. The sides of the cut are parallel and the kerf width can be adjusted by a change of laser power or gas flow. There appears to be little gain in using inert gases such as nitrogen or helium in the gas assist as air has the desired quenching effect. Wood is not easily cut without a gas jet assist.

There would seem to be little economic advantage to using lasers for simple cutting operations: band and jig saws are cheap, easily maintained, and can cut at comparable rates. Complex machining operations as required, for example, in the preparation of jigs for paper box manufacture may, however, be more easily accomplished using a CO_2 laser cutter. A device of this sort has been used commercially.

Textiles. Most varieties of textiles can be easily cut with the CO_2 laser. The combination of computer control of cutting patterns together with the other advantages of laser cutting provides a system that has been referred to as "the first major advance in apparel manufacturing since the invention of the sewing machine" (Eleccion, 1972). Many layers of material can be cut simultaneously and an early problem of lateral penetration of the gas jet between layers, which produces discoloration and charring at the bottom of the stack, has apparently been overcome (Harry and Lunau, 1972). One distinct advantage with synthetic textiles is that the edge of the cut is sealed by the heat from the laser, thus eliminating the frayed edges typical of knife cuts. A commercial laser cutting system has been developed by Hughes Aircraft Co. for the clothing industry.

Paper and Cardboard. Some attractive features of paper cutting with high-power CO_2 lasers have been listed by Miller and Osial (1969):

(1) No contact between the cutting tool and the paper, eliminating the replacement of tools.

(2) The paper is vaporized and not cut away, resulting in a superior edge quality.

(3) No dust is generated by the cutting process.

Despite these advantages, there has been little interest in this process mainly because the powers required seem to be prohibitively large. Table 6.8 lists maximum cutting speeds for different types of paper attainable with a 250-W cw CO_2 laser (Miller and Osial, 1969). Maximum speeds seem to be less than or about 1000 ft/min and this rate is attained only with the thinnest paper. Conventional cutting operations involve rates of 2000–7000 ft/min. Furthermore, up to 20 slitters may be used on a single machine.

Since the required power and the cutting speed are directly related [Eq. (16)] we can estimate the powers required to slit paper at a rate of 7000 ft/min from Table 6.8 simply by multiplying 250 W by $7000/v$, where v is the cutting speed at the low-power level. For example, to cut newsprint at this rate would require $7000 \times 250/530 \simeq 3.3$ kW. With 20 slitters on a high-speed winder a total laser power of about 70 kW would be necessary. This power is within the capability of present-day laser technology but such machines are still in the prototype stage. The alternative would be to use 20 individual 3.3-kW lasers. This is obviously impractical. One therefore has to conclude that the enormous material removal rates inherent in paper cutting at speeds approaching 10^4 ft/min do not seem capable of

Table 6.8

Maximum Cutting Speeds for Paper with a 250-W cw CO_2 Laser[a]

Type of paper	Thickness ($\times 10^{-3}$ in.)	Rate (FPM)
Bond[b]	1.5	700
	2	1000
	3.5	200
	4	350
Graph paper	2	600
Newsprint	3	530
Coated paper	5	200
Forbes cover stock	4.5	300
Laminate	10	130
Bond (3 layers)	4.5	130

[a] After Miller and Osial (1969).
[b] Different types.

being met by lasers of the types that are currently available. However, there may be other more specialized paper cutting operations in which cw laser cutting provides a viable alternative to conventional technology. Some suggestions have been made by Miller and Osial in their article.

Plastics. Most plastics have substantial absorption at the wavelength of the CO_2 laser. This makes them easy to cut, although a major application of the CO_2 laser may lie instead in the welding of plastics (see below). Lunau *et al.* (1969) have published the results of an interesting parametric study on the gas-assisted cutting of perspex. Under standard conditions little difference in penetration of cuts in perspex was noted as the composition of the impinging gas assist was varied. Surprisingly, oxygen and helium gave almost identical penetration depths. It was concluded that an air gas assist was the best compromise.

The penetration was found to be greater with a gas assist only at high incident laser powers. However, the quality of the cuts produced was significantly better with the gas assist even at low laser powers. Little increase in penetration was produced by an increase in gas flow above a threshold value. As predicted from Eq. (16), the maximum cutting speed increased linearly with the incident laser power.

The removal of teflon insulation from wires with a CO_2 laser has been reported by Tencza and Angelo (1969). Conditions could be varied so that the insulation was removed without affecting the strength of the wire.

Welding of plastics with the CO_2 laser has been reported by Ruffler and Gürs (1972) and Duley and Gonsalves (1972). A side view and cross section through such a weld are shown in Figs. 6.23 and 6.24 (Gonsalves, 1973). This weld was produced in 0.44-mm stock polyethylene at the rate of 60 cm/min with a cw laser power of 50 W. Such welds are strong and are free from imperfections.

Rubber. Most interest in laser processing of rubber has been directed not toward cutting but to drilling of fine holes. The CO_2 laser is well suited to this application since, unlike wavelengths in the visible, 10.6-μm wavelength radiation is strongly absorbed by rubber. One of the first applications of CO_2 lasers reported in the literature involved the puncturing of rubber nipples for baby bottles. Three holes were drilled simultaneously using optics to divide the incident beam. A pulsed CO_2 laser could perform this task at the rate of 250 parts per minute (Barber and Linn, 1969).

A more sophisticated application of the CO_2 laser in the drilling of rubber has been reported by Longfellow (1970). The requirement was to produce an extensible matrix of fine (80–90 μm in diameter) holes in thin rubber sheet to be used for the vacuum handling of semiconductor chips. This

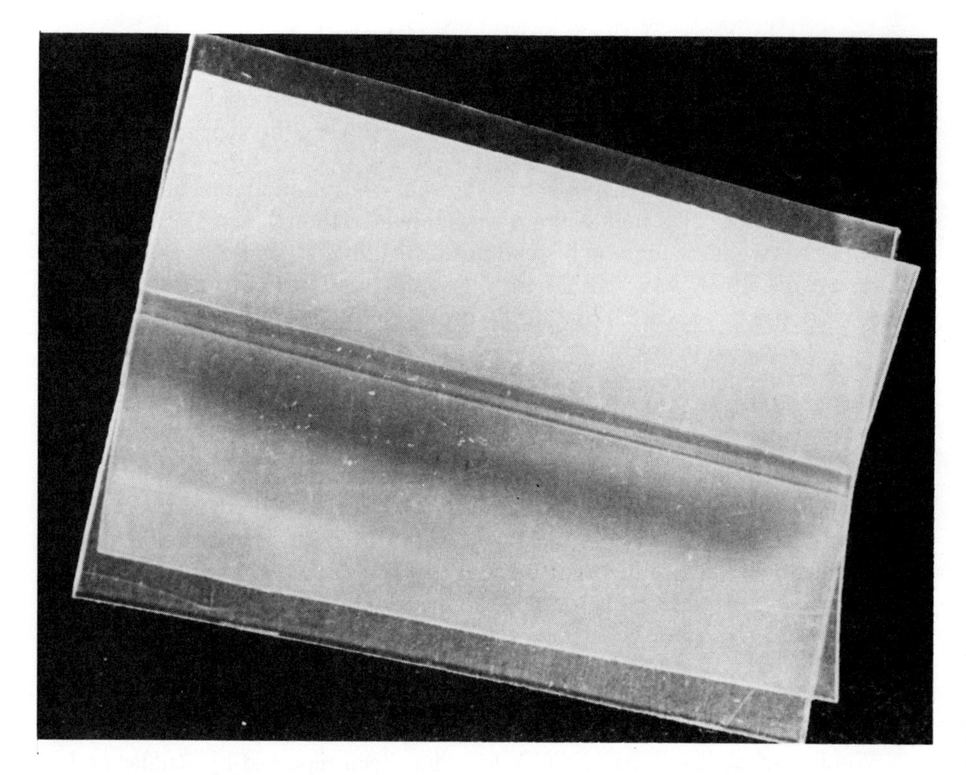

Fig. 6.23. Welded seam in 0.44-mm polyethylene sheet with the cw laser. Side view.

was accomplished with a 250-W cw CO_2 laser pulsed electronically at 25 Hz. A gas jet was used to remove excess rubber. A total of 31,400 holes could be drilled in a 5-cm diameter circle in an operating time of 38 min.

Ice. An interesting but somewhat speculative application of CO_4 lasers in the puncturing of ice to assist ice breakers has recently been suggested by Clark *et al.* (1973). From their experiments they give 8 cm^2/sec/kW for the ratio [depth of cut $\times$ speed/power]. Thus laser powers required to effect a deep cut (1 m or more) at speeds approaching 1 kt are prohibitively large. Clark *et al.* suggest, however, that it may be sufficient to produce a relatively shallow groove, which can induce cracking of the ice under pressure from the ice breaker. In this case, smaller powers could be used (50–100 kW to give a cut 8 cm deep at a rate of 1 kt). Lasers oscillating in the visible or near infrared region of the spectrum might be able to induce stresses within a block of ice by the explosive evaporation of material within the block. Unfortunately, CO_2 laser radiation is not

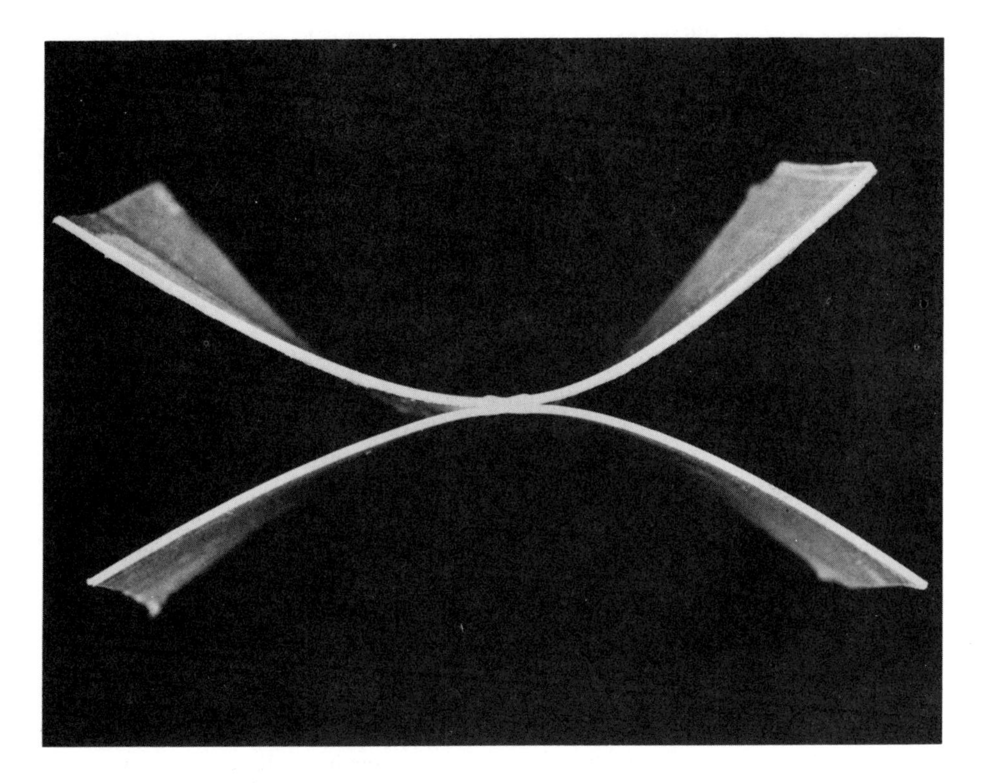

Fig. 6.24. As in Fig. 6.23. End section.

suited to this application since it is absorbed strongly at the ice surface. Nd–glass or Nd–YAG lasers would be more effective.

6.6 SCRIBING AND CONTROLLED FRACTURE

A number of important brittle materials may be separated rapidly by scribing or controlled fracturing with a minimum of surface damage and relatively low laser powers. In the scribing process, a small groove is removed by focusing the laser output on the surface of the material as it moves rapidly through the focal region. Conditions are adjusted so that the amount of material vaporized is small. The groove acts as a fault, which promotes fracture along this line when the material is subsequently stressed. Repetitively Q-switched Nd : YAG lasers and the cw CO_2 laser whose output is strongly absorbed by most insulating materials are both suitable scribing sources. Silicon, glass, and various ceramics have all been successfully scribed (Gagliano *et al.*, 1969; Lumley, 1969). Both authors report the scribing and separation of silicon transistor wafers and thin-film circuits. Scribing rates of 15 in./min and more in silicon are easily obtained with focused Nd : YAG or cw CO_2 lasers.

Absorption of laser radiation at the surface of brittle insulating materials such as some ceramics and many glasses results in localized stresses. These stresses in turn cause the material to fracture. If the material is moved under the focused laser beam, a crack will propagate in an opposite direction to that in which the material is translated. Since the stresses are always localized, fracture is controllable and complex shapes can be generated simply by moving the focal spot over the desired profile (Lumley, 1969). Furthermore, little material is removed during this process so that high separation rates are possible with low laser powers. It has been found advantageous in some cases to focus the output to a line using a cylindrical lens. This is reported to minimize surface damage. Some data reported by Lumley (1969) are given in Table 6.9. These data are quite conservative,

Table 6.9

Controlled Fracture Separation Rates Using a cw CO_2 Laser[a]

Material	Thickness (in.)	Focus	Diameter or length (in.)	Rate (IPM)	Power (W)
99+% Alumina	0.027	Spot	0.010	12	8
	0.040	Spot	0.010	2	16
	0.027	Spot	0.015	12	7
Microcrystalline alumina	0.017	Spot	0.010	12	5
	0.025	Spot	0.010	12	7
	0.035	Spot	0.010	12	11
Glass	0.047	Spot	0.015	12	3
	0.062	Spot	0.020	12	9
Glass (soda lime)	0.039	Spot	0.020	12	3
	0.039	Line	0.50	12	10
Sapphire	0.048	Line	0.015	3	12
Crystal quartz	0.032	Line	0.015	24	3
Ferrite sheet	0.008	Line	0.015	44	2.5

[a] From Lumley (1969).

as Lumley's article shows that parting rates of 60 IPM can be obtained in 0.027-in.-thick high-alumina ceramic and 0.039-in.-thick glass with CO_2 laser powers of less than 40 W. Surprisingly, the separation rate for given laser powers, focusing conditions, and sheet thickness depends sensitively on the width of the sheet. The largest fracture rates were obtained in the narrowest pieces.

Laser heat has been used in cleaving single crystals (Gagliano *et al.*, 1969). Thin diamond foils have been prepared using this technique (Ritter and Murphy, 1970).

6.7 MICROMACHINING

Since the wavelength of the CO_2 laser is much longer than that of readily available high-power lasers, which operate in the visible and ultraviolet, the minimum spot size attainable on focusing the output of CO_2 lasers is correspondingly larger than that obtained with shorter-wavelength devices. This factor seriously limits possible applications of CO_2 lasers in micromachining and microwelding. Nd–YAG, Nd–glass, He–Ne, and argon lasers have, however, found some application in certain areas of micromachining technology. Reviews on this subject have been published by Cohen and Epperson (1968), Gagliano *et al.* (1969), and Ready (1971).

One of the first comprehensive studies of laser micromachining was reported by Cohen *et al.* (1968). Using a *Q*-switched Nd–YAG laser, 6-μm wide grooves were cut in a 3000 Å thick gold layer coated on sapphire and 2.5-μm wide grooves could be cut in a 2000 Å thick layer of nichrome on quartz. Lines 1 μm wide were scribed in tantalum nitride, titanium, and nichrome films. Scribing speeds were less than about 2 mm/sec and were limited by the 400-Hz pulse repetition frequency.

Brisbane and Jackson (1968) showed that cuts of various widths could be produced in thin metallic films by control over the focusing conditions. Under standardized conditions, linewidths were greatest in nichrome and tantalum and least in nickel and aluminum films. Complex patterns were scribed by translating the sample on a tape-controlled *X–Y* table. Using an optical method known as "conjugation of pupils," complex patterns have been scribed in thin metallic and insulating layers without the necessity of translating the workpiece (Boyer *et al.*, 1970).

A Nd : YAG laser machining system capable of generating gold conductor patterns on ceramic substrates at a rate of 17 cm^2/sec with 14-μm resolution has recently been discussed by Weick (1972). The pattern to be scribed is obtained from a code plate that is read by an auxiliary laser to give timing signals that drive the Nd : YAG laser.

The use of holographic lenses instead of conventional optics in focusing the output of lasers for micromachining has been shown to offer the possibility of producing three-dimensional patterns with a single laser pulse (Moran, 1971a). Furthermore, complex arrays of microwelds could be performed simultaneously. Some initial problems due to differences in wavelength between the beam used to record the hologram and that of the machining laser (Moran, 1971b) have been overcome (Latta, 1971). Machining experiments using a modulated zone plate to focus the laser beam have been reported by Engel *et al.* (1974). This method can also be used to machine complex patterns and contours without the necessity of moving the workpiece.

A novel application of laser micromachining has been described by Hokanson and Unger (1969). A problem in the adjustment of quartz crystal resonators involving alterations in resonator geometry and electrode mass loading has been solved by the selective removal of material using a Q-switched Nd : YAG laser. Frequency adjustments greater than one part in 10^8 were shown to be feasible.

Chapter 7

Applications of Laser-Induced Evaporation

7.1 INTRODUCTION

We have seen in earlier chapters that high power CO_2 and other lasers can evaporate any known material. This chapter explores some applications of this effect that are perhaps a little more sophisticated than drilling, cutting, and welding. Laser-induced evaporation will be shown to be a process with wide application in many areas of physics, chemistry, and engineering. Industrial applications to be discussed include the development of the laser microprobe for the spectrochemical analysis of small samples, the use of laser-induced evaporation to trim resistors to precise values in situ, and the use of the laser-induced emission of electrons and ions to trigger high-voltage electrical spark gaps. Some areas in which industrial applications have not yet developed to any great extent but which are worthy of future investigation include the use of high-power lasers to clean surfaces in vacuum, the preparation of thin films via laser deposition, and the study of chemical systems at elevated temperatures through mass spectrometric analysis of evaporation products.

7.2 LASER DEPOSITION OF THIN FILMS

Since a laser beam can be directed into a high-vacuum system through a window to heat a component inside the system, laser heating has found some application in the deposition of thin films. Material to be deposited can be heated selectively without the necessity of heating a container to a corresponding temperature. Thus contamination of the system vacuum and the thin-film substrate by outgasing or evaporation of the container or the heat source can be minimized. Furthermore, the possibility of reactions between the deposition material and the crucible in which it is heated can be reduced. Since laser evaporation can be made to occur at very high temperatures, deposition rates with laser heating are often larger than those attainable with conventional heating methods. However, evaporation at high temperature in general results in a different vapor composition and the tendency for the sample to eject relatively large particles of material. As a result, many studies of laser deposition have focused on a comparison between the structure and composition of thin films produced with laser and conventional heating sources. Table 7.1 gives a list of some materials evaporated with pulsed or cw lasers and some properties of the thin films produced.

The initial work of Smith and Turner (1965) showed that while *Q*-switched or normal pulse ruby lasers were suitable for depositing thin films of many materials, the tendency for liquid droplets or even small particles of solid to be ejected resulted in films that were often of poor quality. Although the deposition rate can be exceedingly high [10^5–10^6 Å/sec in the work of Schwarz and Tourtellotte (1969)] the thickness attainable with a single millisecond laser pulse is limited to a few thousand angstroms even at high pulse energies. This factor requires that films of thickness greater than this value be deposited by the superposition of laser pulses. A discontinuous deposition may result in imperfections in the resulting film and can lead to the trapping of impurities from the ambient gas in the vacuum system between pulses. The deposition process can be made continuous by the use of either cw Nd or CO_2 lasers. In this case, however, the deposition rate is orders of magnitude lower even when the cw laser power is in the 100-W range.

As first shown by Groh (1968), the cw CO_2 laser is well suited to the deposition of thin films of many nonmetallic materials. This is due in part to the high absorption of 10.6-μm radiation in most insulators and semiconductors. As an example, Hass and Ramsey (1969) report that SiO can be evaporated at a rate of 150 Å/sec using a laser power of only 60 W. Metals can also be evaporated with low cw laser powers, but this is accomplished only by minimizing the effects of thermal conduction by heating

Table 7.1

Summary of Materials Evaporated with Pulsed and cw Lasers

Material	Refractive index	Laser	Comments	References
Sb_2S_3	2.7	Ruby, 10^6–10^8 W/cm^2	100–3000 Å thick film per laser pulse	Smith and Turner (1965)
As_2S_3	2.4			
Fuchsine	—			
Se	2.4			
Ni–dimethyl gloxime	—			
ZnTe	2.7			
Te	5.0			
MoO_3	2.0			
$PbCl_2$	1.8		Carbon coating required	
PbTe	5.0			
Ge	3.8			
SiO		cw CO_2, 25 W	Rate: 4000 Å/min	Groh (1968)
ZnS			Rate: 4000 Å/min	
ZnSe			Rate: 4000 Å/min	
PbF_2			Rate: 4000 Å/min	
Na_3AlF_6			Rate: 3000 Å/min	
SiO_2			Rate: 2000 Å/min	
MgF_2			Rate: 1500 Å/min	
Si_3N_4			Rate: 200 Å/min	
$LaAlO_3$			Rate: 100 Å/min	
TiO_2			Rate: 35 Å/min	
Al_2O_3			Rate: 20 Å/min	
SiO	1.55–2.0	cw CO_2	Rate: 150 Å/sec	Hass and Ramsey (1969)
SiO_2	1.46		Rate: 400 Å/min	

Table 7.1 (*continued*)

Material	Refractive index	Laser	Comments	References
MgF_2	1.38		Rate: 1000–1500 Å/min	
Al_2MgO_4	1.70		Low evaporation rate	
Pt		cw Nd–YAG, 20 W	Rate: 0.2 Å/min	Hess and Milkosky (1972)
Cr, W, Ti, C		Nd:glass, 80–150 J 2–4 msec pulse	Rate: 10^5–10^6 Å/sec	Schwarz and Tourtellotte (1969)
Sb_2S_3			Rate: 10^5–10^6 Å/sec	
ZnS				
$SrTiO_3$				
$BaTiO_3$				
Ge		Ruby 10 J	Rate: 10^6 Å/sec	Zavitsanos and Sauer (1968)
GaAs		0.5–0.6 msec pulse		
SiO_2		cw CO_2 100 W	Rate: 2500 Å/min	Madami and Nichols (1971)
Al_2O_3			Rate: 50 Å/min	
Ir		Ruby, 100 J, 0.5 msec pulse	Rate: 10^6 Å/sec	Samson *et al.* (1967)
GaP		cw CO_2, 50 W	Rate: 10^2–3×10^2 Å/sec	Ban and Kramer (1970)
GaAs				
GaSb				
$CaTiO_3$			No evaporation	
Al_2MgO_4			No evaporation	

small volumes of the metal isolated from any heat sinks. Hess and Milkosky (1972) have evaporated platinum from the tip of a thin platinum wire to produce a film at the rate of 0.2 Å/min with a cw Nd–YAG power of less than 20 W.

The cw laser deposition of thin nonmetallic films has been shown to yield films of good mechanical and chemical stability (Groh, 1968). The infrared, visible, and ultraviolet optical properties of laser-evaporated films of SiO, SiO_2, and MgF_2 have been found to be almost identical to those deposited by conventional means (Hass and Ramsey, 1969), although an attempt to produce MgF_2 coatings on Al mirrors with high reflectivity at a wavelength of 1216 Å was unsuccessful.

Zavitsanos and Sauer (1968) have made a careful comparison between the structure of Ge and GaAs thin films produced with a pulsed ruby laser with those produced by conventional means. They noted that the degree of crystallinity obtained with laser-deposited films was attainable by conventional means only by heating the substrate to 200–400°C. Furthermore, electron diffraction patterns of GaAs films showed that GaAs was deposited without disproportionation (see also Poltavtsev *et al.*, 1972). A similar conclusion was reached by Schwarz and Tourtellotte (1969) in the laser deposition of barium titanate and strontium titanate films. It is uncertain at the present time whether dissociation of the parent molecules occurs on laser impact but is followed by recombination on the target with the same stoichiometry as the parent material or whether individual molecules are transported intact from the source to the substrate. Evidence in favor of dissociation has been given by Mirkin (1973), who found that the hardness of $A^{III}B^{V}$ semiconducting crystals such as GaP is drastically reduced at the point of laser impact. This observation together with X-ray structural analysis pointed to the presence of the group III metal (in this case, Ga) at the laser focus. Since Ga is much less volatile than P it would appear that this enrichment of the metallic component arose because of the selective evaporation of the volatile component. Ban and Kramer (1970) have found that congruent evaporation of III–V compounds occurs when a ruby laser is used, but not when a low-power cw CO_2 laser is used as the heat source.

Since many competing processes occur during evaporation with high-power lasers, it would be understandable if significant differences in chemical composition existed. This problem was first examined quantitatively by Baldwin (1970). By collecting the vapor ejected from brass samples of standard composition, it was established that the Zn/Cu ratio was considerably greater in the ejecta collected than that which characterized the original sample. The enrichment of Zn in the vapor was about 30% and did not seem to depend in any simple way on the energy or duration of the laser pulse. Heating thin brass foils and collecting the ejecta from the rear side of the foils resulted in samples that were enriched with Cu. It was found that the Zn/Cu ratio in the vapor correlated well with that of the equilibrium ratio at the melting temperature.

Kliwer (1973) performed similar but not identical experiments on brass, tool steel, and a wide variety of other materials. In this case, the Zn/Cu ratio in the condensate from laser-excited brass was within a few percent of that of the source material. This result was taken as evidence that congruent evaporation is attainable using laser pulse heating. Kliwer's result was further discussed and extended by Baldwin (1973), who demonstrated that the stoichiometry of a laser-deposited sample depends strikingly on the incident laser intensity and on geometrical factors such as the relative attitudes of the evaporating source and the collecting substrate. The enrichment of Zn in the vapor collected from brass that was 400% under low laser intensity excitation decreased to 75% as the laser intensity increased by a factor of 10. This result was obtained using normal pulses from a Nd : glass laser. With Q-switched pulses from the same laser, the enrichment of Zn dropped to about 30%. When all the ejecta were collected with normal pulse excitation, the Zn/Cu ratio was found to be identical to that of the source. Hence it appears that placement of the collecting substrate can affect the stoichiometry of the resulting film when normal pulses are used for evaporation. This geometrical effect occurs because liquid droplets can be collected if the substrate is placed off the optic axis. These droplets are known to be ejected at an angle with respect to the direction of propagation of the laser. Since the composition of the vapor and the liquid droplets differs from each other and also from that of the bulk material, it must be concluded that formation of an evaporated film of the same stoichiometry as that of the target when heating with normal laser pulses is rather a "hit or miss" proposition. This problem should not be as great when Q-switched pulses are used since there is less tendency for liquid to be ejected. Cw lasers, yielding a lower evaporation temperature and little if any ejection of a liquid phase, would seem to be more suitable for the production of films having compositions similar to that of the parent material.

In another application, the CO_2 laser has been used effectively in chemical vapor deposition (*Metals and Materials*, 1973). Reaction between a vapor and a surface occurs only in the region heated to the prescribed temperature by the focused laser beam. In the initial experiments, carbon, silicon, and silicon carbide have been deposited on aluminum using this technique. A related work reports the use of laser radiation to inhibit condensation of gold to form periodic structures (Little *et al.*, 1971). Gold is deposited on the substrate only at the nodes of a standing wave pattern produced by laser radiation on the substrate. This yields a periodic line structure of gold filaments separated by insulating regions.

A novel method of preparing pure superconducting films of Ag, Au, and Cu alloys with germanium has been reported by Alekseevskii *et al.* (1970,

1971). Films were produced by pulsed laser evaporation in a cryostat. This process was shown to result in the formation of new phases of these alloys that, while superconducting at temperatures in the 1–2°K range, did not retain their superconducting properties on warming to room temperature and recooling.

Laser sampling has been used to investigate the chemical composition of irradiated uranium oxide fuel rods (Adams and Tong, 1968). Samples of about 10^{-8} g were collected by laser deposition on glass substrates placed just over the laser-excited area of the target. These specimens were then studied by standard nuclear techniques to obtain the distribution and composition of isotopic species in the fuel rod.

7.3 SURFACE STUDIES

Conventional methods of cleaning surfaces in high vacuum systems include chemical etching, sputtering, electron beam desorption, and bulk heating. High-power laser pulses have also been shown to be effective in this application (Bedair and Smith, 1969; Gauthier *et al.*, 1969; Ertl and Neumann, 1972; Chen and Chang, 1972; Kuznetsov and Shchuka, 1972). Some advantages of laser desoprtion have been listed by Bedair and Smith. The most important of these is that the laser source is "clean" in the sense that no foreign species are introduced into the vacuum system by the heat source. On the other hand, scattered light can simultaneously degas other surfaces in the system, resulting in the production of a pressure pulse that may contaminate the sample. This effect can be minimized by careful control over focusing and by the provision of a port through which the specularly reflected beam may leave the system.

It has been pointed out by Bedair and Smith that the localization of the heating effect with laser excitation due to focusing and the short duration of a laser pulse means that only a surface layer on the sample is subjected to heating. Thus, impurities are not able to migrate into the surface layer from the bulk after the surface has been cleaned.

Chen and Chang (1972) investigated the desorption of Na and Cs from Ge substrates with both *Q*-switched and normal pulses from a ruby laser. With the same energy, *Q*-switched pulses are significantly more effective in producing desorption than are normal pulses. For a given initial surface coverage (less than one monolayer), the coverage decreases continuously with the number of laser pulses incident on the substrate to a limiting value that is attained after 4–10 pulses depending on the adsorbate and the initial coverage. In contrast to normal thermal desorption measurements, Cs is more effectively desorbed than Na with both Q-switched and normal pulses. It was suggested that a fundamental difference exists between the mechanisms of laser and thermal desorption.

The systems O_2 on Ni and S on Ni were studied by Bedair and Smith (1969). Surfaces were systematically exposed to fluxes that increased from 10 to 120 mW/cm², and the surface damage and change in O_2 coverage were reported. 60 MW/cm² was required to reduce the O_2 coverage on Ni significantly. No extensive surface damage with the exception of the presence of small surface craters was noted at this intensity after 10 laser pulses. At an intensity of 120 MW/cm², O_2 was completely desorbed, but this was accompanied by extensive surface damage. A similar effect was observed in the desorption of S from Ni. The attendant surface damage on degased substrates could not be removed by annealing. Adsorbed gases such as N_2, CO, H_2, CO_2, and H_2O could be removed effectively by much lower intensity pulses, typically 30 MW/cm². Strongly chemisorbed gases would seem, however, to require laser intensities above the damage threshold for efficient desorption.

Laser desorption of adsorbed gases such as H_2 and CO from chromium and tungsten surfaces has been reported by Kuznetsov and Shchuka (1972). The residual gas spectrum in a closed vacuum system was analyzed both before and after laser desorption. The bulk gas content in metal films on insulating substrates has been analyzed using a similar technique by Winters and Kay (1967, 1972). In this process, the laser is used to drill a hole in the film and the change in partial pressure of the gases in the system can be related to the gas content in the film. Selective gettering was used to remove certain molecules from the gas in the system, resulting in improved sensitivity for the other components. Noble gas and nitrogen concentrations in a wide variety of materials were determined. The ultimate sensitivity was reported to lie in the parts per billion to parts per trillion range for the inert gases and nitrogen. A similar system developed by Ivanovskii *et al.* (1968) and Ivanovskii and Varnakov (1969) had a sensitivity for nitrogen $\simeq 5 \times 10^{-4}$ wt. %.

7.4 THE LASER MICROPROBE

The ability of the laser to be focused to small areas and to subject these areas to intensities high enough to bring about evaporation has led to an application of lasers in the spectrochemical analysis of small samples. A practical laser microprobe instrument was first reported by Brech and Cross (1962). Since spectral lines emitted by the plume itself are often resonance-broadened and are also weak, it was found advantageous to combine laser excitation with an auxiliary spark, which discharges through the plume (see, however, Marich *et al.*, 1970). This spark is initiated by the passage of plume material between the pole pieces. A detailed description of a conventional laser microprobe system has been given by Rasberry *et al.* (1967a). A block diagram of their system is shown in Fig. 7.1. The spark source operated with the following parameters: voltage, 1500–2200 V; inductance, 0–155 μH; resistance, 0–10 Ω; capacitance 5–10 μF. Electrodes are usually spectroscopic-grade graphite and the gap between them should be as small as possible ($\leq$2 mm). In this system, the emission from the spark was recorded photographically on a 6.4-m Wadsworth-mount grating spectrograph using Kodak 103-0 plates. The grating had 600 grooves/mm and was blazed at 4500 Å. Strong lines from abundant elements could be recorded after only one excitation of the target but several pulses were required for weak lines. Using intense lines, metals have been detected at concentrations in the 10^{-11}–5×10^{-11} g range.

The proximity of the auxiliary spark electrodes to the sample necessary for effective coupling between the plume and the spark leads to the problem that the spark tends to contaminate a larger area of the sample than that sampled by the laser beam. The contamination is in the form of a stain, which often prevents visual observation of the target over an area of several square millimeters around an excited region (Rasberry *et al.*,

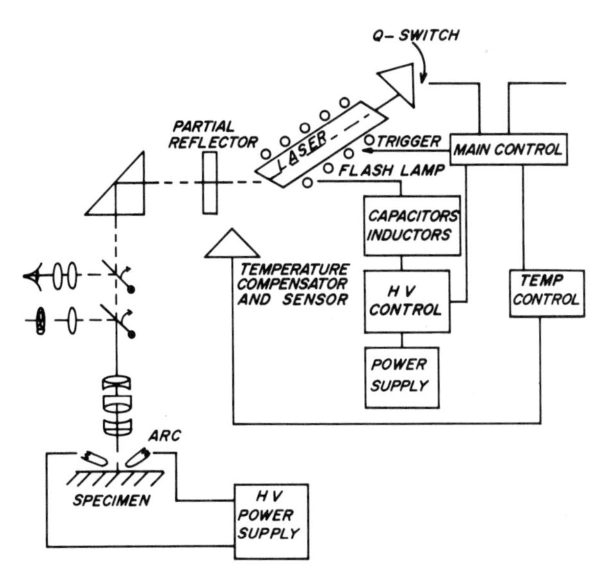

Fig. 7.1. Laser microprobe system of Rasberry *et al.* (1967a).

1967a,b). Contamination can be minimized by shielding all but the area to be excited with paper (Rasberry *et al.*, 1967a) or by a modification of the spark electrode geometry (Beatrice *et al.*, 1969). Schroth (1972) has demonstrated in a study of laser sampling of various metallic alloys, oxides, and sulfur compounds that elemental concentrations are most accurately determined using *Q*-switched as opposed to normal pulse excitation.

Improvements in the laser sampling system have been described by Peppers *et al.* (1968) and details of the modifications required for photoelectric detection of emission features have been given by Beatrice and Glick (1969).

Discrimination against background radiation emitted from the laser plasma itself has been accomplished by using time differentiation (Treytl *et al.*, 1971b) to reject the plasma continuum. Delay times $\lesssim 1$ μsec in measuring an integrated line intensity following the initiation of the 20-nsec *Q*-switched pulse were shown to significantly increase the signal/background ratio. This ratio was shown to depend not only on the time delay, but also on the laser pulse energy. Increases in the signal/background ratio of up to 2000% were possible when the time delay and laser pulse energy were optimized. In a later paper, Saffir *et al.* (1972) performed a statistical analysis of the interrelationship between spectral line intensities, background levels, and laser energy output for iron, zinc, and calcium in a variety of samples, using time discrimination. It was concluded that no significant increase in accuracy in determining concentrations of these elements was obtained by correcting the spectral line intensities for the background emission.

A strong matrix effect on the intensity of spectral line excited with the laser microprobe has been reported by Cerrai and Trucco (1968). Samples of Zircaloy, uranium, and an aluminum–manganese alloy exhibiting a variety of grain structures were probed by normal pulses from a ruby laser. With the Zircaloy sample, the 3457.56 Å Zr line was found to be extremely sensitive to the grain size in the excited region. The intensity of this line was 10 × larger when fine grained areas were probed than when the probed area had a coarse-grained structure. A clear correlation was noted between the intensity of the Cr 3360.3 Å line from type 304 stainless steel and the strain in prestressed samples. These effects were not noted in electron probe microanalysis of the same samples. No simple explanation of the dependence of elemental line intensities on the metallurgical properties of metallic samples would seem to be possible. However, Cerrai and Trucco's results do indicate that metallurgical structure may be reflected in spectral line intensities, and thus that the laser microprobe may in time become a useful tool in structural studies.

A matrix effect in laser probe microsampling of biological samples has been observed by Marich *et al.* (1970). They found that elemental metal concentrations above a certain threshold value in samples tended to decrease the emission line intensity of these elements in the gas phase. In a later paper Treytl *et al.* (1971a) found that both the intensity of spectral lines and the signal/background ratio depended strongly on the ambient atmosphere, although no systematic dependence on atmosphere and laser energy could be found. In both of the above experiments an auxiliary spark source was not used and only light from the plume was sampled.

Some other applications of laser microprobe sampling that have been reported in the literature include the determination of Fe, Mg, Mn, and Ca concentrations in garnets (Blackburn *et al.*, 1968), the investigation of meteorites (Nikolov *et al.*, 1970), the analysis of rare earth elemental concentrations in a number of materials (Ishizuka, 1973), and the determination of boron concentrations in steel (Webb and Cotterill, 1968).

7.5 MASS SPECTROMETRIC STUDIES OF LASER-INDUCED EVAPORATION

At the same time as interest was growing in the laser microprobe technique, it was realized that direct sampling of the vapor ejected from a sample irradiated with a laser pulse using a mass spectrometer was also possible. This approach offers the possibility of studying a wide range of evaporation conditions and the effect of these conditions on the chemical composition of evaporated species. One of the more interesting applications of such a system involves the possibility of studying the composition of vapor over solids at temperatures that exceed those attainable with conventional means.

The time of flight (TOF) mass spectrometer (Fig. 7.2) is well suited to

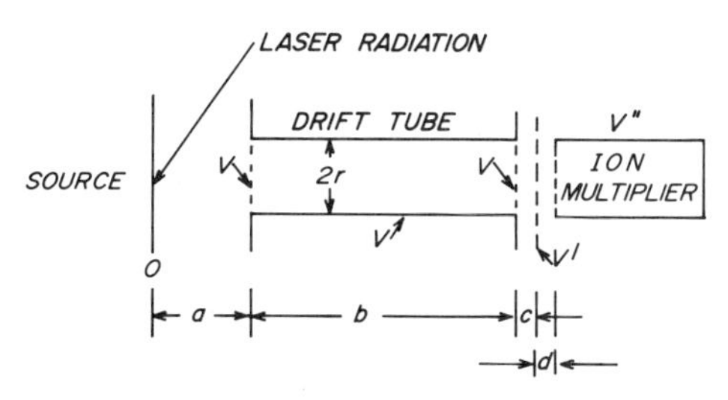

Fig. 7.2. Electrodes and voltages in a TOF mass spectrometer (after Bernal *et al.*, 1966).

studies of laser-induced evaporation, since with Q-switched laser pulses the ions (or neutrals, which are subsequently ionized) can be considered to be created instantaneously at $t = 0$. TOF mass spectrometers especially designed for laser evaporation studies have been described by Fenner and Daly (1966) and by Bernal *et al.* (1966), although the Bendix 12-107 TOF mass spectrometer has been used successfully by several groups (Vastola and Pirone, 1968; Zavitsanos, 1968; Knox, 1968). The design criteria for such an instrument have been reported by Bernal *et al.* (1966). Figure 7.2 shows a schematic of the electrode structure and voltages in such a device. The total time of flight

$$t = t_a + t_b + t_c + t_d$$

where

$$\begin{aligned} t_a &= 1.439(am^{1/2}/\epsilon)[(E_0 + \epsilon)^{1/2} - E_0^{1/2}] \\ t_b &= 1.439bm^{1/2}/2(E_0 + \epsilon)^{1/2} \\ t_c &= 1.439(cm^{1/2}/\epsilon')[(E_0 + \epsilon)^{1/2} - (E_0 + \epsilon - \epsilon')^{1/2}] \\ t_d &= 1.439(dm^{1/2}/\epsilon'')[(E_0 + \epsilon - \epsilon' + \epsilon'')^{1/2} - (E_0 + \epsilon - \epsilon')^{1/2}] \end{aligned}$$

are the times spent by an ion of mass m in each of the four regions, where E_0 is the initial energy of the ion, $\epsilon = eV$, $\epsilon' = eV'$, and $\epsilon'' = eV''$. The units of a, b, c, and d are centimeters, while those of m and t are atomic mass units and microseconds, respectively. Since t_b is usually much larger than any of the other times, $t \simeq t_b \propto \epsilon^{-1/2}$ when $\epsilon \gg E_0$. Typical values of the parameters might be $V = -1000$ V, $V' = 0$, $V'' = -400$ V, $a = 1.5$ cm, $b = 100$ cm, $c = 0.3$ cm, $d = 0.6$ cm, and $2r = 1.5$ cm. The drift time for constant values of these parameters will then depend only on m/e of the ion and on its initial energy E_0. In the regime where E_0 is comparable to ϵ, a range of initial ion energies will result in broadening of the detected current peaks. When the broadening due to this effect is greater than that produced by inhomogeneities in the accelerating field, the widths of a peak may be used to obtain information about the initial ion energies. Ions with initial energies of several tens of keV have been observed to be emitted from solids at relatively low incident laser intensities (Ready, 1971; see also Section 7.6).

The number of ions passing through the spectrometer to be detected can be estimated from simple kinetic and geometrical considerations. The result is (Bernal *et al.*, 1966)

$$n = n_0 r^2/[v_0^2(t_a + t_b)^2]$$

where n_0 is the total number of ions leaving the surface and v_0 their initial speed. n/n_0 may be as high as 10^{-4}, although Fenner and Daly (1966) report a value of 10^{-8}.

The vapor over graphite is known to contain a wide variety of polymeric carbon species (Berkowitz and Chupka, 1964, and references therein). This system was studied by Zavitsanos (1968) using a 15-J normal pulse ruby laser. Time resolution was 0.1 msec and samples could be obtained throughout the laser pulse. This and mass loss data were used to calculate an effective heat of vaporization $\Delta H_v = (44 \pm 9)$ kJ/g and an average molecular weight for the ejected species $MW_{av} = 18 \pm 4$. At the boiling point of graphite, ΔH should be 25.5 kJ/g, while $MW_{av} = 32.1$. Thus, it was concluded that chemical equilibrium was not established in the vapor during excitation. The time-resolved mass spectra showed that C_3 dominates in the vapor during the first part of the laser pulse and after the pulse is terminated. Toward the end of the laser pulse, C and C_2 are most abundant. Time-integrated mole fractions of carbon species over graphite were $X_C = 0.49$, $X_{C_2} = 0.24$, $X_{C_3} = 0.19$, $X_{C_4} = 0.03$, and $X_{C_5} = 0.05$. Other polymeric compounds up to C_{10} were also observed. These results differ significantly from those of Berkowitz and Chupka (1964), although the incident laser intensity was larger in the work of Zavitsanos (1968). Berkowitz and Chupka found that the abundances of ions with odd numbers of carbon atoms were higher than those with even numbers of carbon atoms up to C_8^+. C^+ and C_9^+ did not fit into this trend.

Knox and his collaborators have obtained a wealth of quantitative data on the species ejected from a wide variety of solid materials. The systems studied include Se (Knox, 1968), Bi–Se (Knox *et al.*, 1968), As–Se (Knox and Ban, 1968), Sb and Te (Ban and Knox, 1969), Bi compounds with group VIA elements (Ban and Knox, 1970a), and As and Sb compounds with group VIA elements (Ban and Knox, 1970b). By the addition of a secondary electron source to provide ionization, neutral as well as ionized species ejected under laser impact could be analyzed.

Atomic and molecular species observed over elemental Se, Sb, and Te by Knox (1968) and Ban and Knox (1969) are summarized in Fig. 7.3. These spectra were recorded about 0.6 msec after the start of a normal ruby laser pulse. The focused laser intensity was $\simeq 10^7$ W/cm^2, and spectra were reported to change as a function of time both during and after the laser pulse. The mass spectra recorded in Fig. 7.3 show that, contrary to expectation, a significant fraction of the ejected materials is in the form of complex molecules and molecular ions. Conventional thermal excitation of Te, for example, generates only Te and Te_2, accompanied by no ionic species or complex Te_n molecules. Ban and Knox (1969) suggested that the observation of complex species under laser evaporation could be accounted for if the laser flux heated these materials to temperatures near their critical temperatures. This, together with the pressure exerted by the evaporation

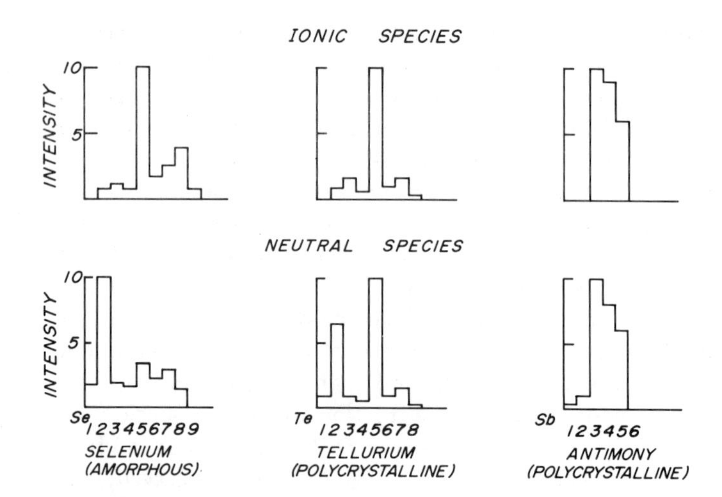

Fig. 7.3. Mass spectra of species ejected from Se, Te, and Sb under laser excitation [after Knox (1968) and Ban and Knox (1969)].

of material, could ensure that vaporization occurred close to the critical temperature. Evaporation at or near the critical temperature would lead to the production of a number of vapor species that cannot be produced in abundance at lower temperatures. Indeed, it is a well-known principle of high-temperature chemistry that the complexity of the vapor over a material increases rather than decreases as the evaporation temperature rises.

It has been suggested by Knox *et al.* (1968) that rapid evaporation as produced by a pulsed high-power laser may yield vapor species whose structure reflects that of the structural units within the solid. This effect was first noted in Knox's (1968) study of laser–induced evaporation of several different crystalline and amorphous forms of Se. The mass spectra of the ejected species showed a strong dependence on the structure of the parent solid and were even different for excitation on different crystal planes of the same crystalline sample.

In their studies of the chemical systems listed above, Knox *et al.* noted another significant difference between laser and conventional thermal evaporation mechanisms. It was found that ionic species never noted in thermal evaporation appeared in quantity during the laser pulse.* Toward the end of the laser pulse and subsequent to it, the ion current decreased

* The pulse duration was $\simeq$1 msec.

drastically and neutral species similar to those evaporated from conventionally heated solids were observed. It was suggested that the ionic species were produced in a "thermal shock" process similar to that expected with a *Q*-switched laser and perhaps involving the explosive removal of material. The neutrals could be produced by a quasi-normal boiling of the solid after the initial rapid heating by the laser pulse. Although this explanation is plausible, differences were noted between the composition of the neutral vapor and that produced by conventional heating (see Ban and Knox, 1970b) and this indicates that even at the end of the pulse evaporation is still far from "normal." In addition, the sampling process for neutrals, which involved ionization with low-energy (15-eV) electrons, may have contributed to some chemical changes in the species actually sampled by the mass spectrometer.

The laser-excited mass spectra of some organic solids have been investigated by Vastola and Pirone (1968) under similar experimental conditions. Ionic species were again seen only during the peak of the laser pulse, while neutrals were emitted even after the pulse had terminated. Ionic spectra of some conjugated aromatics showed predominantly mass peaks of the simply ionized parent ion and a few more massive ions. Those of some alkyl aromatic compounds and one amino acid showed parent ions, heavier ions, and fragments of the parent ion. To promote vaporization of these samples, many of which are transparent or translucent at the ruby laser wavelength, a thin layer of flakes of pyrographite was spread over the sample surface.

Geological materials have been studied by laser mass analysis (Scott *et al.*, 1971). Scott *et al.* used a modified double-focusing mass spectrometer together with a rapidly pulsed Nd laser and report that their system is especially sensitive to the alkali metals. Table 7.2 lists limits of detection for a number of elements. Samples were ground into powder form and compressed into pellets with or without a graphite binder. The graphite was reported to improve detection sensitivities for certain elements.

Megrue (1967) reports on the separation of isotopic mixtures of the rare gases from samples of meteoritic material by volatilizing microgram quantities of the material with a pulse from a ruby laser. The evolved gases were first separated cryogenically before analysis in a static mass spectrometer. In a related experiment, a *Q*-switched ruby laser has been reported to generate micromole quantities of O_2 on excitation of fused quartz (Biscar and Miknis, 1971) although in this case it is uncertain as to whether the O_2 was liberated from trapping sites within the quartz matrix by dissolution of the matrix under the effect of the laser pulse, or whether the laser initiated a chemical reaction that generated O_2.

Table 7.2

Detection Limits for Various Elements in Geological Materials by Laser Mass Analysis[a]

Element	Detection limit (ppm)	
	Without graphite binder	With graphite binder
Li	$\simeq 0.05$	$\simeq 0.05$
Na	$\ll 0.05$	$\simeq 0.05$
Mg	100	100
Si	20,000	200
K	$\ll 0.01$	$\ll 0.01$
Ca	20	20
Cr	100	25
Ti	50,000	200
Fe	200	20
Rb	<0.05	<0.1
Sr	50	15
Cs	≤ 0.1	$\simeq 0.1$

[a] After Scott *et al.* (1971).

Cw CO_2 laser-induced pyrolysis of $BaSO_4$ and BaS_2O_3 has been followed on a TOF mass spectrometer by Vanderborgh *et al.* (1971). Vapor ejected from solid samples of these materials was ionized by 100-eV electrons before passing into the mass spectrometer. Surprisingly, Ba^+ ions were not seen and the dominant mass peaks corresponded to those of SO^+, SO_2^+, and SO_3^+.

7.6 LASER-TRIGGERED SWITCHING

There has been sustained interest in the use of high-power pulsed lasers to trigger high-voltage spark gaps over the past ten years. The advantages of laser triggering of spark gaps have been summarized by Guenther and Bettis (1967, 1971). Principal advantages over conventional triggering mechanisms include:

(a) no electrical coupling between the voltages on the spark gap and the triggering source,

(b) the low delay and jitter associated with laser switching,

(c) a capability to switch spark gaps at high-pulse repetition frequencies while retaining small jitter,

(d) the possibility of synchronously switching a series of spark gaps with high temporal resolution.

In this section, some of the advances in laser-triggered switching made in the past ten years will be discussed. Further details are contained in the review articles by Guenther and Bettis (1970, 1971).

The initial charges responsible for subsequent breakdown of a laser-triggered spark gap may be produced in two ways. Figure 7.4 shows some methods of introducing the laser beam to effect this ionization. Focusing the laser output on one electrode of the spark gap yields a surface plasma that expands away from the electrode and produces further charge carriers by impact ionization of the atoms and molecules of the gas in the spark gap. Focusing the laser pulse within the gas in the spark gap can lead to direct production of a breakdown plasma at points removed from the electrode surfaces. When a high-power pulse traverses the gap to impinge on one electrode, a volume charge will be produced along the path of the laser beam through the gas, which conditions the gas so that an arc breakdown occurs along the path defined by the beam. This results (Guenther and Bettis, 1967) in single-channel arc breakdown with an attendant decrease in the time delay for breakdown over that attainable with conventional triggering mechanisms. It is evident then that laser impact can have the double effect first of producing a plasma to initiate breakdown, and second

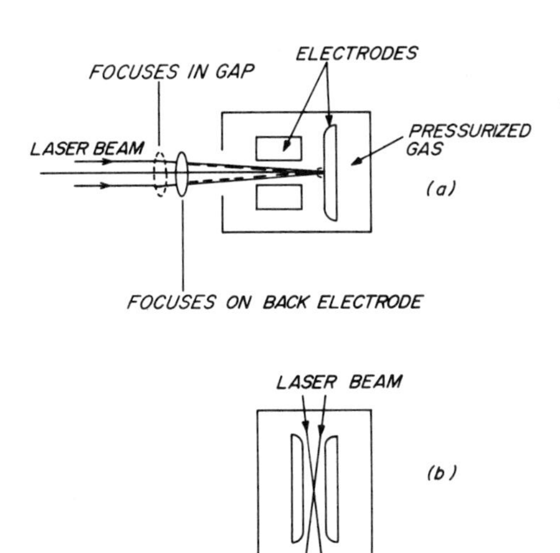

Fig. 7.4. Two methods of laser triggering of spark gaps. (a) Direct impact on electrode surface, (b) volume breakdown in gap.

of creating a path for the arc discharge to propagate between the electrodes of the spark gap. Both of these effects tend to increase the control over breakdown conditions and promote a well-defined breakdown current pulse.

Guenther and Bettis (1971) have modified the classical theory of gas breakdown in a spark gap to include the effect of laser ionization at one electrode. Their result for the time delay Δt_d between the creation of charge and the initiation of breakdown is given by

$$\Delta t_d = \frac{\ln n_c - N_0}{\alpha v} + \frac{d - \chi_c}{S} \tag{1}$$

where

α = Townsend first ionization coefficient $\alpha p[E/p]^m$
p = gas pressure in gap
E = field strength
m = constant
v = avalanche velocity (10^5–18^8 cm/sec)
n_c = critical number of electrons attained after avalanche propagates a distance χ_c, $= N_0 \exp(\alpha\chi_c)$
χ_c = distance at which avalanche converts to a streamer
N_0 = number of electrons initially produced at the cathode due to laser impact.
d = separation between electrodes.
S = streamer velocity (10^8–10^9 cm/sec)

The first term in Eq. (1) represents the time taken for the avalanche discharge to travel χ_c cm. The second term is the time for streamer propagation over the remaining distance $d - \chi_c$ to the anode. Breakdown first occurs via the formation of an avalanche discharge beginning at the cathode in which the initial N_0 charges are increased through electron impact to a charge n_c. Up to this stage, the discharge moves across the gap at a relatively low speed (10^5–10^8 cm/sec). When the number of charges reaches n_c, propagation proceeds via photoionization and a streamer is formed. The streamer propagates at a much higher speed (10^8–10^9 cm/sec) to terminate on the anode and result in massive breakdown between the electrodes.

The parametric dependence of Δt_d on p, E, N_0, etc., in Eq. (1) has been substantiated in a variety of experimental investigations (Pendleton and Guenther, 1965; Guenther and Bettis, 1967; Deutsch, 1968; Bettis and Guenther, 1970). Delay times approaching 1 nsec have been reported (Guenther and Bettis, 1967). Some data on the performance of laser-triggered spark gaps are collected in Table 7.3. A few generalizations from this and other work (Pendleton and Guenther, 1965; Steinmetz, 1968;

Table 7.3

Representative Data on Laser-Triggered Switching

Gas	N_2	Ar	85% Ar, 15% N_2	50% Ar, 40% N_2, 10% SF_6	Air	50% Ar, 50% N_2	N_2	50% Ar, 40% N_2, 10% SF_6
Pressure	5–10atm	5.8 bar	8 bar	24.5 kg/cm^2	to 30 atm	1200 Torr	11 atm	20 atm
Voltage	6 kV	12 kV	97 kV	550 kV	to 1.1 MV	34.5 kV	19 kV	3.05 MV
% of SBV[a]		95	85	97	80	92	95	94
Gap width		4 mm	8 mm	2 cm	0.75–3 cm	1.13 cm	$\simeq$0.5 mm	11 cm
Focusing		In gap or on electrode	In gap or on electrode	On electrode	On electrode	On electrode	On cathode	On electrode
Δt_d (nsec)				8	2	20	1	10
Jitter (nsec)	1	±0.5	±0.9		1	1	1	
PRF (pps)				0.01		50		
Laser power (MW)	0.5 (CO_2)	0.9	1	10	250	3.5		160
Reference	Nurmikko (1971)	Deutsch (1968)	Deutsch (1968)	Strickland *et al.* (1973)	Guenther and Bettis (1967)	Guenther and Bettis (1967)	Alcock *et al.* (1970)	Guenther and Bettis (1971)

[a] SBV: static breakdown voltage of gap.

Ujihara, 1968; Bradley *et al.*, 1969; Guenther *et al.*, 1970; Bettis and Guenther, 1970; Ujihara and Kamiyama, 1970) can be summarized as follows:

(a) Moderate laser powers (generally <10 MW) are sufficient to induce switching. These powers are easily attainable from conventional ruby, Nd, and pulsed CO_2 lasers.

(b) Under fixed conditions in the gap, delay and jitter both decrease with increasing laser power until a threshold is reached, at which point both of these parameters remain constant with increasing laser power.

(c) When Δt_d is less than the duration of the laser pulse, the jitter is minimized, although exceptions to this rule have been noted (Guenther and Bettis, 1971).

(d) The delay time Δt_d varies linearly with $1/p$ for constant E/p as predicted from Eq. (1).

(e) Favored electrode materials for laser impact initiated breakdown are Ta, W, Al, brass, and stainless steel, in roughly that order.

(f) A mixture of 90% Ar, 10% N_2 is favored for low jitter ($<\pm 0.1$ nsec; Bettis and Guenther, 1970).

(g) Switching can be achieved at rates of up to 50 pps with a jitter of ± 0.1 nsec.

(h) Voltages of up to 3 MV have been switched using laser triggering.

Bradley and Davies (1971) have described a useful modification of the usual method of laser triggering of spark gaps. In their method, a streamer is produced by conventional means, but then a synchronized pulse from an N_2 laser preionizes the gas in front of the propagating streamer. This causes its propagation speed to increase greatly, decreasing the overall delay time between the initiation of the discharge and the time at which breakdown occurs. The laser pulse traverses the gas parallel to the electrode surfaces.

Triggering can also be performed in a liquid dielectric (Marolda, 1968) and in solid state systems using lasers (Guenther and Bettis, 1971). Some applications of laser-triggered switching in quantum electronics have been reported by Michon *et al.* (1969), Ernest *et al.* (1966), and DeMaria *et al.* (1966).

7.7 LASER TRIMMING OF RESISTORS

We have seen in Section 6.7 that lasers may be used effectively in the micromachining of thin films on substrates. A logical extension of this fundamental work lies in the area of trimming thin-film resistors and capacitors to precise values using controlled deposition of heat from a pulsed laser. It is safe to say that trimming of resistors constitutes one of the widest applications of lasers in industry at the present time. This section outlines some of the benefits and problems associated with the use of lasers to trim thin- and thick-film electrical components. Some review articles on this subject are Gagliano *et al.* (1969), Thompson (1970), Ready (1971), Torrero (1972), Gagliano and Zaleckas (1972), Britton (1973), and Willis (1974).

Adjustments of the value of a thin-film resistor using laser heating may involve one or more of the following processes. The resistor may be trimmed by drilling a series of holes in the thin film at well-separated points (Fig. 7.5a) or by producing a continuous cut to remove part of the resistance element from the conduction path (Fig. 7.5b–d). Alternatively, the heat from the laser may be used to effect a thermally induced change in the resistivity of parts of the conducting element. The first two of these processes can only lead to an increase in the value of the resistance of the element; the third process may also make it possible to decrease the resistance in certain materials.

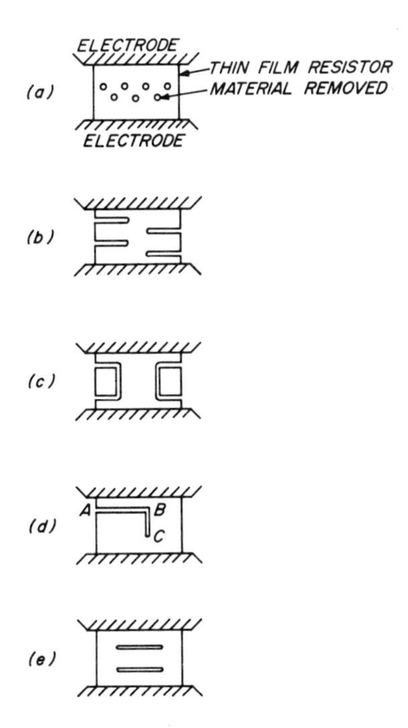

Fig. 7.5. Some methods of trimming thin-film resistors by laser evaporation.

An example of resistor trimming using the first technique has been reported by Unger and Cohen (1968). Tantalum nitride (Ta_2N) thin-film resistors formed on alumina substrates were trimmed by the evaporation of small holes using a *Q*-switched Nd : YAG laser. The diameter of these holes could be adjusted from 8 to 40 μm and an adjustment precision of $\simeq$0.01% per hole was reported when the number of holes was kept small. One immediate conclusion reached in the work of Unger and Cohen (1968) was that a given overall resistance change is best obtained by the evaporation of a small number of relatively large diameter holes, rather than by a large number of small holes. This effect occurs because the total heat-affected zone in the resistance film scales as the number of holes drilled and is relatively independent of their diameter. It was found that areas that had been heated to some extent changed their resistance, and furthermore, this change was found to be time dependent, so that the overall resistance drifted somewhat after trimming. Posttrimming drift was minimized when the trimming was accomplished using as small a number of holes as possible. For extremely high-tolerance trimming, a three-stage trim–drift–trim process may be more suitable. A study on the morphology of holes produced in thin resistive films has been reported by Stoyanova *et al.* (1972).

The production of continuous cuts in a thin-film resistor has also been shown (Thompson, 1970; Gagliano and Zaleckas, 1972) to be an effective method of trimming thin-film resistors. The cuts may be separate as in Fig. 7.5b,e or may be joined together to remove relatively large volumes of the resistive element as in Fig. 7.5c. Thompson (1970) points out that greatest sensitivity is obtained using the method shown in Fig. 7.5d. The initial cut $A \rightarrow B$ produces a relatively large $\Delta R/\Delta l$ where ΔR is the resistance change by removing the length Δl and yields poor sensitivity, in addition to increased heating during conduction at points in the film near B. By cutting in the direction $B \rightarrow C$, $\Delta R/\Delta l$ is smaller and the final resistance needed can be approached with greater sensitivity. Thus as small a cut as possible is made in the A–B direction, only enough to bring the total resistance into the range where the final value can be reached by a cut B–C, which is shorter than the distance between the electrodes. Obviously, the machining operations in Fig. 7.5c and 7.5d are equivalent.

It has been reported (Gagliano and Zaleckas, 1972) that posttrimming drift is less of a problem when the material is removed in continuous strips as shown above. Apparently this is due to a significant reduction in the heat-affected area when individual holes are caused to overlap.

An example of resistor trimming by laser-induced heating in the absence of vaporization has been described by Braun and Breuer (1969). It was found that laser heat could be utilized to anneal small areas in a chromium–silicon monoxide cermet resistor and thus to effect a *decrease* in resistance. A laser fluence of about 100 J/cm^2 incident for $\simeq$150 μsec was required to achieve the annealing temperature of 1000°C. Further studies on laser-induced resistivity changes in cermet resistors have been reported by Hardway and Callihan (1968) and Berg and Lood (1968), in silicon by Narasimha Rao (1968), and in beryllium films by Avotin *et al.* (1972).

A comparative study of laser trimming and air abrasive trimming has been published by Thompson (1970). Thompson points out that air abrasive trimming has the advantage of low cost and familiarity from many years of commercial use. Laser trimmers, on the other hand are more expensive, but may offer advantages in high-speed trimming and a cleaner operating environment. Certainly, laser trimmers are advantageous when the trimming of encapsulated components is required. With regard to a choice of lasers, precision trimming involving the removal of very small volumes of resistor limits consideration to those lasers (ruby, argon ion) with short-wavelength outputs that can be focused to the smallest possible spot sizes. YAG lasers are to be preferred over CO_2 lasers when the material to be trimmed reflects strongly at 10.6 μm. On the other hand, CO_2 lasers may be more effective in trimming thick-film devices. Since the depth of focus with CO_2 laser beams on focusing is intrinsically larger than that possible with short-wavelength lasers, CO_2 laser trimmers require less careful maintenance of the focusing lens–target distance.

Chapter 8

Spectroscopy and Laser-Induced Reactions

8.1 INTRODUCTION

The advent of the tunable laser represents a development that is likely in time to revolutionize spectroscopy. Until recently, the tunability of lasers was limited to wavelengths in the near infrared and visible. With the development of the spin–flip Raman laser, a variety of diode lasers, and two-photon techniques, the tuning range moved into the middle and far infrared. It is now likely that devices of this sort will eventually replace conventional light sources and spectrometers for high-resolution spectroscopic studies in this spectral region. This chapter discusses some aspects of the continuously developing area of high-resolution spectroscopy with lasers.

An area that will benefit greatly from the availability of tunable infrared lasers involves the optical separation of isotopes by selective excitation of vibrational levels leading to sensitized photocatalytic reactions of the irradiated isotopic species. Isotope separation can also be accomplished by the radiation pressure of laser light brought into resonance with a vibration–rotation line of a particular isotopic species. The economic benefits of a simple method of isotope separation with lasers are manifold and much work is proceeding on the development of suitable laser isotope separation systems.

A somewhat more prosaic but not unrelated application of lasers is described in the sections on laser-induced chemical reactions at surfaces and directly in the gas phase. A surprising and possibly important application of high-power cw CO_2 lasers, the gasification of hydrocarbon fuels such as coal, will be discussed.

8.2 LASER-INDUCED REACTIONS AT SURFACES

In this section we will consider two main types of reaction initiated by the focusing of intense laser light on solid surfaces. The first of these involves the use of a laser to create a plume of evaporated solid in vacuum or in a reactive gas. Reactions between the plume material and/or the heated substrate and the ambient gas will then lead to the production of further chemical species. Products of a reaction initiated in this way are expected to differ from those occurring when the solid is heated using more conventional means. Differences will be due to (i) the high temperatures possible with laser heating, (ii) the transient nature of the heating process, which makes attainment of true thermodynamic equilibrium unlikely, and (iii) rapid cooling of the reacting gas, which may quench in high-temperature reaction products.

The second type of laser-induced reaction to be considered involves the use of a laser strictly as a heat source to effect the degradation or pyrolysis of a chemical system. Here lasers offer the possibility of studying these processes at very high heating rates and at higher temperatures than attainable with conventional heating techniques.

The vapor over laser-heated graphite is known to consist of many different types of C_n species (Berkowitz and Chupka, 1964; Zavitsanos, 1968). The reaction of these molecules with gas phase molecules should yield a wealth of chemical compounds. Namba *et al.* (1969) have studied the species produced by laser heating graphite in hydrogen, ethylene, methane, ethane, and cyclopropane. After the laser-induced reaction had occurred, the product gases were identified by gas chromatography. Similar experiments were conducted by Schaeffer and Pearson (1969) and Blaxell *et al.* (1972). Acetylene was found to be the primary species generated. It was suggested that the reaction scheme was dominated by C_2 molecules ejected from the target. However, the work of Zavitsanos (1968) indicates that while C_2 is abundant after the laser pulse is terminated, C_3 is the most important gas phase molecule during the laser pulse, and the time integrated mole fraction of C is greater than that of either C_2 or C_3. Spectroscopic observations (Howe, 1963; Ferguson *et al.*, 1964; Mentall and Nicholls, 1967) of carbon flames produced in air show emissions from C_2 (Swan bands $A^3\Pi$-$X'^3\Pi$) and from CN ($B^2\Sigma$-$X^2\Sigma$ violet system). The Swan bands of C_2 were also seen on excitation of graphite in a hydrogen atmosphere (Namba *et al.*, 1969). It has been pointed out by Asmus (1971) that a carbon–hydrogen system in equilibrium at a temperature of 2000–4000°K has C_2H_2 as the primary product. Thus, pulsed laser heating of graphite in a hydrogen atmosphere would seem to yield primarily C_2H_2 as predicted from equilibrium thermochemical considerations.

Asmus (1971) has also considered the economic feasibility of producing C_2H_2 via cw CO_2 laser heating of graphite in hydrogen. Although it is concluded that such a process would not be competitive with more conventional means of producing C_2H_2, some advantages perhaps of importance in more economically attractive reaction schemes were noted. First, the temperature at which the reaction occurs and the atmosphere in the reaction chamber are independently variable and can be defined with some precision, since the heat source is external to the reaction chamber. Second, the time to quench the reaction and to bring the products back to room temperature can be orders of magnitude smaller with laser heating because of the high thermal gradients and small heated areas possible with focused coherent light. This effect is expected to minimize the effects of the competing reactions that may be of importance at temperatures lower than that at which the reaction of interest occurs. To these positive aspects of laser heating one must add the disadvantage that the laser beam must be brought into the reaction chamber through the reacting gas. At high flux levels, the incident radiation may induce gas phase dissociation or even breakdown and may in this way interfere with the production of the desired chemical compound.

The related subject of the pyrolysis of coals using high-power pulsed or cw lasers has been discussed in the literature by Sharkey *et al.* (1964), Karn *et al.* (1967, 1969, 1970), Shultz and Sharkey (1967), Karn and Singer (1968), Karn and Sharkey (1968), Joy *et al.* (1968, 1970), and Asmus (1971).

High-temperature volatilization of coal yields large quantities of methane and hydrogen. The methane–acetylene conversion $2CH_4 \leftrightarrow C_2H_2 + 3H_2$ is favored by high temperatures and there has thus been much interest in the use of high-power lasers as heat sources for the carbonization of coals. As early as 1964, Sharkey *et al.* (1964) began investigating the products evolved from coals heated with pulses from a ruby laser. The laser heating process was shown to produce gases richer in acetylene, carbon monoxide, and hydrogen cyanide than those possible with conventional high-temperature carbonization techniques.

Studies of the species emitted from coals during irradiation with a ruby laser pulse (Joy *et al.*, 1968, 1970) using a TOF mass spectrometer with a time resolution of 0.2 msec showed an enormous variety of radicals with little relation to the known cracking patterns of the light hydrocarbons released on normal coal carbonization. The principal hydrocarbon peak in these spectra was that of acetylene, although some polyacetylene species were also noted.

The effect of gas composition of the incident laser intensity (Karn *et al.*, 1969) showed that the number of moles of gas produced in a single laser pulse increased only slowly with laser intensity once a threshold value ($\simeq$50 kW/cm^2) was exceeded. A 10-W cw CO_2 laser focused to yield an intensity of 0.2 kW/cm^2 produced little volatilization. By assuming chemical equilibrium was reached during heating for C_2H_2 and CH_4, the equilibrium constant for the reaction

$$2CH_4 \rightarrow C_2H_2 + 3H_2$$

could be calculated from the measured gas concentrations and then compared with equilibrium values to estimate the temperature of the system. The temperature worked out in this way was $\simeq$1350°K and was more or less independent of laser intensity for intensities $\gtrsim$50 kW/cm^2. The temperature calculated for irradiation with the 10-W cw CO_2 laser was $\simeq$830°C. There should, however, be no problem in achieving any required volatilization temperature with currently available cw CO_2 lasers. The economics of large-scale gasification of coal with a gas dynamic CO_2 laser have been investigated theoretically by Asmus (1971).

The related problem of obtaining hydrocarbon fuels from oil shale has been studied by Biscar (1971). With laser pyrolysis, acetylene is again the major product. Other products are methane and ethylene. It was shown that a linear relation exists between the Fischer assay yield of samples and the quantity of acetylene liberated by a laser pulse. The laser technique of measuring the hydrocarbon content of oil shales would seem on the basis of this work to offer an attractive, faster method of assay than the conventional Fischer method.

Modifications to commercial gas chromatographs to permit immediate sampling of the products arising from the degradation of organic solids by laser pulses have been reported by Folmer and Azarraga (1969), Guran *et al.* (1970), and Ristau and Vanderborgh (1970, 1971). In these systems laser radiation passes through a window to impinge on a sample directly in the gas-chromatographic stream. The gas flow continues throughout the period for which the sample is irradiated and for some seconds afterward. Subsequently the gas flow may be diverted to pass directly to the chromatograph, allowing the sample to be changed. To aid in absorption of laser light by the sample, it may be coated with powdered graphite or carbon black (Folmer and Azarraga, 1969; Folmer, 1971). An alternative approach was suggested by Fanter *et al.* (1972), which involved coating a blue cobalt glass rod with the material to be pyrolyzed. When the layer was thicker than a few tenths of a millimeter, the pulsed laser produced no vaporization of the glass. However, absorption of laser light occurred at the sample–glass interface and this was found to be where pyrolysis occurred.

Degradation of many aromatic compounds by focused ruby laser radiation has been shown to lead primarily to the products methane and acetylene (Wiley and Veeravagu, 1968; Ristau and Vanderborgh, 1971). The ratio of methane to acetylene is low for polycyclic aromatics and high for monocyclic aromatics. While the formation of acetylene from aromatic compounds is understandable, the quantities of methane produced are not subject to such a simple explanation, although methane is formed on conventional thermal degradation of these compounds. In addition to these low-molecular-weight compounds, heavier compounds are also produced on laser degradation. It has been suggested (Ristau and Vanderborgh, 1971) that these compounds are formed by direct fragmentation of the parent species. The heavier molecular weight compounds are not thought to be stable in the plume itself and thus must be ejected at oblique angles away from the heated surface. Low-molecular-weight compounds are, on the other hand, apparently created in the plume by recombination of smaller fragments. There is a clear analogy here with the observed evaporation mechanisms that are observed in the erosion of metal surfaces with high-power normal laser pulses (Section 5.2). With metals, atomic fragments are ejected along with droplets of liquid metal. Droplets may be ejected almost parallel to the target surface, while vaporized species move mainly back along the optic axis. One could then identify the low-molecular-weight mass fraction in laser degradation experiments with the vapor ejected from a metal surface. The high-molecular-weight fraction would correspond in analogy to liquid droplets.

Laser pyrolysis of some polymers has been shown to yield degradation products that are similar to those expected from 1200–1500°K thermal pyrolysis. The main degradation products of polystyrene were acetylene, styrene, benzene, ethylene, methane, and toluene. Polyethylene yielded ethylene, acetylene, methane, pentene, hexane, benzene, and octane. In the polystyrene pyrolysis, acetylene was the principal product at all incident laser energies, while ethylene and styrene were produced in quantity only at low incident energies.

Thermal degradation of an epoxy using a 100-W cw CO_2 laser as a heat source was followed thermogravimetrically by Vlastaras (1970). The laser was used to heat a small platinum crucible to temperatures in the range 300–500°C. The volatilization of the epoxy contained in the crucible could be discerned by its mass change as measured on the electrobalance. Complete volatilization of Union Carbide type ERL-4221 epoxy resin cured with hexahydrophthalic anhydride was accomplished by 2–7 min of heating to a temperature of from 373 to 455°C. Degradation products were analyzed on a gas chromatograph, and mass spectrometrically. Infrared spectra of the undegraded polymer and the degradation products were compared. Spectral features due to water, carbon dioxide, methyl formate, and acetone were seen in the ir spectrum of the degradation products. Additional products noted in the mass spectrometer spectra included toluene, pyridine, hexatriene, methylacetylene, and butadiene.

A comprehensive study of some of the factors that affect the reproducibility of laser pyrolyses of organic materials has been reported by Folmer (1971). A number of polymeric materials were pyrolyzed using direct-sampling gas-chromatographic analysis of the degradation products. It was found that good reproducibility was obtained if the samples were strongly absorbing at the ruby laser wavelength or if they were mixed with carbon powder to increase their absorption. Carbon was, however, found to have an effect on the pattern of fragment peaks produced, and it was suggested that care should be taken in comparing the spectra of samples that do not have the same carbon content. In this regard, the work of Ristau and Vanderborgh (1972) offers some interesting insights into the effects of carbon loading on the degradation products from laser photolysis. A number of inorganic metallic salts were irradiated with and without the presence of carbon powder. The degradation products showed marked changes when carbon was included in the samples. As an example, Ag_2SO_4 irradiated in the pure state gave SO_2, O_2, and metallic Ag as degradation products. Mixing with carbon resulted in the formation of CO, O_2, and CO_2 in addition to metallic Ag. There was no evidence of sulfur compounds in the gas phase, although elemental sulfur was left in the pyrolysis tube. Thus the composition of the degradation products was completely altered by the presence of a small amount of carbon. Changes of this sort are relatively easy to follow in inorganic systems because degradation products containing carbon can be assumed to be generated from some reaction involving the carbon filler. In organic systems, this effect will act to change the C/H ratio in degradation products and thus may be more difficult to distinguish from true changes in the degradation products. The need to modify samples to make them absorbing at the laser wavelength should be less important with pulsed or cw CO_2 lasers because many organic materials absorb strongly at 10.6 μm.

Reactions between sulfur and hydrocarbons were studied by Miknis and Biscar (1972) using a sulfur substrate irradiated with pulses from a *Q*-switched ruby laser to generate sulfur species in a hydrocarbon gas. The only product molecule containing both C and S was CS_2. This molecule can be formed in the plume via the C atom insertion reaction

$$C + S_2 \rightarrow CS_2$$

S_2 may be formed by direct evaporation or by the dissociation of a S_n polymer. C may be formed by gas breakdown at the target (Adelman, 1966).

The laser-induced degradation of a variety of copper and nickel carboxylic acid salts and the subsequent reaction of the decomposed fragments with simple hydrocarbons has been investigated by Kim *et al.* (1971). Inoue *et al.* (1973) describe a direct imaging process that involves the ruby laser decomposition of metal halides. The process of direct deposition of metallic layers on substrates by the laser or electron beam decomposition of some inorganic oxides has been discussed by Martin *et al.* (1968). Decomposition will occur at a temperature such that the partial pressure of O_2 over the oxide exceeds the ambient O_2 pressure. However, decomposition with removal of the oxygen to leave an adhering metallic layer on the substrate is a much more complex process and only certain oxides would appear to be suitable. Some data given by Martin *et al.* on the most suitable systems for this process are listed in Table 8.1. A primary consideration is that the decomposing compound must not be highly volatile at the decomposition temperature. Data in Table 8.1 are listed in descending order of preference as determined by the above considerations.

8.3 LASER-INDUCED REACTIONS IN THE GAS PHASE

Lasers may be used to induce gas phase reactions among a number of components in a variety of ways. If the laser wavelength coincides with that of an atomic or molecular transition of a component of the mixture, then this species may be selectively excited by the absorption of laser energy. This excitation may simply be radiated away in the form of one or more quanta of energy, in which case a reaction may not occur. Alternatively, it can be transferred in whole or in part to another component of the mixture via collision. Such collisions can also lead to the formation of new chemical species. If the laser excitation is into a level that causes the absorbing molecule to dissociate, then the products of this dissociation may undergo further reactions. Photoionization of an atom or molecule

Table 8.1

Temperature Range in Which Various Metallic Oxides Can Be Thermally Decomposed on a Substrate to Deposit a Metallic Layer[a]

Oxide	Minimum decomposition temperature (°C) at $P_{O_2} = 10^{-6}$ atm	Maximum permissible (°C) decomposition temperature at[b]			Allowable temperature (°C) range $T_{max} - T_{dec}$ at[b]		
		10 mm/sec	100 mm/sec	1000 mm/sec	10 mm/sec	100 mm/sec	1000 mm/sec
Gold	—	1910	2210	2610	—	—	—
Silver	<150	1370	1620	1940	1220	1470	1790
Rhodium	590	2690	3050	3680	2100	2460	3090
Platinum	230	2660	3100	3560	2430	2870	2330
Palladium	280	2050	2400	2880	520	810	960
Copper	1130	1650	1940	2090	520	810	960
Nickel	1330	1900	2120	2440	570	790	910
Lead	1130	1000	1190	1480	—	60	350

[a] From Martin *et al.* (1968).
[b] Producing metallic line of 25-μm width and 10-μm thickness.

may occur due to single- or multiple-photon absorption. The resulting fragments will also be capable of undergoing further reaction.

At high incident laser intensities, the gas can break down electrically with the formation of a spark, which releases quantities of ions and electrons as well as short-wavelength radiation into the background gas. Needless to say, such a process will result in the generation of other chemical species either through direct reaction with neutral or charged radicals in the spark or through photochemical processes initiated by the ultraviolet light emitted from the breakdown plasma.

Conventional photochemistry involving direct excitation of electronic states several eV above the ground state in a gas phase system is not possible with CO_2 lasers because of the small energy ($\simeq$0.1 eV) of a quantum of CO_2 laser radiation. However, vibrational transitions can be directly excited, and this may lead to the formation of molecular species having high degrees of vibrational excitation through upward cascading driven by the absorption of several low-energy quanta. These species can then undergo chemical reactions. The products of such reactions are expected to be similar to those occurring in thermal reactions, but the quantity of reaction products will depend not on free-energy differences as in conventional thermally induced reactions but on the absorption coefficient of the reactants as in a photochemical reaction (Yogev *et al.*, 1972).

Next we will discuss some reactions produced in laser-induced gas breakdown and the question of photochemistry with infrared lasers. One of the first studies of the chemical species produced in gas breakdown of organic vapors was reported by Adelman (1966). A *Q*-switched ruby laser was used and breakdown thresholds corresponded to laser intensities in the 10^7–10^8 W/cm^2 range. CCl_4, $CHCl_2$, CH_3OH, hexane, and acetone were irradiated and spectral emission from the resulting spark showed the presence of C_2, C, C^+, and C^{2+} in all systems together with Cl^+ and O^+ in the systems containing these elements. Compounds present in the CCl_4 and $CHCl_3$ systems following the decay of the excitation included tetrachlorethene, hexachloroethane, hexachlorobenzene, and octachloronapthalene. Similar experiments (Wiley and Reich, 1970) on the degradation of gaseous aliphatic hydrocarbons and cyclopropane presumably in the absence of laser breakdown yielded methane, ethylene, and acetylene as the primary gas phase reaction products. When breakdown occurs in methane, the primary products are C_2H_6, C_2H_2, C_4H_4, and C_3H_4 (Epstein and Sun, 1966). In the absence of breakdown the compound 1,4-dioxane decomposes when subjected to a flux of *Q*-switched ruby radiation to give hydrogen, ethylene, carbon monoxide, and a trace of formaldehyde (Watson and Parrish, 1971). It was suggested that the initial decomposition in this case was due to a multiphoton absorption to a dissociating state of the irradiated molecule. Breakdown of oxygen gas containing small amounts of the sulfur compounds thiacyclobutane and thiacyclopentane with a *Q*-switched ruby laser pulse has been shown to yield the products CO_2, SO_2, H_2S, H_2O, COS, CS_2, and C_2H_2 (Miknis and Biscar, 1971). Although the mechanisms of the reaction with *Q*-switched pulses could not be accurately defined, this reaction did not occur when a normal laser pulse was passed through the mixture.

A *Q*-switched ruby laser pulse passed through a vacuum system containing residual gases at a pressure of 10^{-9} Torr produced the ions CH_2^+, $C_2H_n^+$, and $C_4H_n^+$, with $n \simeq 6$, due to multiphoton ionization of residual organic impurity molecules (Evans and Thonemann, 1972). This indicates that the initial stages of reactions initiated by gas breakdown may be dependent on minute amounts of organic molecules that act as sources for the first few electrons and ions, which subsequently promote total breakdown of the gas. It further illustrates the ease with which molecules in high-energy states can be created in a nominally transparent gas through the processes of stepwise excitation through single-photon absorption and through direct excitation of higher electronic states via multiphoton absorption. Since stepwise excitation and multiphoton processes will depend greatly on the wavelength of the incident laser radiation, a change in wavelength may very well occasion a change of reaction products in laser breakdown of a particular gaseous system. For this reason, the reaction products reported above may no longer be those that dominate when the same chemical systems are irradiated with high-power CO_2 laser radiation.

A number of gas phase molecules that absorb energy strongly at wavelengths emitted by the CO_2 laser (NH_3, SF_6, C_2H_4) exhibit intense fluorescence when irradiated with relatively low cw laser fluxes. This fluorescence can extend shortwards from 10.6 μm through the infrared into the visible region of the spectrum or to longer wavelengths into the far infrared. Radiation emitted to the long-wavelength side of 10.6 μm can be due to rotational transitions of the absorbing molecule or to vibration–rotation bands of the absorber or a chemical compound produced from the absorber. Transitions on the short-wavelength side of 10.6 μm, which at first glance might seem to be in violation of conservation of energy laws, can occur when several 10.6-μm quanta are absorbed in a stepwise process resulting in subsequent relaxation through emission of more energetic quanta. Short-wavelength radiation ($\lambda < 1$ μm) should really be termed chemiluminescence, since in these systems it is usually due to the emission by species that are excited as a result of chemical reactions.

Initial studies of the emission from NH_3 gas excited with a cw CO_2 laser

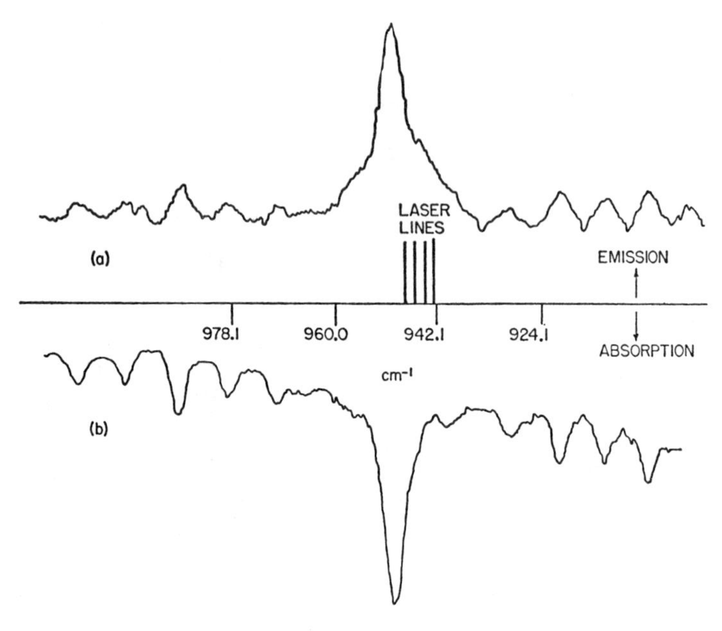

Fig. 8.1. Spectra of ethylene at 50 Torr in the cell described in the text. (a) Emission spectrum, (b) absorption spectrum. Exciting laser lines are located at 945.96, 944.18, 942.35, and 940.49 cm^{-1} as indicated in the figure (from Ronn, 1968).

(Rigden and Moeller, 1966; Bordé *et al.*, 1966a) showed that significant dissociation of NH_3 was produced with cw laser fluxes as low as a few hundred watts per square centimeter. NH_2, the product of this dissociation, emitted strongly in the visible near 6000 Å when the NH_3 pressure was greater than about 50 Torr. Intense infrared fluorescence at 10 μm (Ronn, 1968; Suzuki and Suzuki, 1968) and at 30–50 μm (Suzuki and Suzuki, 1968) from NH_3 has also been reported. The 10-μm emission from NH_3 is due to emission from the first excited vibrational state of this molecule to the ground state.

Ethylene (C_2H_4) also absorbs strongly at the CO_2 laser frequency. In this case absorption is due to the excitation of the ν_7 (b_{1u}) mode (Herzberg, 1945). Both visible (Bordé *et al.*, 1966b) and infrared (Ronn, 1968; Robinson *et al.*, 1968) light are emitted from C_2H_4 under excitation with a cw CO_2 laser. Figure 8.1 shows a comparison between the emission and absorption spectrum of C_2H_4 in the vicinity of the CO_2 laser frequencies (Ronn, 1968). Most rotational transitions in the ν_7 band are seen in emission at the pressures used (50 Torr) since the time for thermalization of rotational levels is several orders of magnitude shorter than the vibrational relaxation time. Some ethylene is converted by the action of the CO_2 laser radiation into acetylene (Quel and de Hemptinne, 1969) and an explanation of this effect together with a discussion of the dependence of conversion rates on chopping frequency under ac irradiation has been proposed by de Hemptinne (1973). Other compounds formed by the degradation of C_2H_4 with a cw CO_2 laser beam (Cohen *et al.*, 1967) are hydrogen, methane, butadiene, benzene, and diacetylene.

The infrared emission spectra of a wide variety of gaseous hydrocarbon molecules during excitation with a cw CO_2 laser were investigated by Robinson *et al.* (1968). Surprisingly, emission was seen even from those molecules (i.e., CH_4) that have no significant absorption at the CO_2 laser wavelength. Robinson *et al.* suggested several means by which excitation of molecules can occur in the absence of direct resonance between energy levels of the system and the incident laser wavelength. However, it was later demonstrated by Bailey *et al.* (1971) that emission by molecules such as CH_4 can be sensitized by the presence in the gas phase of small quantities of an absorbing species. Absorption of laser radiation by the sensitizing molecules acts as a mechanism whereby excitation may be transferred to other molecules in the system that have no absorption at the laser wavelength. These molecules can then radiate in the normal way to dispose of their excess energy. Despite the observation that direct excitation is unlikely to be the cause of infrared emission from nonabsorbing molecules, the thesis of Robinson *et al.* (1968) that CO_2 lasers may be used as an analytical tool in the identification of trace amounts of gas phase organic molecules through the initiation of infrared emission is still valid, since in real chemical systems there are often background impurities present that can provide the necessary means of energy transfer to excite nonabsorbing species.

Absorption of CO_2 laser radiation by gaseous components such as SF_6 and BCl_3 followed by transfer of this energy to other species has been used as the basis for a laser-modulated mass spectrometer by Kaldor and Hastie (1972).

The visible luminescence noted previously in many organic systems irradiated with the cw CO_2 laser is also seen with pulsed TEA CO_2 laser excitation at intensities below the threshold for breakdown (Isenor and Richardson, 1971). Isenor and Richardson show that this emission is localized along the path of the beam but may extend both backward and forward from the focal volume along the beam. When breakdown sparks occur in these systems, the spark is approximately 10^3 times more intense than the luminescence excited prior to breakdown and extends over a larger volume. The spark spectrum may include the Swan bands of C_2, but atomic and ionic lines are most prominent. The luminescence spectrum of pure CCl_2F_2, pure C_3H_8, and CH_4 sensitized by SiF_4 showed the Swan bands. SiF_4 luminesced at 4368 Å in the α band of SiF. A study of the question of the probability of multiphoton dissociation of gas phase molecules excited with high-power CO_2 laser pulses has recently been made by Pert (1973). It appears that the dissociation observed by Isenor and Richardson (1971) can be explained by this process.

A quantitative study of the photochemical reactions of limonene and isoprene induced by a cw CO_2 laser has been reported by Yogev *et al.* (1972). Two pressure regimes, low (<3 Torr) and high (>3 Torr), were investigated. Reaction products were found to depend on the pressure of the absorbing gas and this was taken to indicate that reaction mechanisms differ in the two pressure ranges. At 1 Torr, isoprene underwent reactions that led to the formation of benzene, toluene, ethylbenzene, methylethylbenzene, and isomers of allocimene and dihydrolimonene, as well as low-molecular-weight compounds such as C_2H_2, C_4H_4, and C_4H_6. No reaction was observed at pressures in the range 3–30 Torr, but above 30 Torr dimeric products of uncertain structure were formed. In the low-pressure regime, the concentration of reaction products peaked at a gas pressure of about 0.05 Torr. An analysis of activation and deactivation rates for isoprene showed that successive absorption of photons was possible in the low-pressure regime. The reaction was tentatively ascribed to photochemical processes initiated by isoprene molecules that had absorbed several laser quanta. At high pressures (>30 Torr) the concentration of reaction products increased continuously with an increase in pressure. Since isoprene becomes optically thick at pressures in this range while collisional deactivation severely limits the concentration of molecules that have absorbed more than one quantum, the incident beam acts only to heat the gas. The reaction products should be those characteristic of a normal thermally induced reaction.

In an attempt to describe the mechanisms involved in CO_2 laser decomposition of molecular gases, Bailey *et al.* (1974) have examined the decomposition of ethyl chloride (EtCl). The thermal decomposition of EtCl has been extensively studied (see references in Bailey *et al.*, 1974) and thus much supporting data on possible reaction mechanisms are available. At a pressure of 80 Torr or greater, EtCl was found to decompose immediately upon exposure to the flux from a 200-W cw CO_2 laser to yield the products C_2H_4, HCl, CH_4, C_2H_2, H_2, C_6H_6, and larger aromatics. Below 80 Torr a delay in the decomposition was noted, which depended on gas pressure and laser power. Time-resolved infrared spectra of the gas and monitoring of the cell pressure showed that while the HCl concentration grew rapidly during the first few seconds of irradiation, C_2H_2 and C_2H_4 were not seen until after a delay of several seconds. The HCl emission grew to a maximum value and then decayed as the C_2H_2 and C_2H_4 concentrations increased. A strong emission at 1300 cm^{-1} due to overlapped features of EtCl and CH_4 was observed to build up during the first few seconds and then subsequently to decay as $[C_2H_2]$ and $[C_2H_4]$ increased. These results were taken to indicate that the species HCl and C_2H_4 were generated directly from EtCl, while C_2H_2 came from the decomposition of C_2H_4. It was tentatively suggested that CH_4, which was produced under these conditions but not in conventional thermal decomposition, may be produced via a selective excitation of the EtCl.

8.4 SPECTROSCOPY WITH INFRARED LASERS

Two approaches may be adopted in studies of materials using infrared absorption spectroscopy. Simply stated, wavelength discrimination can be achieved either by tuning the source that provides the radiation absorbed by the sample, or by tuning the detector while exposing the sample to the light from a continuum source. Conventional infrared spectrometers can be used in either of these ways. In the first, the sample is exposed only to a narrow range of wavelengths as determined by the spectrometer, which acts as a tunable source. In the second, the sample is exposed to light from a continuum source and the spectrometer acting as a tunable detector analyzes the light transmitted by the sample. Spectral resolution in both of these configurations is limited by the spectrometer and the low intensities available from conventional infrared sources. The development of tunable infrared laser sources that replace both the conventional radiation source and the spectrometer has largely overcome both of these problems. A comparison of conventional and laser infrared spectrometer systems is shown schematically in Fig. 8.2. Some tunable infrared laser sources include the spin–flip Raman laser, a family of diode lasers based on $Pb_{1-x}Sn_xTe$ (Hinkley, 1970), parametric oscillators pumped by Nd : YAG (Wallace, 1970; Goldberg, 1970) or ruby radiation (Yarborough *et al.*, 1969; Johnson *et al.*, 1971), and a method of mixing CO_2 laser radiation with a variable microwave frequency developed by Corcoran *et al.* (1970).

The linewidth of tunable laser sources can be as small as 10^{-6} cm^{-1} but the spectral resolution that this implies cannot always be obtained because spectral linewidths in gases are often Doppler broadened to widths that are orders of magnitude larger than this. Nevertheless, even with the obscuring effect of Doppler broadening, infrared spectra obtained with tunable laser

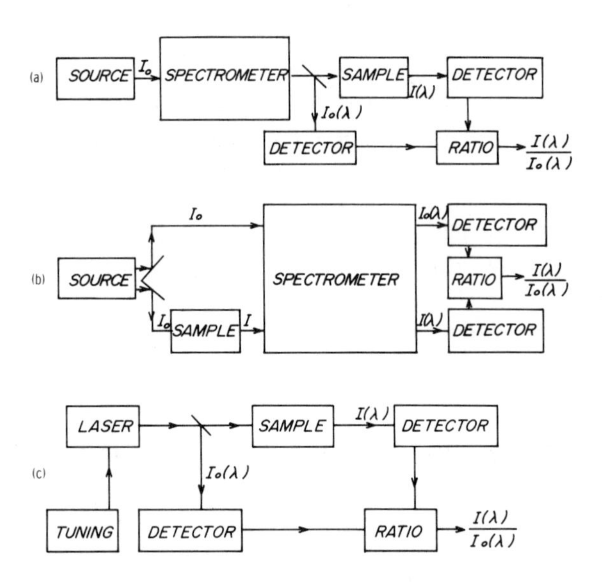

Fig. 8.2. Conventional (a, b) and laser spectrometers (c).

sources (particularly diode laser sources) reveal much more structure than those obtained with the best conventional infrared spectrometers. A revealing comparison between the capabilities of the tunable diode laser with those of a conventional grating spectrometer in resolving infrared spectra has been published by Ewing (1972).

Spectral studies performed with the spin–flip Raman laser (Patel *et al.*, 1970; Wood *et al.*, 1972; Ganley *et al.*, 1974) show that the linewidth available from this device is often >0.01 cm^{-1} or several times larger than the Doppler width of spectral lines in gases at room temperature ($\simeq 10^{-3}$ cm^{-1}), although a direct measurement of the linewidth (Patel, 1972) indicated <1 kHz. Limitations on this linewidth provided by the spin–flip Raman mechanism have been discussed by Patel *et al.* (1970), Hinkley (1971), Brueck and Mooradian (1971), Brueck and Blum (1972), and Colles *et al.* (1974).

Figure 8.3 shows a block diagram of a spin–flip Raman system using frequency doubled CO_2 laser radiation as the pump (Wood *et al.*, 1972). This system was used in an absorption study of NO gas in the 5–6 μm region. The crystal used was n-type InSb pumped with 50-W peak power pulses at $\lambda = 5.15$ μm while at 10°K in a magnetic field of 2–7 kG. After filtering to remove the 5.15-μm pump frequency, the Raman scattered radiation was split into two beams, one of which passed through the sample cell while the other was passed into the reference channel. Path lengths in

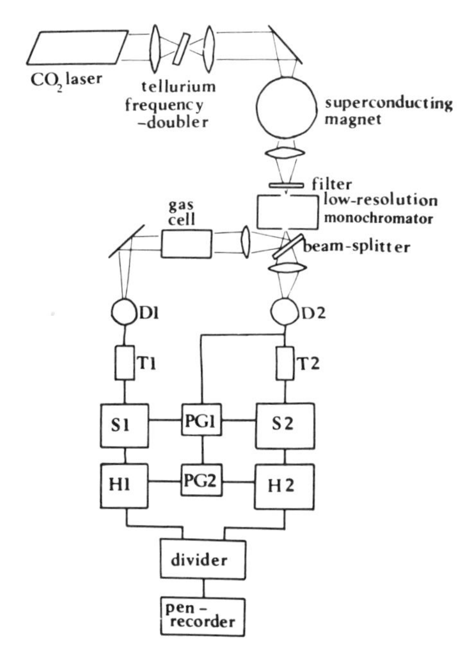

Fig. 8.3. Schematic diagram of experimental apparatus, showing arrangement of detectors (D1 and D2), delay lines (T1 and T2), pulse stretchers (S1 and S2), sample-and-hold units (H1 and H2), and pulse generators (PG1 and PG2) (Wood *et al.*, 1972).

the two beams were adjusted to compensate for atmospheric absorption. The pulse from detector D2 was used to trigger pulse generators PGl and PG2, which responded with a 100-nsec risetime. PG1 triggered the pulse stretchers S1 and S2, which converted the detector pulses into 10^{-5}-sec duration pulses whose amplitude was proportional to that of the original detector signals delayed by 400 nsec in T1 and T2. This delay was necessary to compensate for the 100-nsec risetime of the trigger generators. After stretching, the pulses in each channel were converted to dc levels by H1 and H2. The ratio of these two signals could then be recorded on a chart recorder. By comparing I and I_0 in this way, the effect of instabilities in intensity of the laser output can be largely eliminated. However, one requirement that must be met in order to benefit fully from the noise-suppressing properties of this system is that the pulse amplitude must be such that saturation of the measured transitions does not occur.

When resonances exist between infrared laser lines and molecular absorption lines it is often possible to use the laser source to excite fluorescence from the absorbing gas. This fluorescence, which can extend over a wide spectral range, can be analyzed spectroscopically to gain further information about the energy levels of the absorbing molecule. Examples of CO_2 and N_2O laser-excited fluorescence from polyatomic molecules in the gas phase are given in the article by Chang *et al.* (1970a,b) and Chang and Bridges (1970). Many polyatomic molecules have been found to lase at long wavelengths when pumped with 10-μm radiation.

When no spectral coincidence occurs between laser wavelengths and transitions of an absorbing molecule, it is occasionally possible to generate a coincidence by subjecting the molecule to an electric field. This field will produce a splitting of rotational levels that may be sufficient to bring one of the split components into resonance with the laser frequency. Shimizu (1970a,b) has used this approach in a study of the ν_2 bands of $^{15}NH_3$ and $^{14}NH_3$ using lines from CO_2 and N_2O lasers. The observation of over 90 coincidences between Stark-split levels of $^{15}NH_3$ and laser lines of known wavelength permitted a determination of molecular constants for the ν_2 band of this molecule. Even higher resolution is possible when Stark-split levels are detected using Lamb-dip spectroscopic methods (Brewer *et al.*, 1969; Kelly *et al.*, 1970; Brewer and Swalen, 1970).

Pumping of molecules from rotational levels of the ground vibrational state into rotational levels of an excited vibrational state will produce a strong deviation of the rotational populations from that predicted from the Boltzmann distribution when the pumping signal is strong enough to produce some saturation of the vibrational transition. The lower rotational level involved in such a transition will have its population severely depleted, while the upper-state rotational level will be strongly populated. Collisional processes will tend to reestablish equilibrium and in doing so will transfer the rotational excitation or deexcitation produced in the two perturbed states to other rotational levels of the molecule. The way populations can be redistributed via collisions is determined by a variety of selection rules (see, for example, Oka, 1968). If the system is then probed with microwave radiation, which stimulates transitions between rotational levels of the molecule, the intensity of a particular microwave line may be monitored as the infrared pump is switched on and off. A change in intensity of the microwave transition occasioned by the presence of the infrared pumping radiation then indicates that the rotational levels involved in the microwave transition are coupled in some way to the perturbed levels. This infrared microwave double resonance provides a powerful method of studying rotational energy transfer (Frenkel *et al.*, 1971). The first successful demonstration of this effect was reported by Ronn and Lide (1967) using the $P(20)$ line of a cw CO_2 laser to pump a vibration–rotation transition in methyl bromide. This result was confirmed by

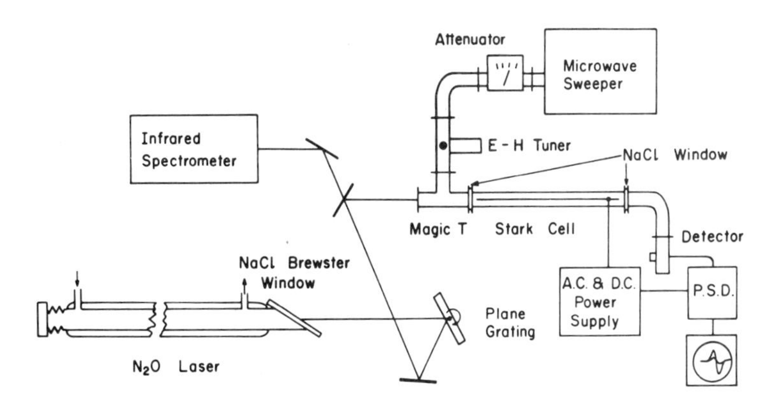

FIG. 8.4. Schematic diagram of the infrared–microwave double-resonance experiment (after Shimizu and Oka, 1970b).

Lemaire *et al.* (1969). Fourier *et al.* (1970) searched for similar double resonances in NH_3 pumped with a CO_2 laser but saw only a small effect, which they attributed to a thermal process involving heating of the gas by the incident laser radiation. Shimizu and Oka (1970a,b) observed a true infrared–microwave double resonance in both $^{14}NH_3$ and $^{15}NH_3$ using the $P(13)$ and $P(15)$ lines of the N_2O laser to provide pumping. Their system is shown schematically in Fig. 8.4. The $P(13)$ line of the N_2O laser was found to coincide almost exactly in wavelength with the ν_2 [$^qQ_-$ (8, 7)] vibration–rotation [see Herzberg (1945) for notation] line of $^{14}NH_3$ providing a strong resonance. As the $P(15)$ line of N_2O was found to lie 332 MHz lower in frequency than the ν_2 [$^qQ_-$ (4, 4)] line of $^{15}NH_3$, it was found necessary to split the lower rotation level using the Stark effect. This was accomplished by applying a dc electric field to the central electrode shown in Fig. 8.4. The energy levels participating in these transitions are shown schematically in Fig. 8.5. Pumping was found to increase the intensity of the (8, 7) line in $^{14}NH_3$, while the (9, 7) and (7, 7) lines decreased in intensity. The $M = 4$ component of the (4, 4) transition in $^{15}NH_3$ increased in intensity while the $M = 3$ component was largely unaffected. It was pointed out that the sensitivity of the measurement was affected by the fact that the narrow laser line is capable of exciting only those molecules whose velocity components v in the direction of propagation of the laser beam satisfy the condition $\nu_0(1 + v/c) \simeq \nu_L$, where ν_L is the frequency of the laser line and ν_0 the center frequency of the vibration–rotation line of the molecule. The laser radiation then "burns a hole" in the Doppler-broadened molecular transition.

A further development in the infrared spectroscopy of NH_3 was reported

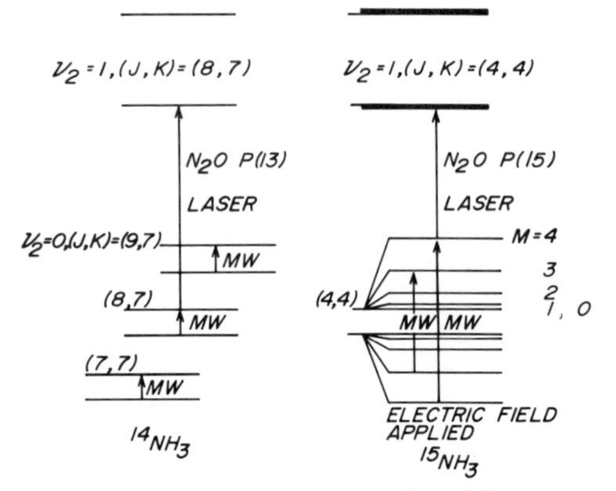

Fig. 8.5. Levels in $^{14}NH_3$ and $^{15}NH_3$ exhibiting infrared–microwave double resonance. MW denotes microwave absorption lines influenced by laser pumping (after Shimizu and Oka, 1970b).

by Oka and Shimizu (1971). It was found that the laser–microwave double resonance can be used to study vibration–rotation transitions whose energies fall in the range $\nu_L \pm \nu_m$, where ν_m is a variable microwave frequency. The absorption mechanism is then a two-photon transition involving the laser frequency and either a sum or difference microwave frequency. Such transitions are possible because of the nonlinearity of the molecular absorption process. Figure 8.6 shows the states involved in the two-photon absorption. By using various molecular laser lines selected wavelength regions can be scanned for vibration–rotation transitions using two-photon absorption. An excellent discussion of other two-photon spectroscopic methods can be found in the review by Moore (1971).

Even with the narrow spectral lines that can be obtained from laser sources, resolution of infrared spectra is ultimately limited by the Doppler width of the individual spectral lines. This broadening, which is always

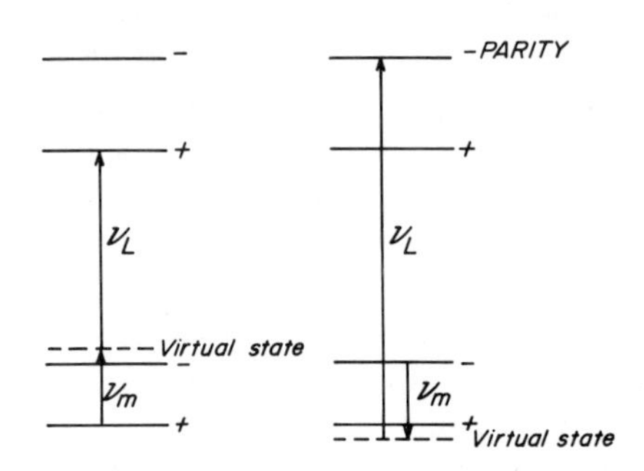

Fig. 8.6. Two-photon microwave–laser transitions.

present at temperatures above absolute zero, conceals much information on the location of vibration–rotation levels, particularly in the spectra of polyatomic molecules where strong overlap within the Doppler width occurs because of the multitude of possible vibration–rotation transitions within a narrow spectral range. When overlap occurs, even high spectral resolution will reveal only a more or less continuous absorption. This problem can be overcome and much higher effective spectral resolution can be obtained by the technique known as "Lamb-dip" spectroscopy (Lamb, 1964). Consider the gas cell shown in Fig. 8.7, which is exposed to a narrow laser line of frequency ν_L. If the gas contains a species that has a Doppler-broadened spectral line centered on a frequency ν_0, then when $\nu_0 \neq \nu_L$ only those molecules with velocities $v_0 = \pm c(\nu_0 - \nu_L)/\nu_0$ in the direction of the laser beam will absorb the laser frequency. When the laser beam is reflected back through the gas, two resonant frequencies within the Doppler-broadened profile will be possible. Now if the excitation rate due to the laser source is much greater than the rate of deexcitation of the upper level due to spontaneous emission and collisional relaxation, the ground state will be partially depleted and the absorption at these resonant frequencies will decrease. Thus dips will appear in the absorption profile

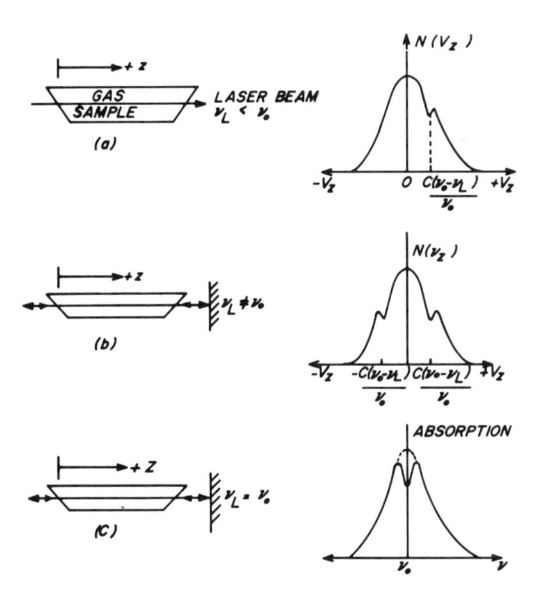

Fig. 8.7. (a) Number of absorbers with velocities v_3 vs. v_3, $N(v_3)$ for laser beam passing once through cell. (b) $N(v_3)$ for standing-wave laser field. (c) Absorption profile of spectral line when $\nu_L = \nu_0$.

within the Doppler-broadened line. As the laser frequency ν_L is tuned to reduce $| \nu_L - \nu_0 |$, these dips will move toward the center of the absorption line, until as shown in Fig. 8.7c, only a single dip is seen at the center of the line. This dip will have twice the area of the individual dips. The width of the Lamb-dip will be a function of the time spent by an absorber in the beam, the natural linewidth of the transition, and the lifetime due to collisions. The advantage of the Lamb-dip method lies, however, in the fact that these sources of broadening usually yield linewidths that are small compared to the Doppler linewidth. Thus two spectral lines ν_{01} and ν_{02} may be resolved, even when $| \nu_{01} - \nu_{02} |$ is much less than the Doppler widths of the individual lines.

The Lamb-dip resonance condition may be detected by a variety of means. Monitoring the intensity of the laser beam after it has passed through the cell, as shown in Fig. 8.7c, will show an increase in intensity as $\nu_L \rightarrow \nu_0$ because of decreased absorption at the center of the line. Alternatively, the sample may be enclosed within the laser cavity itself. If the laser is operated just above threshold, establishment of the resonance condition will yield an increase in laser output. Another method could involve monitoring the fluorescence from the sample cell.

Lamb-dip spectroscopy has been performed on a number of systems using CO_2 or N_2O laser sources. Much attention has been paid to SF_6 (Rabinowitz *et al.*, 1969; Shimizu, 1969; Goldberg and Yusek, 1970); 43 SF_6 absorption lines have been found within 93 MHz of the $P(18)$ line and 24 within about 40 MHz of the $P(16)$ line of CO_2 (Goldberg and Yusek, 1970). Frequencies of the detected lines were said to be accurate to ± 0.1 MHz. At 10 μm wavelength this corresponds to an accuracy of one part in 10^8. This is an improvement of about a factor 3×10^2 over that attainable even with a diode laser used in a conventional absorption experiment (Hinkley, 1970). In the work of Goldberg and Yusek, the minimum frequency separation between resolvable lines was about 1 MHz. In theory therefore, the Lamb-dip method would be able to resolve about 3×10^4 absorption features/cm^{-1} at $\lambda = 10$ μm. The tuning range, which in the previous work was limited by the availability of laser lines, can be extended by using a high-pressure CO_2 laser (Alcock *et al.*, 1973) or by the addition of CO_2 isotopes to the laser mixture (Beterov *et al.*, 1973). Patel (1974) has observed the Lamb-dip resonance in the H_2O line at 1889.58 cm^{-1} using a tunable spin–flip Raman laser. The width of this resonance was $\simeq$200 kHz. This corresponds to a resolution of 3×10^8.

When the Doppler contribution to the linewidth has been removed through the use of the Lamb-dip method, other broadening mechanisms can be studied more precisely. Work has already been reported on pressure broadening in CO_2 (Freed and Javan, 1970) and in CH_4 (Barger and Hall, 1969).

Lamb-dip spectroscopy is just one of the new spectroscopic techniques that have been made possible by the rapid development of laser sources. Many other coherent and nonlinear phenonema have been reported and are discussed in detail in the reviews by Moore (1971), Ewing (1972), and Demtröder (1971).

8.5 ISOTOPE SEPARATION

Perhaps an indication of the possible economic impact of laser methods of isotopic separation can be obtained from the dearth of publications (at least in the open literature) on this subject. There is now little doubt that isotopic separation can be accomplished using the selective excitation of atomic and molecular energy levels by means of lasers but few data on practical systems have found their way into the scientific literature (Mayer *et al.*, 1970; Yeung and Moore, 1972; Pressman, 1971; Guers, 1972; Ashkin, 1973; Letokhov, 1973). In principle, the separation of isotopes is straightforward, given the tunability and narrow spectral bandwidths attainable with presently available lasers. The process is simply to excite selectively an energy level of an isotopic species in a gas or solid containing that species in the normal isotopic abundance. One then arranges a reaction scheme that will trap out only the selectively excited species or the products of its decomposition. Practical problems abound, however, not the least of which is the lack of information on isotopic spectral shifts in complex polyatomic molecules.

Some basic methods by which isotopic separation may in principle be accomplished by laser excitation are (a) selective two-step photoionization, (b) two-step photodissociation, and (c) photopredissociation. These processes have been discussed in some detail by Moore (1973) and only a brief account will be given here.

(a) Selective Two-Step Photoionization

Consider the energy level schemes for two atomic isotopes shown in Fig. 8.8. A tunable laser may be used to generate a photon pulse at an energy $h\nu_1$ that corresponds to the $1 \rightarrow 2$ transition of ${}^nA$ but is out of resonance with respect to the same transition in the isotope ${}^mA$. This will selectively pump the ${}^nA$ isotope. If the sample is now exposed to a second photon flux at energy $h\nu_2$, which can cause photoionization from level 2 of ${}^nA$ but is not absorbed by ${}^mA$, then ${}^nA^+$ ions are produced. These ions may be

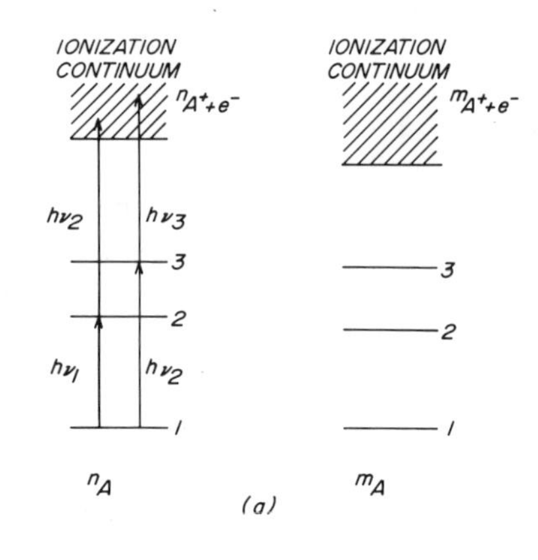

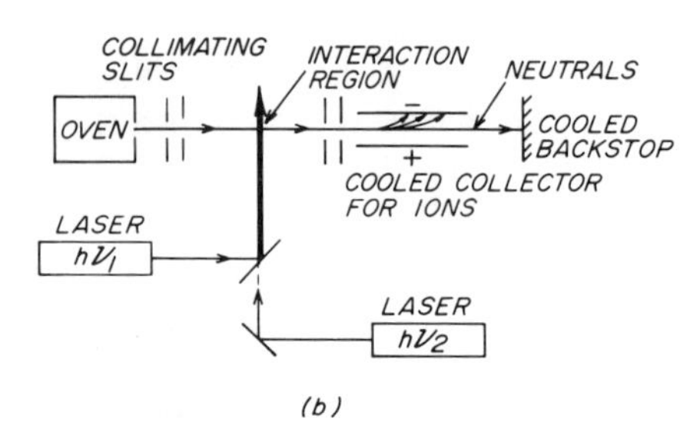

Fig. 8.8. (a) Selective two-step photo ionization. (b) System for isotope separation.

extracted from the system by the application of an accelerating potential as shown in Fig. 8.8. Alternatively, two-photon ionization with level 3 as the intermediate step and photons of identical energy $h\nu_3$ could be used to produce $^nA^+$. The simple system shown in Fig. 8.8b could be operated on a closed cycle by having two ion extraction electrodes symmetrically placed about the interaction region and using an oven in place of the backstop. Material would then be run through in one direction into a cooled oven and then this oven would be heated to reverse the flow. Brinkman *et al.* (1974) have reported on the separation of Ca isotopes using two-step laser photoionization.

(b) Two-Step Photodissociation

In this process, excitation of a molecule into an excited vibrational level of the ground state or into a higher electronic state is followed by inducing a transition into a dissociating level or into an ionization continuum. The products of the dissociation can be removed by chemical reaction or, in the case of ionization, by electrical or magnetic means. The overall reaction scheme would be

$$^{n}AB + h\nu_1 \rightarrow {}^{n}AB^*$$

$$^{n}AB^* + h\nu_2 \rightarrow {}^{n}A + B \qquad \text{or} \qquad {}^{n}A^+ + B + e^-$$

while $h\nu_1$ is tuned so that

$$^{m}AB + h\nu_1 \nrightarrow {}^{m}AB^*$$

Generally $h\nu_1$ and $h\nu_2$ each have to be several eV for the photoionization process, since ionization potentials of most molecules are usually $\gtrsim 8$ eV.

The energy of the first quantum $h\nu_1$ absorbed in the two-step photodissociation should be much larger than kT, where T is the gas vibrational temperature if the process is to be efficient. When $h\nu_1 \lesssim kT$, the thermal population of the upper level involved in this transition may be appreciable in both ^{n}AB and ^{m}AB. In this case, $h\nu_2$ may excite ^{m}AB as well, since the transition is into a continuum. Therefore, $h\nu_1$ optically separates the different isotopes into two groups: those that can absorb $h\nu_1$ and those that cannot. $h\nu_2$ may be absorbed by both isotopes but only produces dissociation in the tagged group. Of course, the photochemistry will be simpler if $h\nu_2$ is absorbed only by one type of isotope, but in principle this requirement is not necessary for the success of this method.

Ambartzumian and Letokhov (1972) point out that if the pulse $h\nu_1$ has a duration $\tau_p \ll \tau_{rot}$, where τ_{rot} is the rotational relaxation time, then only the population in one rotational level of the lowest vibrational level will be transferred to the excited level. When the pulse duration $\tau_p \gg \tau_{rot}$, rtoational relaxation can occur during the pulse and a larger population can be excited to the upper state. An attempt to dissociate HCl, but not to separate the isotopes, using this method was reported by Ambartzumian and Letokhov (1972). It would seem that CO_2 or other infrared lasers may find application in this area (Guers, 1972).

(c) Photopredissociation

Predissociation is a well-known effect in molecular spectroscopy (Herzberg, 1967). In a vibrational progression associated with an electronic transition, predissociation may start quite abruptly at a particular vibrational level of the excited state, making all subsequent higher levels diffuse. The predissociation rate for such levels will be $\gtrsim 10^{10}$/sec. With laser excitation it is advantageous to have a narrower line, which in general implies that the predissociation rate must be $<10^{10}$/sec. Other considerations provide a lower limit for this rate of 10^7/sec (Letokhov, 1972) in practical systems. Hence ideal transitions for laser photo predissociation to yield isotope separation are those in which the predissociation rate is $>10^7$/sec and $<10^{10}$/sec. A successful laser isotopic separation of D and H from formaldehyde and formaldehyde-d_2 has been reported by Yeung and Moore (1972). A 6 : 1 enrichment of D_2 over H_2 was produced from an equimolar mixture of D_2CO and H_2CO. Five percent HD was also produced. The laser was a frequency-doubled ruby. Even in this relatively simple system the photochemistry involved in separation is complex and poorly understood (Moore, 1973). Moore stresses, however, that photopredissociation is both simple and efficient, suggesting that separation factors as large as 10^6 : 1 may be possible under certain circumstances.

Separation of H and D through photodissociation of formaldehyde has recently been reported by Marling (1975) using radiation from a HeCd laser at 3250.3 Å. Separation by absorption of continuum radiation transmitted through an H_2CO or D_2CO gas filter has been observed by Bazhin *et al.* (1975).

^{14}N and ^{15}N have been separated from *sec*-tetrazine ($C_2H_2N_4$) using laser-excited photodissociation by Karl and Innes (1975). ^{12}C and ^{13}C have been separated from formaldehyde by Clark *et al.* (1975) using this technique. A similar separation of ^{79}Br and ^{81}Br from Br_2 has been reported by Leone and Moore (1974). The theory of these processes has been discussed by Karlov (1975) and by Liu (1974).

Light pressure on an absorbing atom or molecule has been suggested as a possible mechanism whereby isotopes may be separated in the gas phase (Ashkin, 1970, 1973; Usikov *et al.*, 1972). Since both momentum and energy must be conserved when a photon is absorbed by an atom or molecule, absorption will result in the transfer of linear momentum in the direction of the incident light beam to the absorbing species. This momentum will be retained on average even after the absorber reradiates its energy, since the radiation emitted by the absorber is isotropic. Ashkin (1970) shows that an atom will experience an average driving force $F\sigma/c$ due to this effect, where F is the incident light intensity, σ the absorption cross section at the center of a spectral line, and c the velocity of light. This expression is valid when the gas pressure is low enough that the incident radiation is only partially absorbed in the sample (sample has small optical depth) and there is no depletion of the ground state of the system. If x_{cr} is the distance required for an atom to travel before it loses its average kinetic energy $mv_{av}^2/2$, then $F'x_{cr} = ma_v{}^2/2 \simeq kT$, where T is the gas kinetic temperature and F' the force. With a constant force, the pressure variation with distance in a cell exposed to F' will be

$$p(x) = p_0 \exp(-F'x/kT) = p_0 \exp(-x/x_{cr})$$

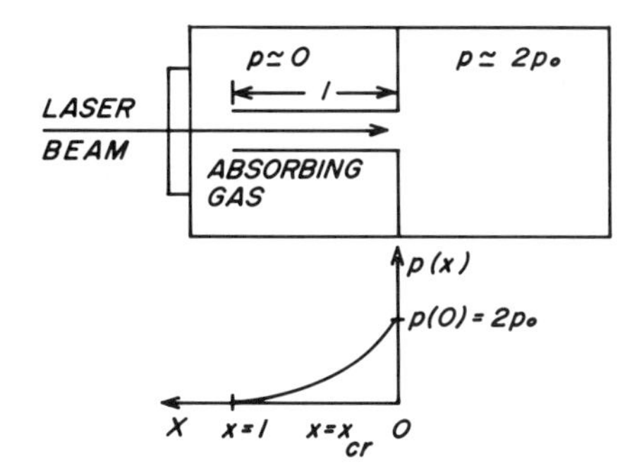

Fig. 8.9. Sample cell for gas separation due to radiation pressure (after Ashkin, 1970).

The geometry is shown in Fig. 8.9. Considering a practical system in which one has absorption saturation as well as Doppler and collisional broadening, Ashkin (1970) derives the following expression for x_{cr}:

$$x_{\mathrm{cr}} = \frac{kT\lambda}{h}\left(\frac{\tau_{\mathrm{n}}\tau_{\mathrm{L}}}{\tau_{\mathrm{n}} + \tau_{\mathrm{L}}}\right)\left(\frac{\Delta\nu_{\mathrm{D}}}{\Delta\nu_{\mathrm{n}} + \Delta\nu_{\mathrm{L}}}\right)$$

where

λ wavelength of transition
τ_{n} natural lifetime of upper level
τ_{L} collisional lifetime of upper level
$\Delta\nu_{\mathrm{D}}$ Doppler width of transition
$\Delta\nu_{\mathrm{n}}$ natural width of transition
$\Delta\nu_{\mathrm{L}}$ Lorentz width due to collisional broadening
h Planck's constant

For Na vapor at a pressure $p_0 = 10^{-3}$ Torr at $T = 510°\mathrm{K}$ in a cell with $l = 20$ cm, Ashkin finds $p(l) = 3.4 \times 10^{-9}$ Torr when the system is buffered with 30 Torr of He gas and $F = 7.6 \times 10^4$ W/cm^2. This would correspond to complete evacuation of one side of the tube shown in Fig. 8.9. By exciting only one isotope in a mixture, this isotope could be driven away from the light beam, resulting in separation. This process would be effective with both visible/uv and infrared lasers.

Recently, the efficiency for separation of isotopic atoms and molecules using radiation pressure and electromagnetic radiation of various wavelengths has been calculated by Gelbwachs and Hartwick (1975). Separation coefficients and efficiencies for excitation in the microwave region are some seven orders of magnitude smaller than for excitation in the visible or UV. Experimental observation of a laser-induced density gradient in Na vapor has subsequently been reported by Bjorkholm *et al.* (1975). Similar experiments involving the creation of a density gradient in SF_6 gas by radiation pressure at a wavelength of 10.6 μm have been performed by Rinehart *et al.* (1976). Separation of isotopes by laser deflection out of an atomic beam has been treated theoretically by Nebenzahl and Szöke (1974). Isotope separation in a Ba atomic beam has been reported by Bernhardt *et al.* (1974).

Another method of separating isotopes using laser excitation, which shows great promise, involves photocatalyzation through selective excitation of a particular ground state vibrational energy level. Species that do not react, or react very slowly, when in their lowest vibrational levels may react readily when one of these species is excited vibrationally. As an example, Moore (1973) reports that the reaction rate

$$H^{37}Cl\ (v = 2) + Br \rightarrow HBr + {}^{37}Cl$$

should occur at a rate 10^{12} times larger than that of the ground state reaction

$$H^{37}Cl\ (v = 0) + Br \rightarrow HBr + {}^{37}Cl$$

Mayer *et al.* (1970) report an experiment in which a mixture of CH_3OH, Br_2, and CD_3OH was excited by wavelengths in the range 2.64–2.87 μm obtained from an HF laser. These wavelengths correspond to excitation of the OH stretching frequency in CH_3OH. Apparently, vibrational excitation of CH_3OH sensitized a reaction with Br_2 that removed methanol from the system, leaving deuteromethanol. The resulting mixture was enriched to 95% CD_3OD from an original 1 : 1 mixture.

In another study (Laurent and Kikindai, 1972) the reaction of NH_3 with CO_2 was followed with and without irradiation with a CO_2 laser. The reaction rate was increased by the absorption of laser radiation and it was suggested that isotopic separation of ^{14}N and ^{15}N might be accomplished by excitation of either $^{14}NH_3$ or $^{15}NH_3$ in the following reactions:

$$CO_2 + 2\,{}^{14}NH_3 \rightarrow CO\begin{array}{l} \diagup\ {}^{14}NH_2 \\ \diagdown\ O^{14}NH_4 \end{array}$$

$$CO_2 + 2\,{}^{15}NH_3 \rightarrow CO\begin{array}{l} \diagup\ {}^{15}NH_2 \\ \diagdown\ O^{15}NH_4 \end{array}$$

Ambartsumyan *et al.* (1973) have also reported on the laser separation of nitrogen isotopes.

Recent results on the separation of isotopes by reactions catalyzed with CO_2 laser radiation have been reported by Ambartzumian *et al.* (1974), Freund and Ritter (1975), and Lyman and Rockwood (1976) (boron isotopes from BCl_3); Lyman and Rockwood (1976) (^{13}C from CF_2Cl_3); Lyman and Rockwood (1976) (^{29}Si from SiF_4); and Ambartzumian *et al.* (1975) and Lyman *et al.* (1975) (^{34}S from SF_6).

These studies, while of intrinsic interest, are obviously peripheral to the areas in which the main research effort on laser isotope separation is being directed. The main interest would seem to center on the separation of ^{235}U, and in the absence of published data one can only assume that while the scientific feasibility of ^{235}U separation by laser excitation in the gas phase has been proven, technological problems associated with obtaining an economically feasible process may be substantial (Farrer and Smith, 1972; Altschuler, 1973).

Chapter 9

Thermal Effects

9.1 INTRODUCTION

The rapid heating and cooling rates possible with laser heating have opened up new areas in high-temperature chemistry and metallurgy. This chapter discusses some of the new metallurgical effects that have been observed with laser heating. One application in the area of high-temperature chemistry involves the growth and purification of crystals using controlled cw laser heating. This work has already led to the discovery of at least one other high-temperature modification of carbon and the development of a means of drawing high-quality fibers for optical communication systems. More developments in this and related areas are to be expected as high-power cw CO_2 lasers become a standard tool in university and industrial research laboratories.

Fundamental research into the measurement of the thermal constants of materials using laser heating techniques and into the generation and propagation of stress waves in condensed materials will also be discussed in some detail.

9.2 MEASUREMENT OF THERMAL CONSTANTS

An elegant method of measuring the high-temperature thermal conductivity of nonmetallic solids has been described by Schatz and Simmons (1972, a,b). High-temperature heat transport in nonoptically thick samples is governed by a combination of lattice conduction and radiative transfer. Since the heat transferred to a particular point in a solid at high temperatures is due in part to radiative transfer from other points in the solid, when the solid is not optically thick, i.e., when the extinction coefficient for thermal radiation $\bar{\epsilon}$ is such that $\bar{\epsilon}L \lesssim 1$, where L is a characteristic dimension of the solid, then all points in the solid may be coupled optically. Thus a calculation of the total heat transfer becomes extremely difficult, if not impossible, and depends strongly on the shape of the sample. The method of Schatz and Simmons is shown schematically in Fig. 9.1. A cw CO_2 laser is pulsed to provide a periodic source of heat on one surface of a slab mounted in a temperature-stabilized furnace. Thermal radiation from the rear face is monitored by a detector that is blind to 10.6-μm radiation. When the sample is optically thick, only radiation from a thin outer layer of the rear surface is detected. On the other hand, when the sample is heated into a range where it becomes optically thin, the detector sees radiation from deeper inside the material. For a periodic heat source incident on the front surface, the radiation emitted from the rear surface will be modulated at the same frequency but with a phase lag due to the finite heat diffusion time from front to back surface. As the optical thickness of the sample decreases, the phase lag will decrease since the detector is seeing further into the sample. The phase lag is a function of the frequency of the heat source, the thermal conductivity, the extinction coefficient, and the temperature of the sample. Schatz and Simmons were able to show that by measuring the phase lag at two different frequencies while keeping other

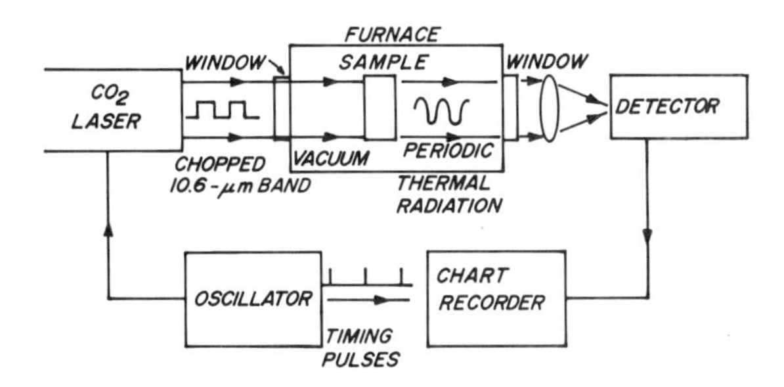

Fig. 9.1. Method of Schatz and Simmons (1972) for measuring thermal constants of materials using laser excitation.

parameters constant, the data could be used to obtain K_L and K_R, the lattice thermal conductivity and radiative thermal conductivity, respectively. Data were obtained for sintered Al_2O_3, sintered Forsterite, single and polycrystalline olivines, and single-crystal enstatite in the temperature range 500–1900°K. It should be noted that the measurements first give κ_L, the lattice thermal diffusivity, and $\bar{\epsilon}$, the mean blackbody extinction coefficient. K_L is then calculated from $K_L = \kappa_L \rho c_p$ and K_R is found independently from $\bar{\epsilon}$. The total thermal conductivity $K = K_L + K_R$.

The thermal diffusivity of a material can be obtained by subjecting a thin slab of the material to a heat pulse over one surface and measuring the time-dependent temperature on the opposite face. The requirements on the thickness of the specimen and the duration of the heat pulse have been discussed by Parker *et al.* (1961), Cape and Lehman (1963), and Taylor and Cape (1964). The theory that suggested that such a method could be used to measure thermal diffusivity was first given by Parker *et al.* (1961). From Carslaw and Jaeger (1959, p. 101) the temperature $T(z, t)$ in a semi-infinite insulated slab with a temperature distribution $T(z, 0)$ at $t = 0$ is given by

$$T(z, t) = \frac{1}{L}\int_0^L T(z, 0)\, dz + \frac{2}{L}\sum_{n=1}^{\infty} \exp\left[-\frac{n^2\pi^2\kappa t}{L^2}\right] \times \cos\frac{n\pi z}{L}\int_0^L T(z,0)\cos\frac{n\pi z}{L}\, dz \tag{1}$$

where L is the slab thickness and κ the thermal diffusivity. Assuming now that the surface is heated instantaneously at $t = 0^-$ by absorption of an energy flux Q (J/cm^2) in a depth Δ,

$$T(z, 0) = \begin{cases} Q/\rho C\Delta, & 0 \le z \le \Delta \\ 0, & \Delta < z \le L \end{cases}$$

Then Eq. (1) becomes

$$T(z, t) = \frac{Q}{\rho CL}\left\{1 + 2\sum_{n=1}^{\infty}\left[\cos\frac{n\pi z}{L}\right]\frac{L}{n\pi\Delta}\sin\frac{n\pi\Delta}{L}\exp\left(-\frac{n^2\pi^2\kappa t}{L^2}\right)\right\} \tag{2}$$

where ρ is in units of g/cm^3 and C is in J/g°C. It is reasonable to take $\sin(n\pi\Delta/L) \simeq n\pi\Delta/L$ since Δ is always small, and terms in the expansion that may arise when n is large will be attenuated by the exponential factor. Then at the back surface,

$$T(L, t) = \frac{Q}{\rho CL}\left[1 + 2\sum_{n=1}^{\infty}(-1)^n\exp\left(-\frac{n^2\pi^2\kappa t}{L^2}\right)\right] \tag{3}$$

Defining

$$\theta(L, t) = T(L, t)/T_{\mathrm{m}} \qquad \text{and} \qquad \tau = \pi^2 \kappa t/L^2$$

where T_{m} is the maximum value of the rear surface temperature,

$$\theta = 1 + 2 \sum_{n=1}^{\infty} (-1)^n \exp(-n^2 \tau) \tag{4}$$

A plot of θ versus τ is given in Fig. 9.2. One sees that $\theta = 0.5$ implies $\tau = 1.37$, and thus one obtains the following simple relationship for κ:

$$\kappa = 1.37L^2/\pi^2 t_{1/2} \tag{5}$$

where $t_{1/2}$ is the time at which the temperature of the back surface of the slab reaches $0.5T_{\mathrm{m}}$. It has been pointed out (Yurchak, 1971) that only the first term in the expansion in Eq. (4) is important for times $t > t_{1/2}$ and little error is introduced by eliminating the other terms. Yurchak suggests that the following expression derived from Eq. (4) with the above approximation may actually yield a more accurate value for κ in a given experimental situation,

$$\kappa = \left[\frac{\ln(1 - \theta_1) - \ln(1 - \theta_2)}{(\theta_2 - \theta_1)}\right] \frac{L^2}{\pi^2} \tag{6}$$

where both θ_1 and θ_2 should be chosen in the range $\gtrsim 0.5$ for good accuracy.

Since κ will in general be a function of the temperature, while there is, by the very nature of the measurement process, a temperature gradient in the sample, an average temperature must be derived theoretically that characterizes the sample temperature encountered by the heat pulse.

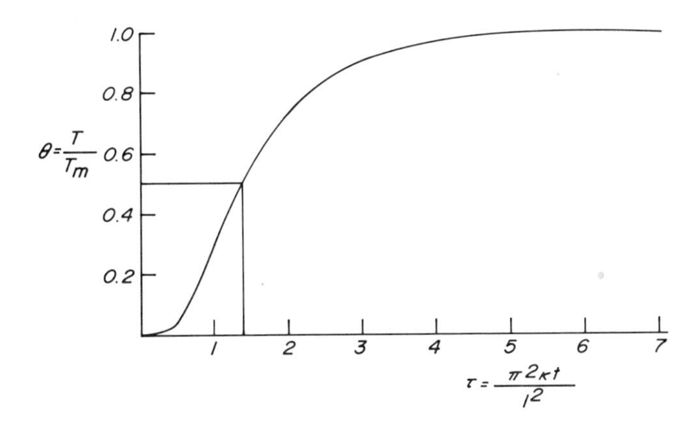

Fig. 9.2. θ vs. τ for semi-infinite slab.

Parker *et al.* (1961) have used the definition that the effective temperature is given by the time average of the mean of the front and back surface temperatures over the time taken for the back surface temperature to reach $0.5T_m$. It can easily be shown that this temperature $T_L = 1.6T_m$. To avoid possible nonlinearities in the heating process, it is important to ensure that the surface temperature never rises to the melting point. Originally a triangular (in time) heat pulse was assumed for the incident heat flux $F(t)$,

$$F(t) = h(1 - t/y)$$

where h and y are chosen to best fit the actual time dependence of $F(t)$. Then $T(z, t)$ can be found from (Carslaw and Jaeger, 1959)

$$T(z, t) = \frac{1}{\rho C(\pi\kappa)^{1/2}} \int_0^t \frac{F(t-s)}{s^{1/2}} \exp\left[-\frac{z^2}{4\kappa s}\right] ds \qquad (7)$$

which gives

$$T_f(0, t_m) = 4hy/3\rho C(2\pi\kappa y)^{1/2} \qquad (8)$$

for the maximum surface temperature T_f occurring at time $t_m = y/2$. Equation (8) can be related to the pulse energy flux through the expression

$$T_f(0, t_m) = 8Q/3\beta\rho C(2\pi\kappa y)^{1/2} \qquad (9)$$

where $Q = \beta hy/2$, with β a correction factor. Although the assumption of a triangular pulse leads to a simple analytic expression for T_f, evaluation of Eq. (7) is quite straightforward even with more realistic pulse shapes. For a general pulse shape, however, Eq. (7) would have to be integrated numerically.

It is obvious that the simple theory given above, which allows κ to be easily obtained from a measurement of the back surface temperature, places severe constraints on the boundary conditions, which must be satisfied if the results are to be accurate. The boundary conditions are

(i) The heat pulse should switch on and off instantaneously and the duration of the heating pulse must be much less than $L^2/\pi^2\kappa$.

(ii) The sample must be uniformly heated over one entire surface and the characteristic dimensions of this surface must be $\gg L$.

(iii) The sample must be thermally insulated.

In practice, samples must be thin to ensure that the temperature rise on the rear surface is sufficiently large to give a good signal/noise ratio during the measurement. Since Eq. (5) is accurate to 1% only when $L^2/\pi^2\kappa \gtrsim 50t_p$, where t_p is the pulse duration (Cape and Lehman, 1963; Taylor and Cape, 1964), measurements on millimeter thick samples with κ in the range 0.01–1 cm^2/sec requires $t_p < 10^{-3}$ for good accuracy. Such pulse lengths are not difficult to obtain from either solid state or CO_2 lasers. However, when the sample thickness and pulse length are limited by other considerations so that $L^2/\pi\kappa \not> 50t_p$ for a particular material, one may use the following more exact expression to relate θ to τ (Cape and Lehman, 1963):

$$\theta = 1 + \frac{2L^2}{\pi^2\kappa t_p} \sum_{n=1}^{\infty} \frac{(-1)^n}{n^2} \exp\left[-\frac{n^2\pi^2\kappa t}{L^2}\right]\left[\exp\left(\frac{n^2\pi^2\kappa t_p}{L^2} - 1\right)\right] \tag{10}$$

In this case, the initial pulse is assumed to be square and of duration t_p, while $t > t_p$. Taylor and Cape (1964) have verified that this expression provides more accurate values for κ in the regime where the laser pulse length is not negligible compared to the thermal diffusion time.

Modifications to the theory to permit the incorporation of nonuniform (but still axially symmetric heating) radial heat flow and a variety of surface boundary conditions have been outlined by Cowan (1963) and Watt (1966). In general, these modifications, while providing more accurate predictions for κ, result in a great increase in complexity of the mathematical analysis needed to extract κ from the $T(L, t)$ curve. The following generalities may be noted, however. When the pulse length t_p is such that it is comparable to the thermal diffusion time across the sample, then the numerical constant in Eq. (5) is increased and the measurement will tend to underestimate κ. Conversely, when the sample loses heat by radiation the constant in Eq. (5) is effectively decreased and the value of κ will be overestimated.

An empirical study of the influence of some of these effects on the accuracy of the results has been made by Schriempf (1972a). In one experiment the sample was exposed to a beam that had an intensity maximum on the sample axis. $T(L, t)$ then increased to a peak value and subsequently decreased. When the beam profile was uniform, the theoretical curve of Eq. (4) was obtained. For a donut-shaped beam, $T(L, t)$ rose rapidly at first, then changed slope to rise more slowly but continuously with t. This behavior is predicted from the theoretical considerations of Watt (1966) but its verification illustrates that care must be taken to ensure a uniformly distributed beam on the target if it is hoped to reduce the data using the simple theory. In another experiment it was determined that no comparable effects arose out of heat losses from the sample.

If one puts $t = \infty$ in Eq. (3), then the term involving the summation vanishes, and since $T(L, \infty) = T_m$,

$$C\ (\equiv C_p) = Q/\rho L T_m$$

Thus, a simple measurement of the maximum value of the back surface temperature suffices (given the approximations inherent in the simple theory) to yield a value for C, the heat capacity of the material. The thermal conductivity K can then be calculated from the relation

$$K = \kappa \rho C$$

It is apparent that all three thermal constants K, κ, and C can be obtained from a material using the laser flash method and a relatively simple measurement of the time-dependent back surface temperature. κ is obtained directly from this measurement, while C requires an estimation of the absorbed laser energy.

One of the first reported users of a laser in flash thermal diffusivity measurements was by Deem and Wood (1962). Graphite, stainless steel, and nuclear fuel specimens were tested at temperatures in the range 200–800°C and the resulting values of K were in good agreement with those measured in conventional ways. Namba *et al.* (1968) measured κ for a variety of metals and some alloys including a sintered Cu ferrite. The latter was examined in the vicinity of the tetragonal–cubic phase transition and also through the Curie temperature. Both showed well-defined features in the κ versus T curve at the appropriate temperatures. This indicates that the laser flash diffusivity method is capable of good temperature resolution. It should be noted that the temperature excursion at the back surface of a thin sample is often only several degrees.

An extensive study of the thermal constants of uranium monocarbide, monophosphide, and monosulfide derived from laser flash measurement of K and C_p at various temperatures has been reported by Moser and Kruger (1965, 1967). The compound UW was investigated by Nasu and Kikuchi (1968).

The heat capacity of sintered alumina has been measured between 20 and 700°C using the laser flash method by Murabayashi *et al.* (1970). Since this requires a careful estimate of Q, the absorbed laser energy flux, a standardization procedure involving the comparison of the high-temperature data with those obtained at 20°C as compared to iron was developed. Deviations between NBS standard values for C_p of alumina and the results of this experiment were less than $\pm 1.5\%$.

The thermal diffusivities of liquid mercury and aluminum were determined by Schriempf (1972b) using a modification of the normal laser thermal diffusivity experiment (Schriempf, 1972a). It was pointed out that the laser method offers the possibility of an increase in accuracy over conventional methods through the elimination of heat transport via convection.

9.3 METALLURGICAL EFFECTS

As discussed previously (Section 5.2) heating rates with pulsed lasers can easily exceed 10^6 °C/sec and rates of 10^{10} °C/sec are not impossible to obtain. What is not quite so obvious is that the temperature may decay upon cessation of the laser pulse at similar rates. With heating and cooling rates of this order it is not surprising that a variety of interesting metallurgical effects can be produced with laser excitation. The most obvious application of this rapid heating/quenching process would seem to lie in the area of the formation and study of new phases of metallic alloys. Phases that are stable only in a limited temperature range may be created by laser heating and then "frozen in" by the rapid quenching that follows the laser pulse.

The Ag–Cu system that satisfies the Hume–Rothery rules for solid solubility but that exists in a two-phase eutectic structure over a wide range of composition (Barrett, 1952) can be quench cooled to form a single-phase structure using laser heating (Elliott and Gagliano, 1972). This work provides conclusive evidence that nonequilibrium phases can be formed with laser excitation. Further studies by Laridjani *et al.* (1972) on the laser heating of a silver–germanium alloy show that, in this instance, the metastable phase formed was identical to that formed by splat cooling. Other experiments by Garashchuk *et al.* (1969), Garaschuk and Molchan (1969), and Baranov *et al.* (1968) on laser welding of dissimilar metals show that the formation of intermediate phases and perhaps intermetallic compounds is a fairly common occurrence. A new phase of the Fe–C system called Baikovite has been produced on laser heating and quenching by Zukov *et al.* (1972). It has been suggested (Longfellow, 1972) that the use of lasers to produce small quantities of materials in intermediate phases or of intermetallic compounds may open up new applications for lasers in metallurgical studies. This is supported by the recent work of Nelson *et al.* (1972), which shows that at least two new phases of carbon are formed during heating with a cw CO_2 laser. However, it is not necessarily true that rapid heating and quenching will always result in the stabilization of high-temperature phases at room temperature. The interesting study by Warlimont *et al.* (1971) on the conditions required to produce quenched in disorder in an Fe–Al alloy shows that the finite time required for reconstitution of the high-temperature phase may not be compatible with the time available above a critical temperature during the laser pulse.

Elliott and Gagliano (1972) were able to make a direct estimate of the cooling rate of 2024 aluminum alloy by comparing the dendritic spacing d obtained with laser heating to that observed with splat cooling (Matyja *et al.*, 1968). The empirical relationship derived by Matyja *et al.*,

$$d(r)^{0.32} = C \tag{11}$$

where r is the cooling rate and C a constant, together with the measured value of $d \simeq 0.35$ μm gave $r = 3.7 \times 10^6$ °C/sec. This rate is only two orders of magnitude less than the highest reported value obtainable with splat cooling (Predecki *et al.*, 1965). Pure metals often do not exhibit dendritic structures on cooling (Barrett, 1952) but recrystallize in columnar grains. The orientation of these grains is usually along important crystal directions. A good example of this structure in recrystallized laser-heated molybdenum is shown in the article by Gagliano and Zaleckas (1972). Very often columnar grains will be surrounded by a region of symmetrical recrystallized grains at the periphery of the resolidified melt. Oriented crystal structures on the surface of laser irradiated steel have been reported by Mirkin (1973a). Murphy and Ritter (1966a) show that surface hardness increases markedly in the vicinity of craters formed in copper.

Rapid heating and cooling rates are inevitably accompanied by thermally induced stresses. When single crystals of copper are irradiated with 1-msec pulses from an Nd laser, this stress is nearly radial and acts to form or move dislocations, which can be later revealed by etching the crystal (Haessner and Seitz, 1971). Murphy and Ritter (1966b) also observed a somewhat similar structure on the surface of Cu irradiated with 80-nsec laser pulses. This structure, which was attributed to thermal etching, took the form of terraces radiating from the center of the focal area. Wu *et al.* (1972) exposed a cleaved zinc crystal annealed at room temperature to pulses of various energy from an Nd : glass laser. A comparison of the dislocation structure before and after laser irradiation showed that appreciable plastic deformation had occurred. The laser damage consisted of deformation twinning, which involves the shearing movement of one atomic plane over another, nonbasal slip, and microkinking. These deformation states were "locked in" to the crystal perhaps, as suggested by Wu *et al.*, by the presence of a thin surface layer of oxide or fine-grained polycrystalline material. Little change in this structure was noted after annealing for 8 months at room temperature.

The strength and dislocation structures of type 7075 aluminum alloy before and after impact of *Q*-switched laser pulses with fluences in the range 40–70 J/cm² have been compared by Fairand *et al.* (1972). The stress due to laser impact was made more uniform by subjecting both sides of thin plates to separate pulses from the laser. In addition, the metal surface was coated with a thin transparent silicate layer and covered with a 1-mm thick glass microscope slide to enhance the surface shock wave

(Siegrist and Kneubühl, 1973). Specimens in the soft solution-annealed and quenched condition prior to laser impact showed the largest ($\simeq$25%) increase in yield strength after shocking. Fully hardened materials showed little change in yield strength. The soft material with relatively few dislocations prior to shocking exhibited a dense tangled dislocation structure after impact. This structure was reported to be similar to that observed after explosive shocking. Warlimont *et al.* (1971) found that the density of dislocations in an Fe–Al alloy increased with both the duration and energy of the laser pulse and that the general appearance of the dislocation structure also resembled that produced by shock loading.

Thin metallic films subjected to irradiation with high-intensity short-duration laser pulses show defect structures that are not necessarily the same as those observed in bulk materials. Metz and Smidt (1971) report that little change in dislocation density or in inclusion size occurs in nickel or vanadium foils irradiated with pulses from a Q-switched ruby laser. However, they found that vacancy concentrations as high as 1 at.% are often produced. Howard and Ross (1972) studied laser radiation effects on thin aluminum foils and found that a typical damage region had the structure shown in Fig. 9.3. The outer edge of this region exhibits a structure that suggests resolidification from a melt in contact with a cold surface (the surrounding film). Columnar grains are seen to converge from this region into an area of network structure that coincides with the center of the focal spot. A similar structure has been observed by Speich and Fisher (1966). Material around the periphery of the outer recrystallized region exhibits localized regions in which islands of large grains are found in the background matrix of fine-grained material.

A novel application of the stress enhancement and embrittlement that occurs in the vicinity of surface areas subjected to laser pulses has been reported by Cervay and Perak (1972). It was shown that defects produced on metal surfaces by the action of a laser pulse can act as centers for the growth of cracks in specimens for mechanical fracture studies. Defects generated in this way on the surface of 7075 aluminum alloy readily acted as crack initiators when the material was subjected to bending. On the other hand, simple pulsing was not effective in producing crack starter defects in steel specimens. It was found necessary to coat the steel surface with graphite oil prior to laser irradiation before such defects could be generated. This interesting observation was explained by the possible hydrogen embrittlement of the steel surface at the point of laser impact. However, it is known that liquid surface layers can drastically enhance laser-produced shock waves (Siegrist and Kneubühl, 1973) and that carbon-containing compounds spread on the surface of steel before laser im-

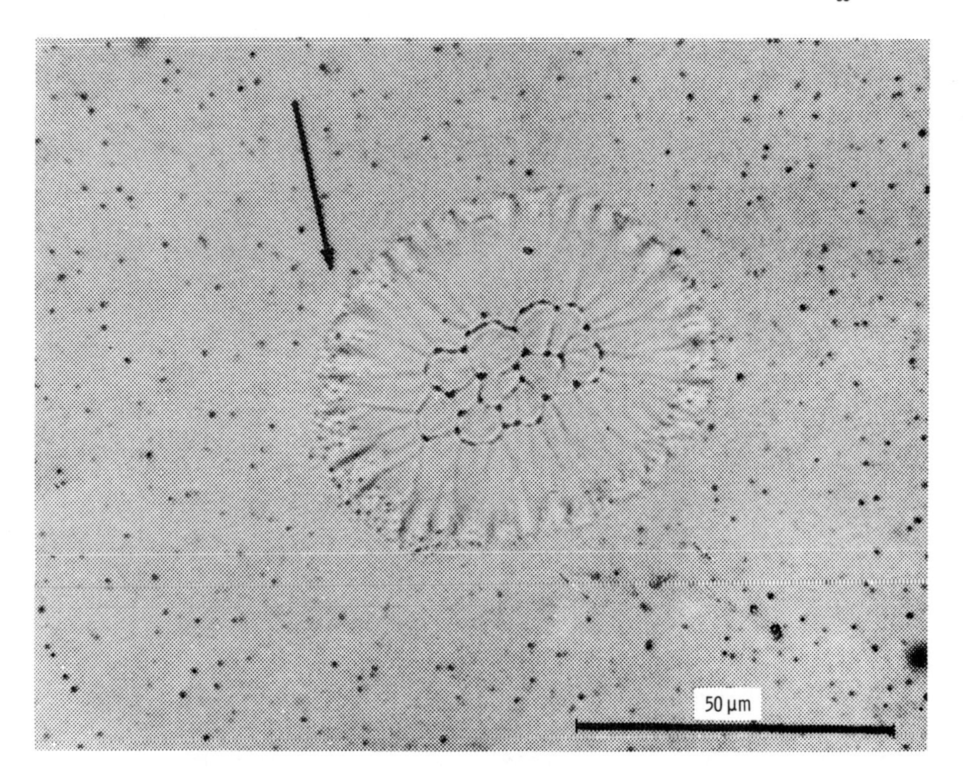

Fig. 9.3. Optical photograph (750×) showing laser damage at 0.025 J in 3140A aluminum film (from Howard and Ross, 1972).

pact result in impregnation of the steel with carbon (Mirkin, 1969). In view of the results of Cervay and Perak (1972) in which a saltwater solution was not effective in yielding crack starter defects in steel while graphite oil, but not dry graphite, was effective, it would appear that either carbon or hydrogen released from the oil combined with the heated steel surface to produce an embrittled layer. Mirkin (1969) shows that a white layer of nonuniform hardness peaking at 1400 kg/mm^2 is formed on the surface of iron coated with carbon-containing compounds. Beneath this lies a heat-worked layer with a hardness of 250 kg/mm^2.

Surface heat treating of large objects with complex profiles with a high-power cw CO_2 laser has been discussed by Locke and Hella (1974). For a scan rate of 470 cm^2/min, carbon steel could be hardened to a depth of about 0.4 mm with a cw laser power in the 20-kW range. Large areas can be case hardened by scanning the laser beam in a slightly overlapping pattern.

Transparent crystals such as NaCl also show evidence of dislocation structures when subjected to multiple pulses from a high-power laser (Aver'yanova *et al.*, 1966). Damage can extend several millimeters away from the point of laser impact and is thought to be due to the rapid heating/cooling that occurs even in transparent materials due to some residual absorption of the laser radiation. The surface layer of some refractory metal carbides has been found to spall away from the bulk material when subjected to Q-switched pulses from a ruby laser (Bastow *et al.*, 1969). The layer fragments into a large number of square or rectangular slabs, which subsequently can be peeled away from the substrate in slabs of constant thickness. The boundaries of these slabs correspond to the intersection of crystal cleavage planes with the surface plane. Damage within the slabs consists of arrays of dense dislocation tangles. Bastow *et al.* suggest the following mechanism for the formation of these slabs. On heating with the laser pulse, the surface of the material will expand but will be under compression due to the effect of the cooler subsurface layers. Above a particular temperature, compressive strains will be relieved by plastic flow. However, on recooling to room temperature, the surface layer will contract more than the sublayers and hence will be under tension, while the sublayers experience a compressive stress. At temperatures below the brittle–ductile transition point, stress relief can occur only by fracture of the surface layer. This forms the initial cracks in planes perpendicular to the surface. When a slab has parted from the remaining surface area in this way, the tensile stress within the slab will cause it to tend to bend away from the surface, promoting a fracture in a plane parallel to the surface. Although this is a plausible explanation of the effects observed, there would seem to be other mechanisms whereby fracture could occur in the manner noted. First, the penetration of visible radiation into insulating materials of this type may be substantial and may result in a higher temperature being obtained inside the material than on its surface (Gagliano and Paek, 1974). Superheating of a subsurface layer would subject the cooler layer above to a pressure pulse in the manner described by Dabby and Paek (1972). This could also lead to fracture. A second fracture mechanism exists in the transient stresses that are known (Maccomber, 1968; Emmony and Irving, 1969; Anderholm, 1970; Steverding, 1970, 1971; Apollonov *et al.*, 1972) to be generated in solid during laser impact.

9.4 CRYSTAL GROWTH

An interesting method of growing crystals of several refractory metal oxides using cw CO_2 laser heating was reported almost simultaneously by

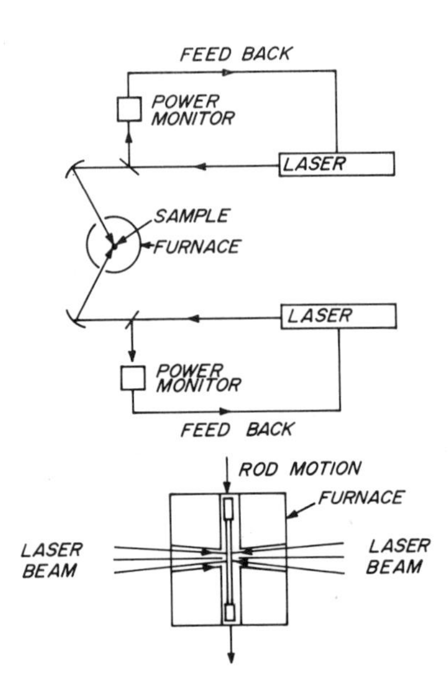

Fig. 9.4. Method for floating zone recrystallization of metal oxides using laser heating (after Cockayne and Gasson, 1970, and Eickhoff and Gürs, 1969).

Cockayne and Gasson (1970) and Eickhoff and Gürs (1969). The method is shown schematically in Fig. 9.4. Basically the technique is similar to that used in conventional floating-zone processes except that the source of heat is obtained from the focused output of two lasers. The oxide to be crystallized is formed into a sintered rod, which is then placed in a furnace that provides a bias temperature and minimizes the effects of thermal gradients during crystal growth. The lasers are then focused to small spots on opposite sides of the rotating oxide rod. The additional heat supplied by the lasers is sufficient to produce a melt zone, which can then be moved through the rod by translating the rod along its length. In the experiments of Gasson and Cockayne (1970) the incident laser intensity could be varied up to a maximum value of 50 kW/cm^2. This intensity together with a bias temperature of 1700°C was sufficient to melt or vaporize all of the oxides investigated. Optically transparent single crystals of Y_2O_3, $CaZrO_3$, $MgAl_2O_4$, and Al_2O_3 could be prepared using this method, although all crystals had residual strains due to the temperature gradients inherent in this process. The surface of the crystals showed a helical structure due to the asymmetry of the heating process. Typical growth rates were 3–5 cm/hour and the rods were rotated at 7.7 rpm.

Several materials were found to vaporize before melting so that no crystals could be formed. These materials were CeO_2, CaO and MgO. Vaporization occurred to some extent in all systems, however, and an investigation of this effect by Cockayne and Gasson (1971) showed that the higher peak powers obtained under ac excitation of the laser were responsible. Conversion to dc operation reduced these vaporization losses by two orders of magnitude.

If the melt is spun rapidly then material is removed in the form of small liquid droplets, which subsequently cool to form spherules of the solid. Nelson *et al.* (1970, 1972) and Mayerstr (1972) have investigated this process. Nelson *et al.* (1970) report that high-alumina tubing with a 250-W cw CO_2 laser generates particles whose diameter lies mainly in the 420–840 μm range. It would appear that this method may develop into a useful process for the production of microspheres of some refractory oxide materials (Topol and Happe, 1974).

The melting and recrystallization of pendant drops of aluminum oxide in oxygen and argon atmospheres produced with a cw CO_2 laser has been studied by Nelson *et al.* (1973). One might expect that there would be little difference in the melting and solidification of Al_2O_3 in the two types of atmosphere, since previous experiments (Diamond and Dragoo, 1966) had indicated that the atmosphere had little effect on the properties of the resulting crystals. A careful study by Nelson *et al.* (1973) showed, however, that quite significant changes were observed when Al_2O_3 was heated and recooled in an oxygen atmosphere as opposed to heating in argon. Some of the notable differences can be summarized as follows:

(i) The decrease in visible light emitted from the drops on the termination of heating showed a smooth decay for about 200 msec, followed by an abrupt rise in emission, and then constant luminosity for $\simeq$400 msec. The amplitude of the abrupt rise was found to be larger in oxygen atmospheres.

(ii) Dendritic crystal growth occurs along veinlike loci on cooling in argon. In oxygen, the crystallization is much more ordered, although the drops were occasionally observed to "shudder" due to the propagation of a type of shock wave through the drop just prior to solidification.

(iii) Drops solidified in argon were found to be considerably smoother than those solidified in oxygen.

(iv) Samples solidified in argon were found to be grey while those solidified in oxygen were white. It was suggested that the grey color in argon may be due to the precipitation of metal from the melt due to oxygen starvation.

(v) $\simeq$20% less laser power was required to just melt drops in oxygen than in argon. A corresponding change in the melting point was noted. The melting point was 2026 $\pm$ 4°C in oxygen and $\simeq$2054°C in argon.

The significance of this work is twofold. First, with regard to Al_2O_3, it points out that ambient atmospheric effects cannot be neglected in the use of this material as a high-temperature pyrometric and calorimetric standard. Second, and more generally, it indicates that laser heating has certain advantages over conventional heating methods in the study of melting and recrystallization of high-temperature materials. These advantages arise because laser heating can be applied to small isolated drops so that optical observations are unobscured by background radiation due to other heated objects (crucibles, etc.). Furthermore, small pendant drops connected to a solid substrate by only a thin filament are little affected by the presence of the substrate and uniform exposure to an ambient atmosphere can be obtained.

An elegant method of growing thin rods of pyrolytic carbon using a cw CO_2 laser has been reported by Nelson and Richardson (1972) and independently by Lydtin (1972). The system (Fig. 9.5) involves creation of a small heated area on a substrate, which is then subjected to a flow of natural gas. Pyrolysis of the hydrocarbons in the gas flow results in the selective deposition of carbon at the heated spot. If the laser focus is then moved by changing the position of the lens, the diameter of the focal area remains constant as a filament of deposited carbon builds up out of the substrate. Since only the tip of this filament is heated, deposition occurs only in this area and a filament of constant diameter can be formed. With a natural gas flow of 5 liters/min and a laser power of 20 W focused to a 0.5-mm diameter spot, a 0.5-mm diameter rod of pyrolytic carbon could be grown at the rate of 20 to 30 mm/hr. The total length of this rod was limited to about 2.5 cm by mechanical vibrations in the system. Substrates of graphite, zirconia, pencil lead, and a carbon/carbon composite were used. The structure of the filaments formed in this way showed that the deposit grows with the *c* axis oriented in the direction of growth. The free surface of the rod heated by the laser is hemispherical.

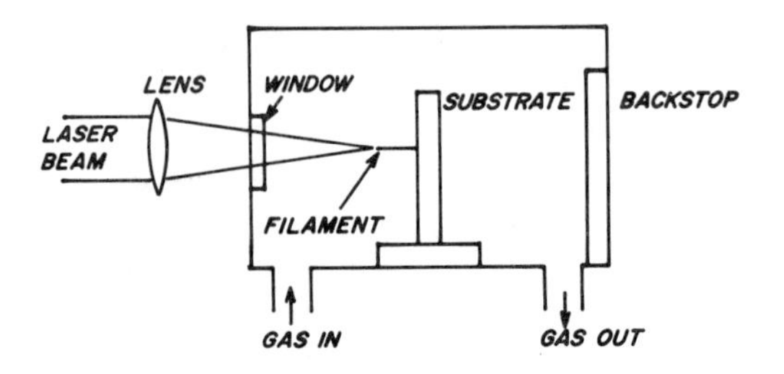

Fig. 9.5. Schematic representation of system for CO_2 laser-assisted growth of carbon filaments (Nelson and Richardson, 1972).

Other aspects of the interaction between high-power cw CO_2 laser radiation and carbons have been reported by Nelson *et al.* (1972) and Nelson (1972). On exposure of several types of graphite and vitreous carbon to laser fluxes in the range 25 kW/cm^2 these materials undergo phase changes leading to the allotrope chaoite and to at least one other previously unidentified modification. There is also some indirect evidence that a liquid phase may be created in the irradiated area. This would be an exciting development since previous indications have been that carbon cannot exist as a liquid at atmospheric pressure. In an attempt to produce liquid droplets, irradiated graphite rods were spun at rates of up to 198,000 rpm. Although direct visual observation of the spinning sample showed what appeared to be waves of liquid moving out from the focal area, no droplets could be collected. However, rods heated in this way exhibited surface features that suggested that liquid had flowed out of the interaction region. This was further supported by observations of the ability of the flowing material to move around corners. This would not be possible, given the geometry of the sample, if vapor deposition were responsible for the observed surface features. It is likely that further experiments in this area will further clarify this process and may require a reexamination of the phase diagram of carbon at low pressures.

The "clean" heat available from the CO_2 laser has recently found application in the preparation of optical fibers (Duley *et al.*, 1973; Jaeger and Logan, 1973; Paek, 1974). By heating the end of a glass rod with the radiation from a cw CO_2 laser, the end may be brought to the melting point and a melt puddle formed. If the melt is then touched with a cool glass rod of small diameter, a fiber will be drawn out of the melt when the rod is removed. The diameter of this fiber will depend on the melt temperature and the drawing speed. For stable drawing of the fiber, the temperature across the melt must have both radial and rotational symmetry and should be lowest at the point where the fiber is being drawn. This places some constraints on the type of focusing that can be used. Figure 9.6 shows a system developed by Jaeger and Logan (1973). Since there is no contact between the melt and any other surface, this method offers the possibility of preparing uniform cladded fibers of high optical quality. Such fibers may be useful in optical waveguide communications systems.

9.5 STRESS PRODUCTION

We have seen that the absorption of an intense laser flux at the surface of an opaque material results in rapid heating or even superheating of a surface layer and the ejection of evaporated material. Both of these effects

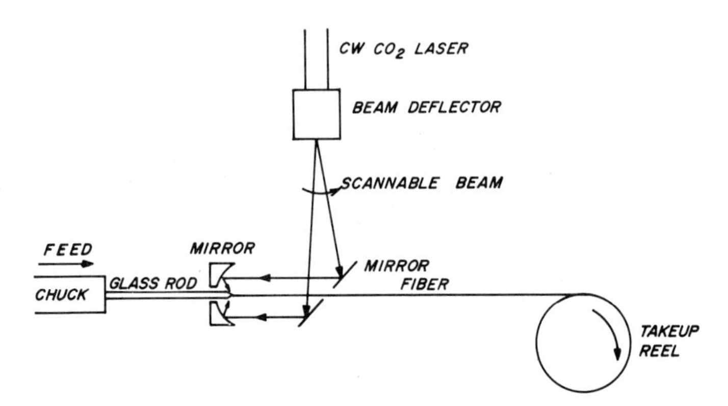

Fig. 9.6. System for drawing optical fibers using a cw CO_2 laser (after Jaeger and Logan, 1973).

can lead to the generation of substantial stresses in the target. Heating produces a differential expansion of the surface layer, yielding large thermal stresses; evaporation generates an impulse loading of the material because of the momentum imparted by the ejected vapor to the target. The first of these processes may occur almost instantaneously, particularly if radiation penetrates some depth into the target. The second process operates on a different time scale, since the temperature must first rise into the region where evaporation is rapid before ejected species can leave the target in quantity. Added to both of these effects is the direct effect of the momentum imparted to the target by the absorption or reflection of incident photons, each of which carries a momentum $=h/\lambda$, and the creation of blast waves by laser heating of the plasma formed in front of the target. It is not surprising, therefore, that significant stresses may be generated in targets during irradiation. Stress waves created at the irradiated surface propagate into the target and can be reflected from free surfaces where they change from compressive to tensile and may lead to spallations of the rear surface. In this section, some measurements of laser-induced stress waves in solids will be discussed and the theory describing these effects will be briefly outlined. One practical application of stress wave generation has already been described in the literature (Yang and Menichelli, 1971; Yang, 1974). Stress waves generated in a thin and metallic layer have been shown (Yang and Menichelli, 1971) to lead to a means of detonating insensitive high explosives.

Two papers by Steverding (1970, 1971) have outlined a simple theory that can be used to describe the instantaneous pressure and impulse generated by the absorption of a short high-intensity laser pulse on the surface of an opaque target. The light pulse, which is assumed to be of constant intensity for a time τ, can be thought of as being divided up into n equal "subpulses" of duration τ/n. Steverding (1970) shows that the average temperature $\tilde{T}_n$ in the surface layer after n of these pulses is obtained from

$$C_v(\tilde{T}_n - \tilde{T}_{n-1}) = E_0(1 - R)/n\rho\delta_{n-1} \tag{12}$$

where $\tilde{T}_{n-1}$ is the temperature after n-1 pulses, C_v the specific heat at constant volume, ρ the density of the material, E_0 the fluence (J/cm^2) integrated over the total pulse length, R the reflectivity, and δ_{n-1} the radiation penetràtion depth after the $(n - 1)$th subpulse. $\tilde{T}_n$ is obtained by iteration using $n = 1, 2, 3, \ldots$. When $\tilde{T}_n$ has been found, the average energy density per unit mass $\tilde{\epsilon}_n$ in the surface layer can be obtained from

$$\tilde{\epsilon}_n - \tilde{\epsilon}_0 = C_v(\tilde{T}_n - \tilde{T}_0) \tag{13}$$

and then the pressure after the nth subpulse p_n becomes, through the Mie–Grüneisen equation of state,

$$p_n - p_0 = G\rho(\tilde{\epsilon}_n - \tilde{\epsilon}_0) \tag{14}$$

where G is the Grüneisen ratio and $G\rho$ a constant for a given material. Then

$$p_n - p_0 = \frac{GE_0(1 - R)}{n} \sum_{i=0}^{n-1} \frac{1}{\delta_i} \tag{15}$$

The penetration depths δ_i to be used in this equation are, in general, dependent on temperature and may be much larger at high temperatures than at 300°K. This has the effect of reducing the peak pressure. Steverding (1970) gives some examples of predicted values of p_n for a 10-μm laser pulse with an intensity of 10^9 W/cm^2 and 10-nsec duration. His values (in kilobars) are

copper: $p_n = 212$, aluminum: $p_n = 121$, beryllium: $p_n = 60$

These are very large pressures indeed, and if sustained may lead to rapid fracture of the material. The critical laser power and the pulse length needed to produce fracture have been estimated by Steverding (1971). The dynamic fracture strength σ of a material is related to its static strength σ_0 through the relation

$$\sigma = \sigma_0 + A(d\sigma/dt)^\lambda \tag{16}$$

where A and λ are constants for the material, $\lambda \simeq 0.5$, and t is the time. Then for a square pressure pulse,

$$t/t^* = [(\sigma - \sigma_0)/(\sigma^* - \sigma_0)]^{(\lambda-1)/\lambda} \tag{17}$$

where σ^* is the theoretical strength of the material and t^* an incubation time or the time for which the pressure pulse must be maintained. Making the approximations $p_n = \sigma$ and $p_{crit} = \sigma^* \simeq E/10$, where E is the elastic modulus, Steverding (1971) obtains the following estimate of the critical intensity that must be exceeded before fracture can be expected to occur:

$$F = \epsilon\delta/15(1 - R)t^*G \tag{18}$$

where δ is now an average penetration depth. Approximate calculations can be performed taking $t^* \simeq 10^{-7}$ sec. Typically, for laser pulses of duration $\tau = t^* \simeq 10^{-7}$ sec, fracture of most metals is predicted to occur when $F \gtrsim 10^8$ W/cm^2. In this range of intensities, however, we have already seen (Section 5.2) that a great variety of other heating and material removal mechanisms become important. A plume may be created, for example, and this may attenuate part of the incident intensity. Certainly, strong evaporation is expected and this will give rise to further momentum transfer to the target. Estimates of the critical intensity required for fracture damage obtained from Eq. (18) must therefore be treated with caution.

Fracture and spallation of surfaces exposed to high laser fluxes has been reported by Anderholm (1970), Fox and Barr (1973), Siegrist and Kneubühl (1973), and Fox (1974). It should be noted that material removal by fracture is a much more efficient mechanism than direct removal via melting or evaporation. It is also a means by which short laser pulses can be effectively used to remove relatively large amounts of material independent of the thermal diffusion length for the laser pulse used.

The shape of the laser pulse has been shown (Fox, 1974) to influence greatly the degree of back face spallation in thin metal samples. Spallation of the back face of an irradiated target was shown to occur when the impulse imparted to the front of the target by ejected material results in the formation of a compressive stress wave that propagates through the target to reflect off the rear face. The reflected wave generates a tensile stress at the back surface, which can result in the separation of part of the surface from the bulk material. This spallation was controlled by the duration and energy of a short prepulse. As an example, a 1-mm thick aluminum target showed little evidence for spallation when subjected to a 8000 $\pm$ 600 J/cm^2 main pulse after conditioning with a 4-nsec, 0.06-J prepulse, but spalled extensively when subjected to the same main pulse preceded by a 23-nsec, 4.4-J prepulse. It is likely that part of the increased efficiency of spallation under prepulsing conditions is due to the creation of a plasma in front of the target that is subsequently heated by the main pulse to produce a shock wave that impinges on the front of the target. Another effect may involve a reduction in reflectivity of the sample by the precursor pulse, which allows more of the energy of the main pulse to be coupled into the target (Chun and Rose, 1970).

Experiments by Anderholm (1970), Jones (1971), O'Keefe and Skeen (1972), Felix and Ellis (1972), and Siegrist and Kneubühl (1973) have demonstrated that any confinement of the surface plasma created by the incident laser flux results in a significant enhancement of stresses in the target. This confinement may be accomplished simply by clamping the target to a transparent plate at its front surface (Anderholm, 1970; Felix and Ellis, 1972; Yang, 1974) or by coating the exposed target surface with a thin layer that is either transparent and quite volatile (O'Keefe and Skeen, 1972) or opaque to the incident laser radiation (Jones, 1971). A quantitative study of stresses induced in aluminum targets with and without thin coatings, showed that stresses were augmented by an order of magnitude in coated targets (O'Keefe and Skeen, 1972). This was attributed to the rapid volatilization of the surface layer at the metal–film interface with subsequent expansion of the trapped vapor. Siegrist and Knuebühl (1973) found that the stresses induced in fused quartz by irradiating the surface in the presence of a thin layer of H_2O or other liquid were sufficient to fracture the quartz. Since this work was done at 10.6 μm, where water is absorbing, it is likely that the stress enhancement was due in this case to the impulse given to the target by the rapid evaporation of the liquid layer.

Time-resolved measurements of the stress generated in laser-irradiated targets have been reported by many groups. A stress wave will be induced in a solid only if the shock transit time in the solid is greater than the duration of the laser pulse. With Q-switched lasers, the rise time and half-widths of laser-induced stress waves are typically $\gtrsim 10$ nsec. Excitation with picosecond pulses (Peercy *et al.*, 1970) has been shown to yield stress waves whose rise times are $\lesssim 1$ nsec and that have a duration of only $\simeq 2$ nsec. Figure 9.7 shows the configuration used by Felix and Ellis (1972) to

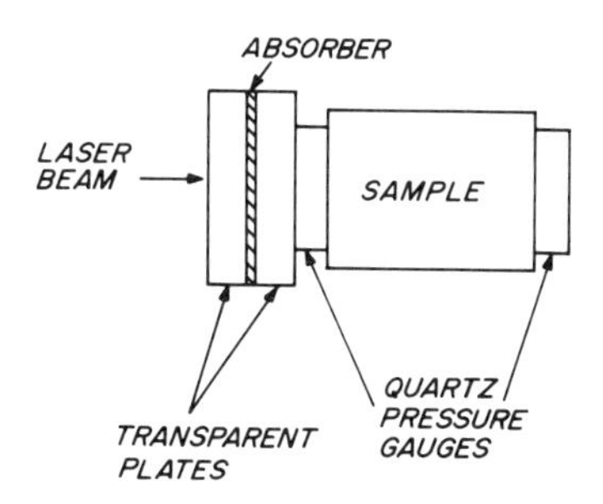

Fig. 9.7. System for time-resolved stress measurements on samples excited by a laser pulse (after Felix and Ellis, 1972).

measure the time dependence of the stress in various solid specimens. The x-cut quartz gauge nearest the absorbing sample measures the stress wave entering the sample, while that at the other end measures the stress wave transmitted by the sample. Using this system, Felix and Ellis were able to show that a stress wave that was nominally compressive before entering developed a tensile tail on propagating through the sample. This dispersion was attributed to the presence of voids in the metal samples used. With water, dispersion was observed only as long as the water contained dissolved air.

Stress pulses as observed in these studies typically have a sharp leading edge, which may rise, as noted above, in <1 nsec. The decay of the pulse is somewhat less abrupt and may have a long tail. This tail occurs because evaporation can continue even after the laser pulse terminates. The study of Fox and Barr (1973b) in which 6061-T6 aluminum was excited directly by 5–30-nsec-duration pulses from a glass laser shows that the peak stress increases with the fluence until a critical point is reached at which point air breakdown appears to shield the surface and the peak stress begins to decrease with increasing fluence. At constant fluence, the peak stress decreases monotonically with the laser pulse duration. The peak stress was about 3–4 kbar for a 30-nsec pulse and a fluence of about 100 J/cm^2. Peak stresses of >20 kbar have been produced in other experiments (Peercy *et al.*, 1970; Anderholm, 1970). Palmer and Asmus (1970) have generated 200-kbar stress waves in particulate-loaded carbonaceous materials.

The results of a comprehensive study of stress wave amplitudes produced in thin metallic films excited with a 15-nsec pulse from a Q-switched ruby laser (Yang, 1974) have been summarized in Table 9.1. In all systems studied, the relation between the maximum stress and the laser fluence was linear for fluences up to 13 J/cm^2. Films were clamped between two glass slabs.

In the excitation regime where strong gas phase energy loss occurs due to laser-supported combustion waves (Stegman *et al.*, 1973), the time-dependent stress shows peaks and dips that follow the attenuation produced by the combustion wave.

The average shock pressure may also be estimated by measuring the momentum transferred to the target as a whole on excitation with an intense laser pulse. The momentum M and average shock pressure $\bar{P}$ are related through

$$\bar{P} = M/A\tau \qquad (19)$$

where τ is the length of the laser pulse and A the area of the target that is excited. Measurements of momentum transferred to a target have been

Table 9.1

Experimental Determinations of Slope of Plot of Peak Stress vs. Laser Fluence for Thin Metal Films[a]

Material	Peak stress (kbar) / Laser fluence (J/cm²)	Film thickness (Å)
Ag	1.30	1500
Al	1.64	1000
Au	1.25	1800
B	1.11	3500–14,000
Bi	1.46	1100–4400
C	1.50	1200–5200
Co	1.3	1150–2300
Cr	1.56	1600
Cu	1.43	1500
Fe	1.30	1750
Ge	1.36	3050–10,050
In	1.5	1100–4400
Mg	1.43	1200–4800
Mn	1.56	1500
Mo	1.34	1500–3200
Ni	1.63	1500
Pb	1.42	
Pt	1.25	1200
Sb	1.36	1050–4200
Si	1.27	4000–11,000
Sn	1.2	1500–600
Ti	1.42	1450–3350
Zn	1.36	1900–6200
Zr	1.56	2300

[a] After Yang (1974).

reported by Neuman (1964), Gregg and Thomas (1966), Skeen and York (1968), Jones (1971), Pirri *et al.* (1972), Metz (1973), Fox and Barr (1973a), Hettche *et al.* (1973), and Lowder and Pettingill (1974). Gregg and Thomas (1966) found that the momentum transfer normalized to the laser pulse energy increased to a maximum as the incident intensity increased and then decreased according to the law

$$M/E_0 = NF^{-n} \tag{20}$$

where N and n are constants for a particular material. For most materials peak values of M/E_0 were reached for $F \simeq 5 \times 10^8 - 10^9$ W/cm². Jones (1971) observed similar behavior when aluminum was excited with 2–3 psec Nd : glass laser pulses. Using a heating model similar to that of Steverding (1970) but including evaporation in which most of the absorbed laser energy is converted to kinetic energy of the ejecta, Jones was able to obtain a simple expression relating M to E_0. His result is

$$M = 2\sqrt{2}[\rho\delta E_0(1 - R)]^{1/2}Q(x)A \tag{21}$$

where

$$x = \rho\delta E_T/[E_0(1 - R)]$$

$$Q(x) = (1 - x)^{1/2} - x^{1/2}\tan^{-1}[(1 - x)/x]^{1/2}$$

where the symbols have the same meaning as above but with E_T a threshold energy (J/g) that can be taken as the heat of vaporization. A plot of M/E_0 versus E_0 should then rise as E_0 increases to attain a maximum value and then decrease. This decrease is due to the incorporation of a threshold energy in the analysis and is not related to any gas breakdown effects. This casts some uncertainty on the interpretation of Gregg and Thomas (1966) concerning their observation that the decrease in M/E_0 at large E_0 was due to decoupling of the incident laser beam by absorption in the plasma formed in front of the target. However, it is now known that absorption in the plume is effective in shielding the surface and reducing the impulse under certain conditions (Stegman *et al.*, 1973), although the blast wave created by extensive laser heating of an ejected plasma may result in increased momentum input to the target at high incident intensities (Pirri *et al.*, 1972; Metz, 1973; Hettche *et al.*, 1973; Lowder and Pettingill, 1974).

Pirri *et al.* (1972) have shown that when a laser-generated detonation occurs in the plasma over the irradiated surface, the impulse M can be described as follows:

$$\begin{aligned} M = {} & 0.7(E'\rho_0)^{1/2}[(A_T/\pi + d^2)^{3/4} - d^{3/2}] \\ & + 2.1(E'\rho_0)^{1/2}d^2[(A_T/\pi + d^2)^{-1/4} - d^{-1/2}] \\ & + 0.6(E'\rho_0)^{1/2}A_T[(A_T/\pi + d^2)^{-1/4} + f(p_0, \rho_0, E')] \end{aligned} \tag{22}$$

where E' is the total pulse energy (J), ρ_0 the ambient density (g/cm^3), A_T the surface area of the target, d the time averaged distance of the detonation point source above the target surface, and f a weak function of p_0, ρ_0, and E', where p_0 is the ambient pressure. This indicates that the total impulse transmitted to the target should be strongly dependent on the total area of the target. This dependence has been observed experimentally (Pirri *et al.*, 1972).

Measurement of the impulse generated at a solid target under conditions in which much of the laser radiation is absorbed in the gas phase in front of the target indicates that impulse coupling coefficients of $\simeq 5 \times 10^{-5}$ N-sec/J can be expected (Hettche *et al.*, 1973; Lowder and Pettingill, 1974) when the target surface area is large. The dependence of the peak pressure on incident laser intensity is less well defined: Pirri (1973) predicts a $\frac{2}{3}$ dependence of p on F, while Hettche *et al.* (1973) find a square-law dependence experimentally and Lowder and Pettingill (1974) obtain $p \propto F^{3/2}$. The origin of some of these differences is discussed briefly by Lowder and Pettingill (1974).

We have seen earlier (Section 6.6) that thermally induced stresses may be effectively used in the machining of materials with cw or pulsed CO_2 lasers (Lumley, 1969; Gagliano *et al.*, 1969). Stresses in this case are generated by the direct effect of thermal gradients in the interaction region. Detailed calculations have been made by Paek and Gagliano (1972) of the stresses surrounding holes drilled in Al_2O_3 ceramic with a ruby laser. These stresses may lead to material fracture during processing or may simply be retained after processing has been completed to act as possible sources of failure of the material at later times. Duley and Young (1974) have studied the residual stresses around holes drilled with a cw CO_2 laser in fused-quartz sheet. The stress appears to be largest at points in the bulk material that lie about $\frac{3}{4}$ of the depth of the hole (Fig. 9.8). These stresses lead to the characteristic form of fracture shown in Fig. 9.9. In addition, there are localized regions of void and crack formation near the base of the hole and spread along the regions adjacent to the surface of the hole at points within the material. Since these defects are due to rapid heating/cooling during drilling, their occurrence can be minimized by careful control over the intensity and duration of the heat pulse. Duley and Young (1974) found that when the intensity is such that heat transfer due to conduction is important (i.e., $F \lesssim 10^4$–10^5 W/cm^2 for insulators) fewer defects are produced and residual stresses are minimized when the laser pulse length is made as large as possible. This tends to reduce thermal gradients in the sample.

This review of both dynamic and static laser-induced stresses has, of necessity, been quite brief. New experimental observations and theoretical descriptions of the effects discussed above are appearing regularly and the literature on this subject is now quite extensive. Further bibliographical references on this subject are Kokodii and Volitov (1969), Alexander and Nurmikko (1973) (effects of radiation pressure), Askar'yan *et al.* (1967), Basov *et al.* (1967), Panarella and Savic (1968), Büchl *et al.* (1969), Emmony and Irving (1969), Thompson *et al.* (1971) (laser-induced detona-

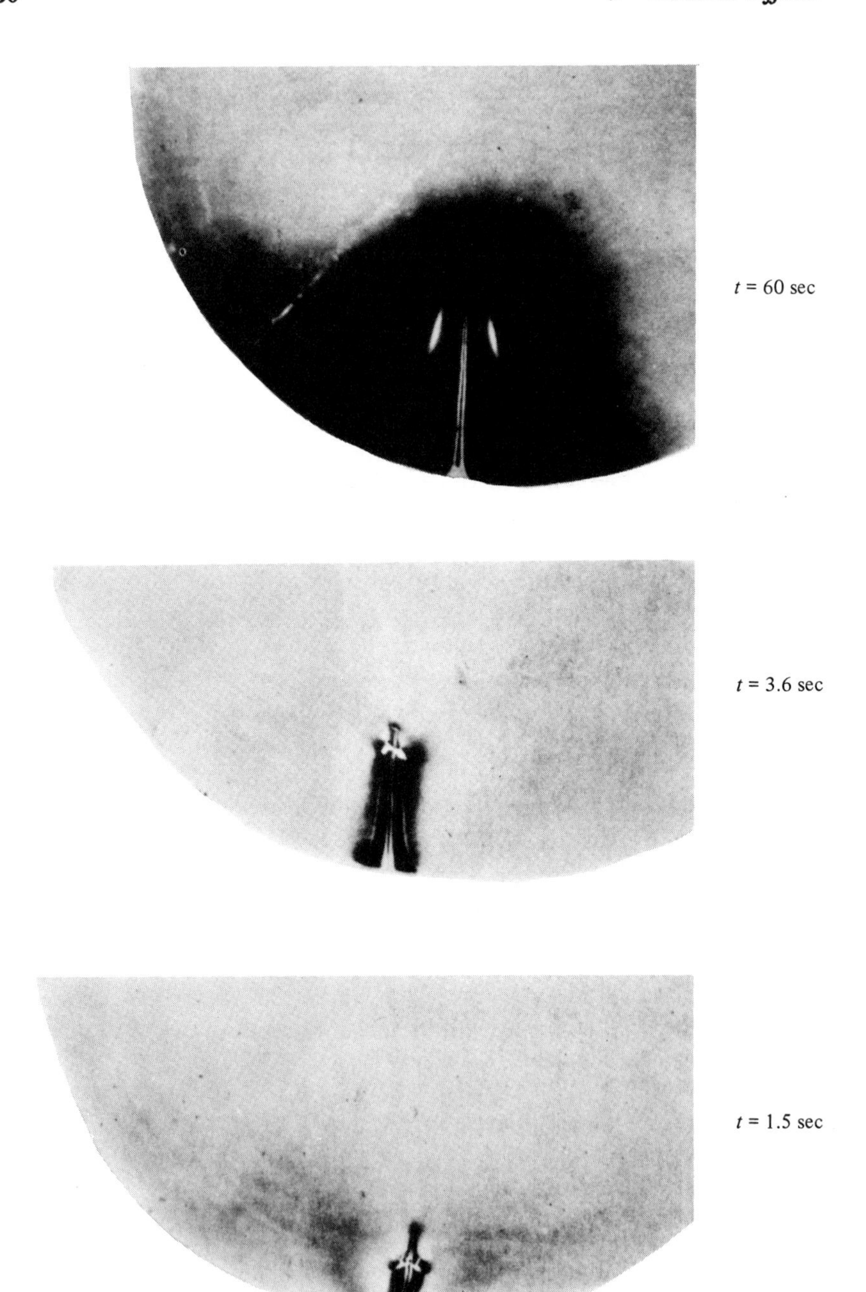

Fig. 9.8. Stress patterns observed in circularly polarized light for holes drilled with a laser intensity of 3×10^4 W/cm^2 (from Duley and Young, 1974).

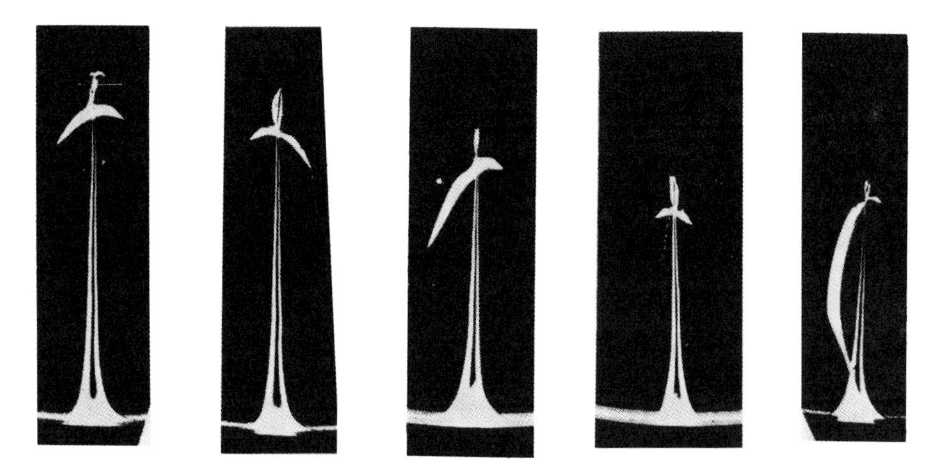

Fig. 9.9. Defect structures observed adjacent to holes drilled in quartz with a CO_2 laser. The left hole is 1.4 cm in depth (from Duley and Young, 1974).

tions), Perceval (1967), Penner and Sharma (1967), Pirri (1973) (theoretical descriptions of laser-induced shock waves in solids), White (1963), Mirkin and Pilipetskii (1966), Bushnell and McCloskey (1968), Mirkin (1970), Ashmarin *et al.* (1971), Anderholm and Boade (1972), Hartman *et al.* (1972), Apollonov *et al.* (1972), Lowder *et al.* (1973), Boling and Dube (1973), Duthler (1974) (experimental and theoretical studies of stress waves and deformations in solids), and Carome *et al.* (1964, 1967), Bell and Landt (1967), Feiock and Goodwin (1972) (laser-induced stress waves in liquids). General discussion may be found in Ready (1971).

Chapter 10

Propagation, Atmospheric Monitoring, and Communication Links at 10.6 μm

10.1 INTRODUCTION

In all but a few applications of CO_2 lasers it is necessary to transmit the beam through an ambient atmosphere to reach a workpiece or a detector. While the attentuation of standard atmospheres is small at 10.6 μm, it cannot be considered zero. Water vapor, while having no strong transitions at 10.6 μm, still absorbs slightly, and CO_2, which is also present in small quantities in terrestrial atmospheres, has a one-to-one correspondence between its absorption lines and lines emitted from the CO_2 laser. The atmosphere also contains particulate matter, which material is responsible for extinction due to absorption and scattering of incident radiation. The presence of all three of these constituents results in the transfer of part of the energy in a propagating laser beam to the molecules along the path of propagation. This heating effect reacts on the beam by causing complex time- and position-dependent distortions in the beam profile and beam bending. In this chapter we consider some fundamental energy transfer mechanisms and the ways this energy transfer affects the propagation of high-power 10.6-μm laser beams through the atmosphere.

Two practical applications of CO_2 lasers involving the propagation of CO_2 laser radiation through the atmosphere are discussed in the last two sections of this chapter. The first of these lies in the area of pollution monitoring, where high-power ultraviolet, visible, and infrared wavelength lasers have provided several diagnostic techniques for remote and laboratory measurements on gaseous and particulate atmospheric contaminants. Section 6 gives a brief discussion of the application of CO_2 lasers to optical communications systems.

10.2 ABSORPTION AND SCATTERING OF CO_2 LASER RADIATION IN THE ATMOSPHERE

CO_2 laser radiation is attenuated on passing through the atmosphere by a combination of absorption in H_2O and CO_2 and extinction by scattering and absorption due to small airborne particles. Fortunately, under normal atmospheric conditions neither of these effects leads to serious attenuation, so that long propagation paths are possible. In this section we will discuss each of these fundamental processes and review experimental measurements made on the propagation of CO_2 laser radiation through real and simulated atmospheres.

10.2.1 Absorption of CO_2 Laser Radiation

In the lower atmosphere, the major absorbers for CO_2 laser radiation are CO_2 and H_2O. Absorption in CO_2 occurs in the 10.4-μm band [$(00^01) \leftarrow (10^00, 02^00)_{\mathrm{I}}$ transition] and in the 9.4-μm band [$(00^01) \leftarrow (10^00, 02^00)_{\mathrm{II}}$ transition]. Although the lower levels involved in these transitions are over 1000 cm^{-1} above the ground state of CO_2, the Boltzmann factor for these levels is $\simeq 10^{-3}$ at 300°K. Thus, $\simeq 0.1\%$ of the CO_2 molecules along the propagation path will be in these levels at 300°K and will be able to absorb incident CO_2 laser radiation [see the discussion by Munjee and Christiansen (1973) on the role played by transitions of the type $(0X^11) \rightleftharpoons (1X^10)$ in the absorption of laser lines in the 10.4-μm band at high temperatures].

H_2O in the vapor phase has several pure rotational lines as well as some lines of the ν_2 band in the vicinity of the 10.4-μm band of CO_2. Some data on these transitions as reported by Ippolitov (1969) are given in Table 10.1. In addition, continuous absorption will be present throughout this region due to the overlapping wings of other strong rotational lines.

Absorption coefficients for attenuation by both CO_2 and H_2O have been reported (Yin and Long, 1968; McCoy *et al.*, 1969) at 10.59 μm. In a

Table 10.1

Wavelengths of Some Lines due to Gaseous H_2O in the Vicinity of 10.6 μm[a]

Wavelength (μm)	Energy of lower level (cm^{-1})	Type
10.639	1114.59	Rotation
10.589	2054.55	ν_2 band
10.583	2322.25	Rotation
10.582	2320.20	Rotation
10.563	842.36	Rotation
10.546	446.66	Rotation
10.544	1327.25	Rotation

[a] From Ippolitov (1969).

standard atmosphere at altitudes below about 9 km, Wood *et al.* (1971) give the following expression for the absorption coefficient due to CO_2:

$$\alpha_C = 1.44 \times 10^{-3}[295/T]^{1.5} \exp[-(970/T) \ln 10] \ (\text{cm}^{-1}) \qquad (1)$$

McCoy *et al.* (1969) find for absorption due to H_2O

$$\alpha_H = 4.32 \times 10^{-11} p(P + 193p) \ (\text{cm}^{-1}) \qquad (2)$$

where T is the temperature in °K, p the partial pressure of H_2O, and P the total atmospheric pressure also in Torr. Table 10.2 gives numerical values for α_H as a function of relative humidity at sea level under standard conditions. The corresponding value for α_C at 10.7°C is $\alpha_C = 5.8 \times 10^{-2}$/km. Thus it is evident that at sea level, absorption at 10.59 μm is dominated by CO_2 absorption at low relative humidities and by H_2O absorption as the relative humidity increases above about 30%. At high altitudes, the absorption due to H_2O becomes much less than that due to CO_2 (Wood *et al.*, 1971). The discrepancy between the values quoted by Wood *et al.* (1971) and McCoy *et al.* (1969) for α_H appears to be due to a misprint in the numerical factor in Eq. (2) quoted by Wood *et al.*

The fate of the energy transferred to CO_2 and H_2O by absorption of CO_2 laser radiation is of great interest in the development of heating and cooling of the gas along the propagation path. The quenching of excitation produced in H_2O is rapid, and absorbed laser energy is almost instantaneously converted to translational energy. On the other hand, the lifetime of the upper CO_2 level (00^01) and the resonant N_2 ($v'' = 1$) level due to quenching collisions is relatively long [$\simeq$1 msec at sea level (Breig, 1972)]. Hence strong translational coupling to the lower CO_2 level, which tends to

Table 10.2

Extinction Coefficient due to Water Vapor Absorption at 10.59 μm, at Sea Level, P = 760 Torr, and T = 10.7°C[a]

α_H (km^{-1})	Loss (dB/km)	Relative humidity (%)
0.0125	0.054	10
0.0338	0.15	20
0.0653	0.28	30
0.107	0.46	40
0.157	0.68	50
0.215	0.93	60
0.284	1.2	70
0.363	1.6	80

[a] From McCoy *et al.* (1969).

maintain the population in this level, results in a momentary cooling of the atmosphere along the laser propagation path. Furthermore, at high intensities stimulated emission from the CO_2 (00^01) level can occur, resulting in amplification of the transmitted beam. Thus complex intensity-dependent heating and cooling effects are expected (Wood *et al.*, 1971; Breig, 1972; Munjee and Christiansen, 1973). These effects and the resulting changes in the characteristics of a transmitted beam will be discussed in more detail in Section 10.3.

10.2.2 Extinction due to Particulate Matter

Consider a single particle with a characteristic dimension a exposed to a plane wave of light of wavelength λ. When $a \simeq \lambda$, the cross section for extinction due to this particle is no longer simply related to the geometrical cross section of the particle. This change in cross section can be allowed for by the introduction of an efficiency factor for extinction Q_{ext}. If the particle is taken to be spherical, then the effective cross section for extinction becomes

$$C_{ext} = Q_{ext}\pi a^2 \quad (3)$$

The units of C_{ext} are area and Q_{ext} are dimensionless. Furthermore, Q_{ext} can exceed unity. Two factors contribute to Q_{ext}: the first is absorption in the particle, which occurs with an efficiency Q_{abs}, and the second, measured by Q_{scat}, is due to light scattered out of the beam. Then

$$Q_{ext} = Q_{abs} + Q_{scat} \quad (4)$$

With regard to the attenuation, we are interested in the ratio of transmitted and incident intensities in the direction of the incident beam. This ratio is given by

$$F/F_0 = \exp[-C_{\text{ext}}Nx] \tag{5}$$

where N is the density (number/cm^3) of scatterers and x the path length.

Q_{abs} and Q_{scat} can be calculated for particles when the refractive index of the particle is known and when the particle geometry is simple [examples of tractable problems are given in van de Hulst (1957) and Kerker (1963)].

For a range of particle sizes, the coefficient of extinction will be

$$k_{\text{ext}}(\lambda) = \int_0^\infty n(a)Q_{\text{ext}}(a,\lambda)\pi a^2\,da \tag{6}$$

where $n(a)$ is the distribution function for the particle size and $k_{\text{ext}}(\lambda)$ is in cm^{-1}. The ratio of transmitted to incident intensities is then

$$F/F_0 = \exp(-k_{\text{ext}}x) \tag{7}$$

Propagation over an atmospheric path involves scattering and absorption by a variety of different types of particle. Some details on types and size ranges are given in Fig. 10.1. In practice, one is mostly interested in the effect of fogs, mist, and rain on laser propagation paths. Extensive calculations of Q_{abs}, Q_{scat}, and Q_{ext} for small particles of condensed water vapor are available (Zelmanowich and Shifrin, 1968), which means that fairly reliable estimates of extinction due to water particles in the atmosphere can be made. Q_{abs} and Q_{ext} at 10.6 μm for spherical water particles are shown as a

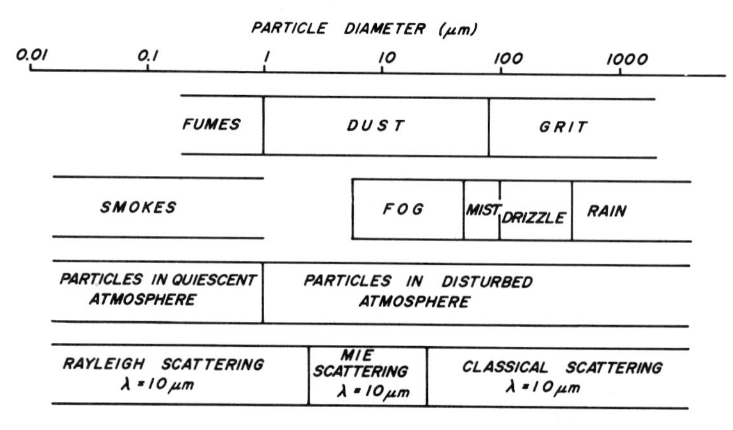

Fig. 10.1. Some size ranges for atmospheric particles and scattering regimes for 10-μm laser radiation.

function of particle radius in Fig. 10.2 (Glickler, 1971). For $a < 10\ \mu m$, one has $Q_{abs} \simeq 1.34a/\lambda$, and for $a \lesssim 1\ \mu m$, $Q_{abs} \simeq Q_{ext} = 1.34a/\lambda$. The limiting values of Q_{ext} and Q_{abs} at large a are $Q_{ext} = 2$ and $Q_{abs} = 1$.

These values can be used to obtain a rough estimate of the relative extinction produced by rain and fog at 10 μm. A heavy rain corresponds to a water content of about 1 g/m³ in particles of radii ≃0.1 cm. In a fog the water content may be 0.1 g/m³ but the particle size will be much less, typically $a \simeq 5\ \mu m$. Then the density of rain particles is ≃250/m³, while in a fog the density can reach $2 \times 10^8/m^3$. Since we assume that all the particles are the same size under each of these conditions,

$$\begin{aligned} k_{ext}\ (\text{rain}) &= N \times Q_{ext}(0.1\ \text{cm},\ 10\ \mu\text{m})\ \pi \times (0.1)^2 \\ &= 2.5 \times 10^{-4} \times 2 \times \pi \times (0.1)^2 \\ &= 1.57 \times 10^{-5}/\text{cm} = 6.8\ \text{dB/km} \end{aligned}$$

$$\begin{aligned} k_{ext}\ (\text{fog}) &= N \times Q_{ext}(5 \times 10^{-4}\ \text{cm},\ 10\ \mu\text{m})\ \pi \times (5 \times 10^{-4})^2 \\ &= 2 \times 10^2 \times 2 \times \pi \times (5 \times 10^{-4})^2 \\ &= 3.14 \times 10^{-4}/\text{cm} = 136\ \text{dB/km} \end{aligned}$$

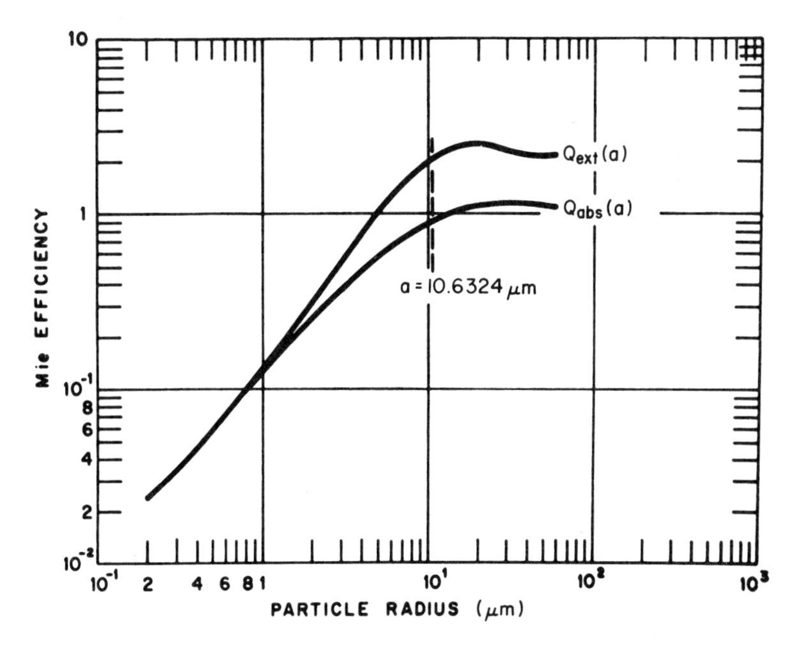

Fig. 10.2. Q_{abs} and Q_{ext} at 10.6 μm for spherical water particles of various radii (from Glickler, 1971).

and it is evident that 10-μm radiation is attenuated by particulate matter much more effectively in fogs than in rain.

Experimental studies on the propagation of 10.6-μm laser radiation through atmospheric precipitation and fogs have been reported by Chu and Hogg (1968), Zuev *et al.* (1969), and Bisyarin *et al.* (1971a,b). Chu and Hogg compared propagation data through rain, fog, and snow using He–Ne (0.63 μm), He–Xe (3.5 μm), and CO_2 (10.6 μm) laser sources. Their data and that obtained by Bisyarin *et al.* are summarized as follows:

Fog. Comparison of the attenuation produced in real and simulated fogs at 0.63 and 10.6 μm showed that the attenuation at 10.6 μm was almost always less than that at 0.63 μm. In real fogs, Bisyarin *et al.* (1971b) found the correlation

$$k_{\text{ext}}(10.6\ \mu\text{m}) = 0.38 k_{\text{ext}}(0.63\ \mu\text{m})$$

between the extinction coefficients in dB/km. In "standard" fogs produced under laboratory conditions, the following relation was found:

$$k_{\text{ext}}(10.6\ \mu\text{m}) = 0.43 k_{\text{ext}}(0.63\ \mu\text{m})$$

for total optical depths $\tau = k_{\text{ext}} x \leq 9$. The maximum value of k_{ext} (10.6 μm) in real fogs was always less than 10 dB/km. Chu and Hogg (1968) found that the attenuation at 10.6 μm in a 2.6-km outdoor path exceeded 10 dB/km 3% of the time over a one-year period. Attenuations as high as 20 dB/km were occasionally noted.

Rain. Bisyarin *et al.* (1971a) found that attenuation coefficients at 0.63 and 10.6 μm during rainy conditions showed good correlation. There was little difference between attenuation at these wavelengths. The highest value of k_{ext} (10.6 μm) noted was 25 dB/km. This occurred during a shower when the rate of rainfall exceeded 1 mm/min. Chu and Hogg found that the attenuation at 10.6 μm was consistently greater than that at shorter wavelengths. The highest attenuation at 10.6 μm occurred during a shower precipitation at the rate of $\simeq$1.9 mm/min. The attenuation in this case was $\simeq$15.4 dB/km. At rainfalls $\simeq$0.4 mm/min, the attenuation at 10.6 μm was about 10 dB/km.

Snow. Bisyarin *et al.* (1971a) obtained the following analytical relation between k_{ext} and the snowfall intensity I in mm/hr:

$$k_{\text{ext}}(10.6\ \mu\text{m}) = 1.5 I^{0.71}, \qquad k_{\text{ext}}(0.63\ \mu\text{m}) = 10.8 I^{0.53}$$

where k_{ext} is in dB/km. Thus, the attenuation at 10.6 μm is consistently greater than that at 0.63 μm during snowfall. The data of Chu and Hogg also support this conclusion.

10.3 THERMALLY INDUCED SPATIAL AND TEMPORAL VARIATIONS IN A 10.6-μm BEAM PROPAGATING THROUGH THE ATMOSPHERE

We have seen that even in the absence of particulate matter, standard atmospheres will attenuate 10.6-μm radiation due to absorption in CO_2 and H_2O. Absorption by both of these species eventually results in the transfer of part of the incident laser beam energy to the atmosphere along the propagation path. The time scale for conversion of radiation absorbed by H_2O to translational energy in the gas is very rapid and can be considered instantaneous. With absorption in CO_2, the energy transfer first results in a cooling of the gas along the propagation path and only some milliseconds later is heating produced. Figure 10.3 shows the ways in which the heating and cooling produced by a propagating beam with a Gaussian cross section can result in focusing or defocusing of the beam. Defocusing produced by heating gives rise to an effect known as "thermal blooming." When the atmosphere moves past the beam or alternatively, when the beam is slewed through the atmosphere, the effect of thermal defocusing produces a beam deflection and distortion of the intensity across the beam profile. Thermal blooming and attendant defocusing effects have been the subjects of extensive investigation by many groups. Some bibliographical references that cover work in this area are Leite *et al.* (1964, 1967), Litvak (1966),

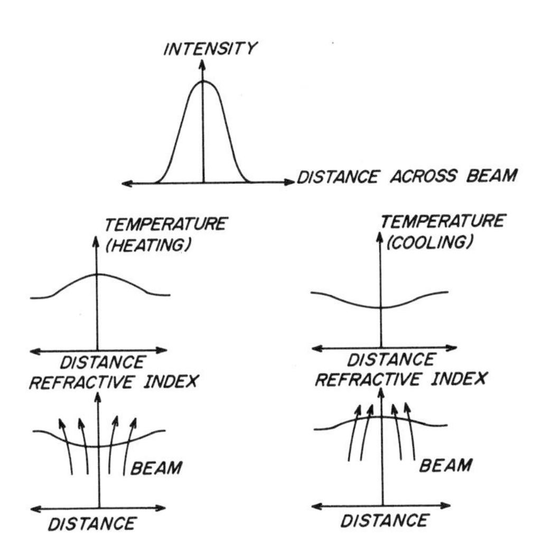

Fig. 10.3. Effect of heating/cooling due to a propagation laser beam on focusing or defocusing along propagation path (adapted from Wood *et al.*, 1971).

Whinnery *et al.* (1967), Akhamanov *et al.* (1968), Carman and Kelley (1968), Inaba and Ito (1968), McLean *et al.* (1968), Gebhardt and Smith (1969, 1971), Glass (1969), Kenemuth *et al.* (1970), Smith and Gebhardt (1970), Wallace and Camac (1970), Kleiman and O'Neil (1971), Livingston (1971), Wood *et al.* (1971), Breig (1972), Hayes (1972), Hayes *et al.* (1972), Buser and Rhode (1973), Munje and Christiansen (1973), Pridmore-Brown (1973), and Bradley and Herrmann (1974).

Breig (1972) has extended the calculations of Wood *et al.* (1971) on the heating and cooling by absorption in CO_2 in the atmosphere to beam intensities of up to 10^6 W/cm^2. At these high intensities, Breig showed that the absorption due to CO_2 saturates as the rate of stimulated emission from the upper level involved in the absorption process approaches the rate at which photons are removed from the beam. If the density of CO_2 molecules in the (00^01) state is X_3 while that for the $(10^00, 02^00)_{\mathrm{I}}$ level is X_1, then the cross section for absorption per molecule is given by

$$\sigma^* = \sigma[1 - X_3/X_1] \tag{8}$$

where σ is the cross section when $X_3 = 0$. As the beam intensity increases, absorption tends to equalize the populations X_1 and X_3, but at the same time stimulated emission becomes large. In the limit when $X_1 = X_3$ the CO_2 no longer contributes to the absorption. Breig points out that X_1 is very small under normal atmospheric conditions and hence the condition $X_1 = X_3$ can be reached at relatively low incident intensities. Calculations of the dependence of temperature on time including this saturation effect and absorption by H_2O and CO_2 showed that both heating and cooling effects can be produced in low- and high-altitude atmospheres. Initially, absorption of laser energy leads to a cooling effect with the amplitude of the temperature drop dependent on laser intensity. In addition, the time at which the lowest temperature is reached decreases as the laser intensity increases. This is due to saturation. At low incident intensities ($\simeq$1 kW/cm^2) and high altitudes where water vapor absorption is not significant, the cooling effect due to the CO_2 absorption may persist for greater than 0.1 sec. Finally, vibrational energy in the coupled CO_2 (00^01), N_2 $(v = 1)$, state gets converted to translational energy and the gas along the propagation path begins to heat.

The cooling effect due to CO_2 can be important even when the concentration of water vapor is such that a heating effect is produced at all times.

The cooling effect due to CO_2 can be important even when the concentration of water vapor is such that a heating effect is produced at all times. Heating increases X_1 in Eq. (8) and hence the saturation intensity. At the same time, an increase in X_1 may result in an increase in the cooling rate.

For time scales less than or about equal to the cooling time, the rise in X_1 may therefore slow down the rate of net atmospheric heating.

Pridmore-Brown (1973) has examined the change in spatial distribution of a high-intensity laser beam propagating in still air containing CO_2 and H_2O under conditions in which the absorption saturates. Since the intensity is usually not uniform across the laser beam, the temperature at different points removed from the optic axis will show different temperature–time characteristics. At the center of the beam, where the intensity is greatest, a heating effect may be produced while the outer parts of the beam are still subjected to cooling. The net result is that the central part of the beam will diverge, while the outer parts of the beam are being focused toward the optic axis. This leads to the formation of an annular ring around the optic axis, where the laser intensity can become very large and whose thickness may be less than the original diameter of the beam. The quantitative calculations of Pridmore-Brown (1973) support these general predictions.

Experimental observations of the development of the distribution of intensity across a laser beam during thermal blooming have been obtained by Carman and Kelley (1968) and Kenemuth *et al.* (1970). McLean *et al.* (1968) have recorded the time variation of the refractive index of a liquid that absorbs part of the energy in a cw He–Ne beam. These studies show that before heating produces significant thermal convection, a Gaussian beam broadens and then develops an annular ring distribution with the region of peak intensity well removed from the optic axis. During this time, the intensity on the optic axis decreases continuously. As convection becomes important, the intensity on one side of the annular ring decreases and the intensity distribution becomes crescent shaped, with the region of highest intensity shifted toward the source of the convectible flow. Theoretical calculations on the distribution of intensity across a propagating beam in the absence of convection (pure thermal blooming) have been made by Akhmanov *et al.* (1968) and Hayes (1972). Figure 10.4 shows schematically how the intensity distribution evolves during thermal blooming.

Smith and Gebhardt (1970) have studied the effect of forced convection on thermal blooming of cw CO_2 laser beams in a wind tunnel. The effect noted above of the formation of a crescent-shaped intensity distribution at low convective flows was verified, but it was also found that large convective flows restored the normal beam intensity distribution. In addition to beam distortion, a beam propagating perpendicular to a wind will bend in the direction of the wind. These effects have elicited considerable theoretical interest and much has been published on the mechanisms by which

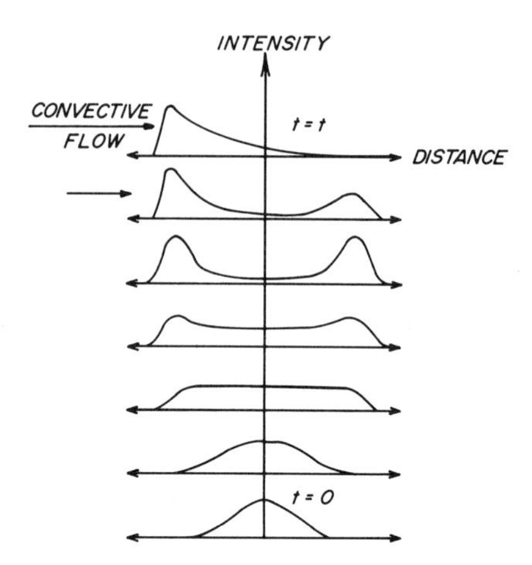

Fig. 10.4. Schematic representation of the development of the intensity profile in a beam during thermal blooming followed by convection.

winds produce distortion and deflection of a propagating beam (Akhmanov *et al.*, 1968; Glass, 1969; Gebhardt and Smith, 1971; Livingston, 1971; Hayes *et al.*, 1972). The development of a crescent-shaped intensity distribution is controlled by two competing thermal lens effects. The first is a focusing of the beam produced by the wind in the direction of the wind; the second is the normal thermal defocusing that occurs perpendicular to the wind direction along the axis of propagation of the laser beam. These two competing effects lead to a narrowing of the crescent-shaped beam with increasing wind speed, and an enhancement in the peak intensity within the crescent. Similar distortions are observed when a cw CO_2 beam is slewed through a stationary atmosphere with weak absorption at 10.6 μm (Kleiman and O'Neil, 1971; Hayes *et al.*, 1972; Buser and Rhode, 1973). Bradley and Herrman (1974) have discussed a method of compensating for thermal blooming with a cw beam.

10.4 INTERACTION OF 10.6-μm LASER RADIATION WITH PARTICLES AND FOG DISSIPATION

On the fundamental level, it is of great interest to determine the effect of high-power laser beams on particles along the propagation path of the beam. At low incident fluxes and short pulse lengths one can reasonably expect that even quite fragile particles such as small droplets of water will be quite unaffected by the absorption of incident radiation. The absorbed radiation may give rise to a momentary rise in temperature within the particle, but this will be slight and will not affect its optical properties. As the incident intensity increases, larger and larger temperature rises will be produced and the particle may start to evaporate. If the flux is maintained at this level and if the particle stays in the beam, then complete removal of the particle can occur through evaporation. In this regard, a cloud of absorbing particles can be thought of as a saturable absorber: at low light levels the extinction produced by the cloud is large, but at high light levels a hole is burned through the cloud, turning it transparent (or less opaque) to the incident laser radiation. Obviously, from the point of view of laser beam propagation through the atmosphere, one would like to estimate the critical laser intensity required for this clearing to occur and the way in which this critical intensity varies with such factors as particle size, particle composition, and path length. From a practical point of view, one can envision using high-power lasers for fog dissipation and the improvement of laser communication links during periods of fog and mist by conditioning the communication link with a high-power laser pulse that clears mist particles from the propagation path.

One of the first experimental studies of fog clearing with a high-power laser beam was reported by Mullaney *et al.* (1968). Laboratory fogs with particle radii in the range 2–7 μm were cleared by pulses from a 100-W cw CO_2 laser. As expected, high laser intensities were more effective in producing clearing than low intensities, but surprisingly the greatest increase in visibility was found for fogs that had a high initial visibility at 0.63 μm.

The interaction of laser light with individual water droplets has been investigated by Kafalas and Ferdinand (1973), Kafalas and Herrmann (1973), Barinov and Sorokin (1973), and Pogodaev *et al.* (1974). Direct observation of the material ejected from particles irradiated with 300-nsec pulses from a CO_2 laser showed that particles with radii $\lesssim 10$ μm heated uniformly in the beam and that material was ejected more or less uniformly from the particles. Particles with radii >10 μm, showed evidence for preferential heating on the surface facing the laser. Material was ejected from the heated surface, while a shock wave generated within the particle gave rise to spallation on the opposite surface. Schlieren photographs during vaporization showed that a shock wave was generated around the particle, which initially expanded at supersonic velocities but then slowed to Mach 1 after $\simeq 2$ μsec. Large particles were found to "rocket" away from the direction of the incident radiation, driven by a jet of vaporizing material. Waniek and Jarmuz (1968) have suggested that this rocketing effect may be used to effect controlled acceleration of microparticles to speeds in the range 10^5 cm/sec). Figure 10.5 shows quantitative data on the energy absorbed by water droplets of various radii for different values of the incident laser fluence (Kafalas and Herrmann, 1973). When the fluence is such that the absorbed energy exceeds that required to vaporize the particle, then the particle explodes and is removed from the beam. At lower fluences the same particle would either dissipate the absorbed energy without vaporizing or would vaporize partially, perhaps to be ejected from the beam by the rocket effect mentioned above. The latter effect is expected to occur mostly on irradiation of particles with radii >10 μm, where the absorbed energy cannot be thought of as being uniformly dissipated throughout the particle.

Weeks and Duley (1974) have studied the interaction of TEA CO_2 laser pulses with particles of carbon black separated according to size in a drift tube. Figure 10.6 shows the time-dependent light emission from an aerosol of these particles excited by the pulse of 10.6-μm radiation shown. The average particle size decreases from I_1 to I_3 due to gravitational separation.

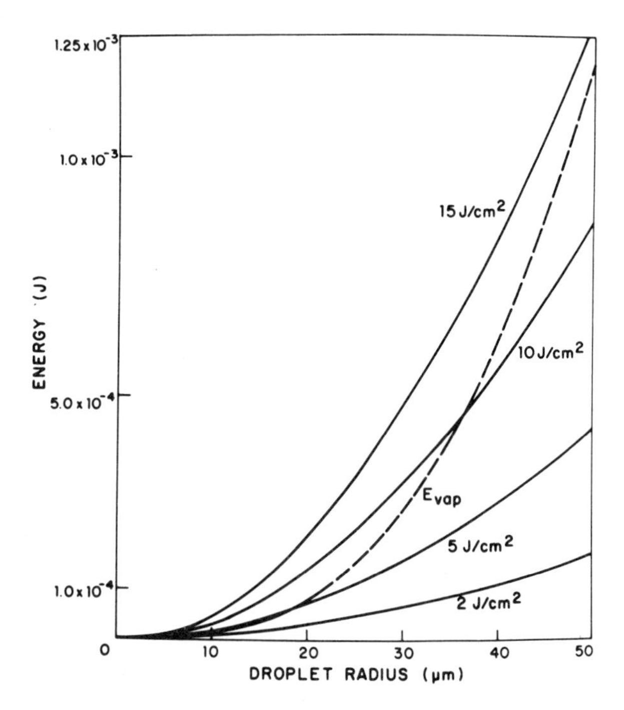

Fig. 10.5. The energy absorbed (solid line) by a water droplet for incident 10.6-μm laser pulses of the indicated energy density. The energy of vaporization E_{vap} (broken line) is also shown for comparison (from Kafalas and Herrmann, 1973).

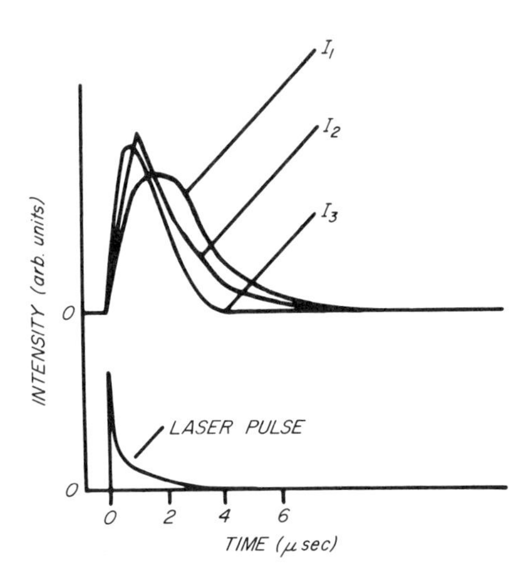

Fig. 10.6. Time dependence of visible light emission from aerosols of different mean size excited by the TEA CO_2 laser pulse shown. Particle size decreases from I_1 to I_3.

It can be seen that the change in average particle size is reflected in the shift of the peak of the visible light emission to shorter times.

Recently, Lencioni and Lowder (1974) have investigated the processes involved in clearing carbon particles with low-intensity high-fluence CO_2 laser pulses. It was found that small particles (radii $\lesssim 1.5$ μm) were cleared by vaporization, while large particles were removed from the beam by the rocketing effect mentioned above. The effect of clearing was to increase the breakdown threshold of the gas along the path of the precursor pulse. This increase in breakdown threshold amounted to a factor of about 3 in intensity when the high-power pulse followed the precursor pulse by $\simeq 10$ μsec. After $\simeq 0.1$ sec the effect of particle clearing by the precursor pulse on the breakdown threshold was no longer noticeable. These interesting results indicate that it is advantageous to clear an atmospheric propagation path of particulate matter before an intense laser pulse is transmitted, if one is to take advantage of the full breakdown pressure. Further discussion on particle-induced gas breakdown has been given by Canavan and Nielsen (1973).

One can obtain some estimate of the laser fluxes required to vaporize small particles in air at atmospheric pressure from the following analysis (Weeks and Duley, 1974). We consider a small spherical particle of radius a and heat capacity C heated by an intensity $F(t)$ incident in a plane wave from one direction. Then for times $t > t_{crit} \simeq a^2/k$ such that the particle can be thought of as heating uniformly throughout its volume,* the particle temperature $T(t)$ can be found from

$$\frac{dT}{dt} + \frac{4\sigma\pi a^2 \epsilon T^4}{C} + \frac{4\pi a^2 \eta_a kT}{C} = \frac{4\pi a^2 \eta_a kT_0}{C} + \frac{\pi a^2 Q_a F(t)}{C} \tag{9}$$

with

- σ Stefan–Boltzmann constant
- ϵ total emissivity of a particle of size a and temperature T
- η_a molecular collision rate (cm^{-2}) with a spherical particle of radius a
- k Boltzmann constant
- Q_a absorption efficiency at 10.6-μm wavelength
- T_0 ambient gas temperature

Simplifying, this equation becomes

$$(dT/dt) + \gamma_1 T^4 + \gamma_2 T = \gamma_3 + \gamma_4 F(t) \tag{10}$$

A TEA CO_2 laser pulse can often be represented analytically by the expression

$$F(t) = F_0[A \exp(-\lambda_1 t) + B \exp(-\lambda_2 t)] \tag{11}$$

where A, B, λ_1, and λ_2 are constants (typical values might be $A = 2$, $B = 1$, $\lambda_1 = 4 \times 10^6$/sec, $\lambda_2 = 0.5 \times 10^6$/sec). The following expression is then obtained for $T(t)$, when it can be assumed that radiative losses (i.e., the term in γ_1) can be neglected:

$$T(t) = T_0 + F_0\gamma_4 \left\{ \frac{A \exp(-\lambda_1 t)}{(\gamma_2 - \gamma_1)} + \frac{B \exp(-\lambda_2 t)}{(\gamma_2 - \lambda_2)} - \exp(-\gamma_2 t) \left[\frac{A}{(\gamma_2 - \lambda_1)} + \frac{B}{(\gamma_2 - \lambda_2)} \right] \right\} \tag{12}$$

A similar expression for a pulse with $F(t) = F_0$, $0 < t \leq \tau$, is

$$T(\tau) = [1 - \exp(-\gamma_2 \tau)][\gamma_4 F_0/\gamma_2] + T_0 \tag{13}$$

and in the limit as τ becomes very large,

$$\lim_{\tau \to \infty} T(\tau) = T_0 + \gamma_4 F_0/\gamma_2 \tag{14}$$

* This assumes that the absorption coefficient of the bulk material $\alpha > 1/a$. When $\alpha < 1/a$, the radiation penetrates into the particle and the particle heats up directly, without the need for heat conduction from exterior to interior.

When $a \lesssim 10\ \mu m$, the following simple expression is available (van de Hulst, 1957) for Q_a:

$$Q_a = -\tfrac{8}{3} x I_m(m - 1) \tag{15}$$

where $x = 2\pi a/\lambda$ and m is the complex refractive index of the particle. Then $T(t)$ can be calculated from Eqs. (12)–(14) when m is known at 10.6 μm. As a numerical example we may ask what laser intensity is required to heat water droplets to 100°C with a square pulse of duration $\tau = 1\ \mu$sec. Then from Eq. (15) with $m = 1.18 - 0.08i$ (Bertie and Whalley, 1967; Irving and Pollack, 1968; Chu and Hogg, 1968) or using the calculated values of Glickler (1971), $Q_a \simeq 1.34a/\lambda$, $C = [4.2\ \text{J/cm}^3] \times (4\pi/3)a^3$, $\eta_a = 3 \times 10^{23}/\text{cm}^2/\text{sec}$, and $T_0 = 20°\text{C}$,

$$T(10^{-6}\ \text{sec}) = 20 + 80^3 a F_0[1 - \exp(-3 \times 10^{-6}/a)] = 100°\text{C}$$

where a is in cm. The laser intensity is found from

$$F_0 = (1/a)[1 - \exp(-3 \times 10^{-6}/a)]^{-1}$$

and thus

$$F_0 = \begin{cases} 3.85 \times 10^5\ \text{W/cm}^2, & a = 10^{-5}\ \text{cm} \\ 3.38 \times 10^5\ \text{W/cm}^2, & a = 10^{-4}\ \text{cm} \\ 3.33 \times 10^5\ \text{W/cm}^2, & a = 10^{-3}\ \text{cm} \end{cases}$$

This analysis does, however, neglect the role of evaporation and therefore underestimates the laser intensity required to effect total removal of the particle through evaporation. Calculations based on more rigorous models, which include evaporation, have been described by Williams (1965), Bukatyi and Pogodaev (1970, 1972), and Zuev *et al.* (1973).

A more difficult problem, but one with many applications in the area of laser radar and communications systems, involves a calculation of the effect of particle evaporation on propagation of laser pulses over long path lengths. Here one would like to know the dependence of laser intensity $F(x, t)$ on both the distance of propagation x and the time t after the pulse is initiated, allowing for the possibility that particle evaporation occurs during propagation. This problem has been discussed by Lamb and Kinney (1969), Sukhroukov *et al.* (1971), and Glickler (1971). Figure 10.7 shows a plot of $F(L)/F_0$ for different values of the incident fluence for a cloud of monodisperse particles with radius 3 μm. Values of δL on the curves shown denote the product of mass density of fog particles and total path length L. The time scale that also appears in this plot refers to the time at which the given ratio $F(L)/F_0$ would be obtained for an incident laser intensity of 10^4 W/cm². We see that below a certain fluence the cloud is opaque to

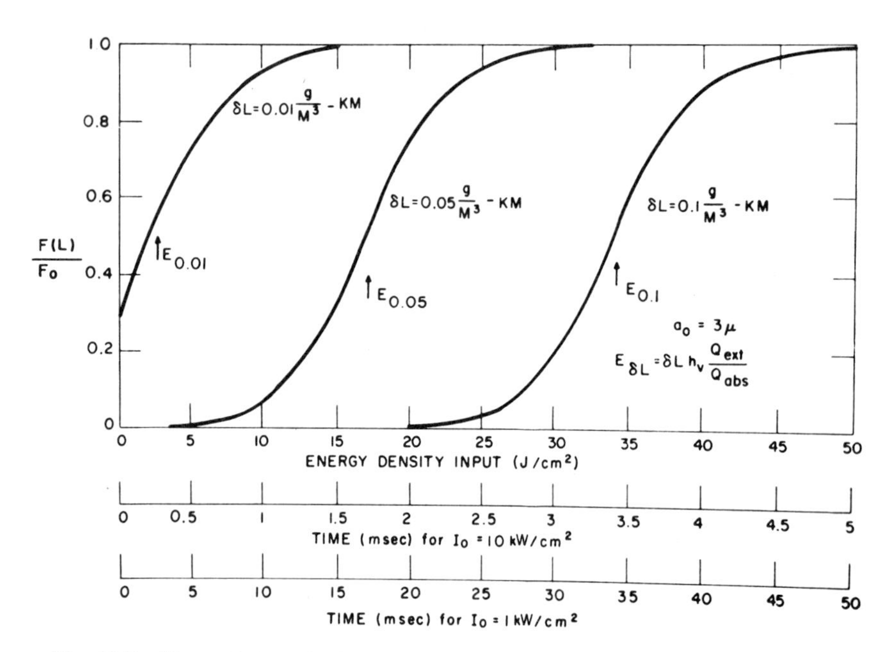

Fig. 10.7. Transmission of a fog of 3 μm radius particles vs. incident laser fluence at 10.6 μm. δL is the product of the mass density of fog particles and the total path length (from Glickler, 1971).

the laser radiation. On reaching a threshold value of $F_0 t$, however, "bleaching" of the absorber begins and the transmission rapidly rises to approach unity. This means that a square pulse of intensity F_0 transmitted through the fog will have a rounded leading edge at the point of detection. It will also exhibit an apparent time delay $t_{th} = E_{threshold}/F_0$, or a pulse of length t_p will be shortened by extinction to $t_p - t_{th}$. The effect of this change in pulse shape is of significance in laser communication links. To date, there seems to be little discussion of this process in the literature.

The analysis of Glickler (1971) assumes that the beam has a uniform cross section. Sukhroukov *et al.* (1971) have extended these calculations to consider the shape of the channel opened by a beam of Gaussian cross section propagating through clouds and fogs.

10.5 POLLUTION MONITORING WITH INFRARED LASERS

In this section we discuss some recent developments in the monitoring of gaseous and solid atmospheric pollutants, which have been made possible by the availability of high-power infrared lasers.

10.5.1 Detection of Molecular Species in the Atmosphere

Figure 10.8 shows some methods that have been used or proposed for the *in situ* detection of trace molecular impurities in the atmosphere. The simple absorption method shown in Fig. 10.8a is limited in sensitivity by the need to keep the sample length small ($\simeq$1 m) to permit portable operation. Hinkley and Kelley (1971) conclude that a practical detection limit for a species having a strong absorption line within the range of a tunable diode laser is $\simeq$0.3 ppm in a 1-m-long cell. Although tunable infrared lasers provide good wavelength discrimination, the problem involved in a sensitive detection system based on absorption lies in the measurement of a small change $(I_0 - I)$ in a large signal I_0. This can be done using synchronous detection techniques, but for low concentrations of impurities the absorption path must be increased. Alternatively, one may substitute a measurement of I/I_0 by one of the absorbed power $I_0 - I$. This can be accomplished by the optoacoustic method (spectrophone) shown schematically in Fig. 10.8b and first investigated using a laser source by Kreuzer (1971).

This technique relies on the fact that vibrational and rotational energy given to molecules in a gas by absorption of laser energy is partially converted to translational energy as collisions quench the excited vibrational and rotational energy level populations. Thus, the absorption of a fraction of the incident energy during a laser pulse will lead to a pressure pulse in the absorbing gas that may be detected with a microphone. Since the spectrophone is a thermal detector, its response is independent of wavelength. Furthermore, the sensitivity of this device should increase with increasing laser intensity up to the point where the laser flux is sufficient to cause saturation of the molecular absorption. Kreuzer (1971) concludes that the optimum laser intensity (maximizing the acoustic signal compatible with saturation) would typically be $\simeq 10^5$ W/cm^2. The ultimate sensitivity of the spectrophone is limited by Brownian motion in the diaphragm of the microphone. Kreuzer suggests that concentrations as low as one part in 10^{13} could be detected under optimized conditions.

Demonstrations of the practicality of the spectrophone as an instrument for detecting low concentrations of pollutants in atmospheric gases have been reported by Kreuzer and Patel (1971), Kreuzer *et al.* (1972), and Hinkley (1972). Sources have included the spin–flip Raman CO_2 laser (Kreuzer and Patel, 1971), fixed-wavelength CO and CO_2 lasers (Kreuzer *et al.*, 1972), and amplitude- or frequency-modulated $Pb_{0.88}Sn_{0.12}Te$ diode lasers (Hinkley, 1972). Experimental data obtained by these groups are summarized in Table 10.3. Kreuzer *et al.* point out that tunable lasers may not be necessary for many systems of practical interest since resonances

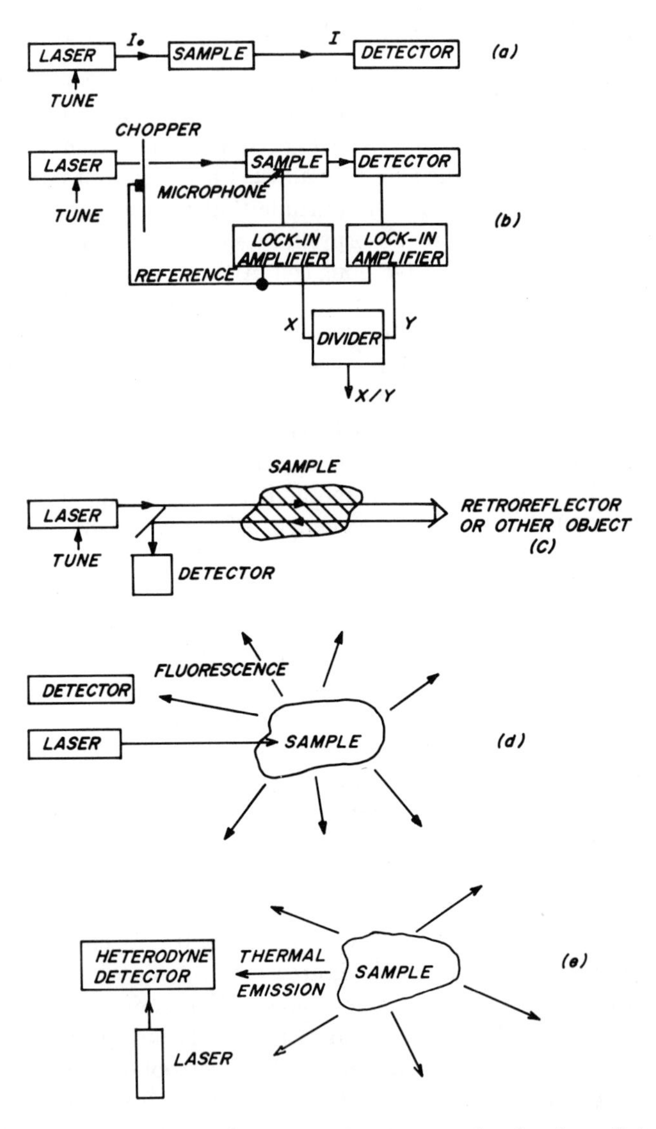

Fig. 10.8. Various methods of detecting the presence of molecular pollutants in the atmosphere using infrared lasers. (a) Direct absorption in laboratory sample, (b) optoacoustic method (Kreuzer, 1971), (c) absorption in remote sample, (d) laser-excited fluorescence, (e) heterodyne detection of thermal radiation from sample.

Table 10.3

Representative Minimum Detectable Concentrations of Some Molecules Using the Spectrophone Technique

Molecule detected	Laser	Wavelength (μm)	Sensitivity	Reference
NO	Spin–flip CO	5.479–5.519	10 ppb	Kreuzer and Patel (1971)
NH_3	CO	6.1493	0.4 ppb	Kreuzer *et al.* (1972)
C_6H_6	CO_2	9.6392	3 ppb	
1–3-butadiene	CO	6.2153	1 ppb	
	CO_2	10.6964	2 ppb	
1-Butene	CO	6.0685	2 ppb	
	CO_2	10.7874	2 ppb	
Ethylene	CO_2	10.5321	0.2 ppb	
CH_3OH	CO_2	9.6760	0.3 ppb	
HNO_3	CO	5.2148	0.4 ppb	
NO_2	CO	6.2293	0.1 ppb	
Propylene	CO	6.0685	3 ppb	
Trichloroethylene	CO_2	10.6321	0.7 ppb	
H_2O	CO	5.9417	14 ppb	
C_2H_4	$Pb_{0.88}Sn_{0.12}Te$	10.535	100 ppm	Hinkley (1972)
	$Pb_{0.88}Sn_{0.12}Te$	10.535	1 ppm[a]	
SO_2	$Pb_{0.88}Sn_{0.12}Te$	8.7	<670 ppm[a]	

[a] Using absorption spectrum through gas.

can often be found between one of the many lines emitted by CO and CO_2 lasers and most common atmospheric pollutant molecules (Table 10.4). When a continuously tunable output is not available, the sensitivity of the spectrophone method is often found to be limited by background absorption due to another infrared active species (this also occurs with continuously tunable laser outputs, but a judicious choice of the exciting wavelength may reduce the sensitivity to background absorption). An example given by Kreuzer *et al.* involves NO detected at $\simeq 5.3$ μm in the presence

Table 10.4

Coincidences between Various Laser Lines and Vibration–Rotation Lines in Several Atmospheric Pollutant Molecules

Molecule detected	Wavelength (μm)	Laser	Wavelength (μm)	Sensitivity[a] (ppm)	Reference
NO	5.1886	CO	5.1887	0.3	Menzies (1971)
	5.316	Doubled CO_2	5.316	0.5	
CO	4.776	Doubled CO_2	4.776	0.05	
SO_2	7.4-μm band	CO	7.376	<1	
		CO	7.441	<1	
		CO	7.4577	<1	
C_2H_4	10.535	$Pb_{0.88}Sn_{0.12}Te$	10.535	several[b]	Hinkley (1972)

[a] For 1% absorption in a 100-m path.
[b] 500-m path.

of H_2O absorption centered at $\simeq$5.8–5.9 μm. In ambient air at 120°F and 100% relative humidity, the background-limited (due to H_2O) sensitivity would be 0.01 ppm. In an automobile exhaust with 10% water vapor, this limit would be raised to 0.1 ppm.

Another sampling technique shown in Fig. 10.8c involves a spectroscopic measurement on a sample of absorbing gas located at a large distance from the transmitter and receiver. Unless a detector can be mounted at a remote location, such a measurement would involve a double pass through the sample provided by a retroreflector or some other reflecting object. Ideally, the laser is continuously tunable over a wide frequency range, so that a true absorption spectrum of the absorbing sample can be obtained. However, coincidences between fixed-frequency laser lines and many pollutant molecules can be found as noted above, which may make an estimate of molecular concentrations possible on the basis of a simple frequency measurement. Some of these coincidences are listed in Table 10.4.

Laser-excited fluorescence (Fig. 10.8d) is another valuable technique in the characterization of atmospheric molecular species through remote sensing. Here the laser output wavelength is absorbed by some constituent of the sample, which then reemits, usually at a different wavelength. The reemitted light can be detected at a frequency or frequencies well removed from that of the exciting line and perhaps in a region of high atmospheric transparency, so that high sensitivity may be achieved. Usually fluorescence is excited by short-wavelength laser radiation that is absorbed in an electronic transition of the molecule (Measures and Pilon, 1972; Menzies, 1971; Gelbwachs *et al.*, 1972). However, fluorescence can also be excited with infrared lasers (Chang *et al.*, 1970a,b; Chang and Bridges, 1970; Robinson *et al.*, 1968; Bailey *et al.*, 1971; Bordé *et al.*, 1966b; Ronn, 1968) and it seems probable that high-power CO or CO_2 lasers may be useful for exciting fluorescence from a variety of atmospheric pollutant molecules.

Menzies (1971) has suggested that the use of a visible or uv laser to excite fluorescence, together with heterodyne detection at an infrared frequency of the excited molecule, should vastly improve the sensitivity of the remote fluorecence technique. Such a system would be as shown in Fig. 10.8e, except that fluorescence instead of thermal emission would be detected. The local oscillator would be a laser generating a line of the species to be monitored (CO, N_2O, CO_2) or a line that was within the receiver bandwidth of an emission line from the sample. In the limit as shown in Fig. 10.8e, one might use heterodyne detection to sample purely thermal emission from the molecule at a remote location. Experiments on the detection of NO, SO_2, and CO_2 using a laser heterodyne receiver have been reported by Menzies (1972).

10.5.2 Detection of Particulate Matter in the Atmosphere

Laser radar or LIDAR systems have been used for many years to study the distribution of particulate matter in the atmosphere, and the literature on this subject is quite extensive (for reviews of work in this area, see Derr and Little, 1970; Collis, 1970; Carswell *et al.*, 1971, 1972; and Landry, 1974).

A basic LIDAR system is shown schematically in Fig. 10.9. Pulses from the laser source are propagated through a cloud as shown, while the light at the laser frequency scattered back toward the laser by the particles in the cloud is gathered by a telescope and focused on a suitable wide-bandwidth detector. The time delay between transmitted and received signals is then used to obtain the distance from the transmitter to the scatterer, while the amplitude of the pulse received at a particular time can be related to the back-scattering efficiency and density of particles within a subvolume of the cloud. Other parameters such as the depolarization produced in the backscattered light when the incident beam is polarized can also be used to obtain information about the size range, composition, and shape of the scattering particles. Most LIDAR systems use ruby or neodymium lasers as the transmitter. One reason for this choice can be seen from calculations of the back-scattering efficiency for typical atmospheric

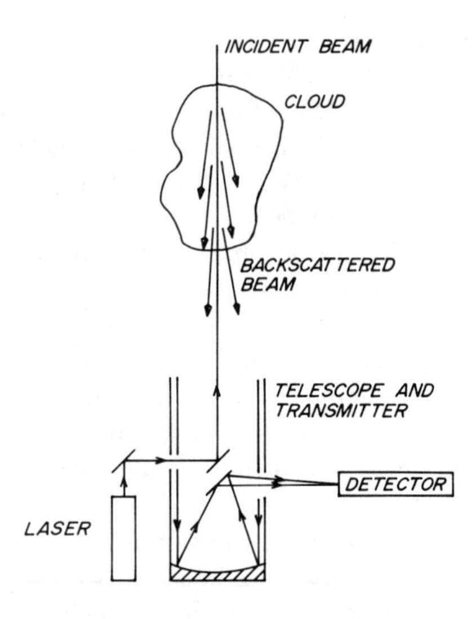

Fig. 10.9. Schematic of LIDAR system.

particles (see, for example, Collis and Uthe, 1972). When $2\pi a/\lambda \simeq 5$, these calculations predict that Q_{scat} (180°) will be larger by several orders of magnitude than when either a or λ is such that $2\pi a/\lambda < 5$. Thus at 10 μm a large back-scattering efficiency will be obtained only for those particles whose characteristic dimensions are $\gtrsim 20$ μm, while at 1 μm this limit is reduced to $\simeq 2$ μm. Full diagnostic capability is then achieved only with lasers oscillating at relatively short wavelengths, and consequently there has been little interest to data in LIDAR studies at 10.6 μm. A parametric study of a 10.6-μm laser radar system has, however, been reported by Brandewie and Davis (1972).

Thermal emission from laboratory aerosols excited with pulsed (Weeks and Duley, 1974) or cw (Young and Duley, 1974) CO_2 laser radiation can also be used to obtain information about the size and composition of particles in the gas phase. At low laser intensities, the time dependence of light emission can easily be related to a heating model that predicts the time of maximum light emission in terms of the size and heat capacity of the irradiated particles (see Section 10.4). At high incident intensities, particles are evaporated and the incandescent vapor monitored spectroscopically yields information about elemental abundances in the particle and hence its composition. Alternatively, the wavelength dependence of thermal emission from heated particles can also be used to determine particle composition.

10.6 OPTICAL COMMUNICATIONS SYSTEMS AT 10.6 μm

A 10.6-μm CO_2 laser beam can be thought of as a carrier at frequency of 3×10^{13} Hz and can be modulated to transmit information in the same general way that rf or microwave frequency carriers are modulated. However, the great advantage of communications systems based on carriers at laser frequencies derives from the enormous bandwidths possible. A system operating at 10.6 μm could, in principle, comprise 10^7 channels, each with a bandwidth of 1 MHz transmitted simultaneously over a single highly directional beam. While information-carrying capacities of this magnitude have not yet been even remotely approached, development of optical communications systems based on CO_2 and other lasers continues at an ever increasing rate. As in other applications, the use of the CO_2 laser has both advantages and disadvantages when compared to other possible laser sources. The purpose of this section is not to investigate the relative merits of communications systems operating with different laser sources, but to describe some of the advances that have recently been made in the transmission of information over 10.6-μm CO_2 laser links. Further details on laser communications systems in general may be obtained from Pratt (1969).

The evolution of practical 10.6-μm communications links has proceeded over the past 6–7 years from laboratory prototypes (Mocker, 1969) to systems capable of unattended operation for over 1000 hours of continuous operation, transmitting over paths of up to 20 miles through a variety of weather conditions (Nussmeier *et al.*, 1974). These and proposed space communications systems all use heterodyne detection (Forster *et al.*, 1972) to achieve near-quantum noise-limited performance (Peyton *et al.*, 1972). The state of the art in this area is best illustrated by the system developed by Nussmeier *et al.* (1974) shown in block diagram form in Fig. 10.10.

Stable single-frequency operation is obtained by using metal–ceramic narrow-bore cw CO_2 lasers in the transmitter and receiver mounted in a temperature-stabilized container. The intracavity CdTe modulator is contained within a thermostated oven and is insulated from its environment by a Fiberglas sleeve. One end of the CdTe modulator is coated to form the output mirror of the laser cavity, while the other is antireflection coated. Oscillation on the center of the $P(20)$ transition of the 10.4-μm band of CO_2 is ensured by a feedback system involving a detector tuned to $P(20)$ and a 7-Hz dither system coupled to the piezoelectrically actuated totally reflecting mirror in the laser cavity. The output of the transmitter is directed through a focusing lens into a telescope. Visible acquisition of the target is provided by the eyepiece.

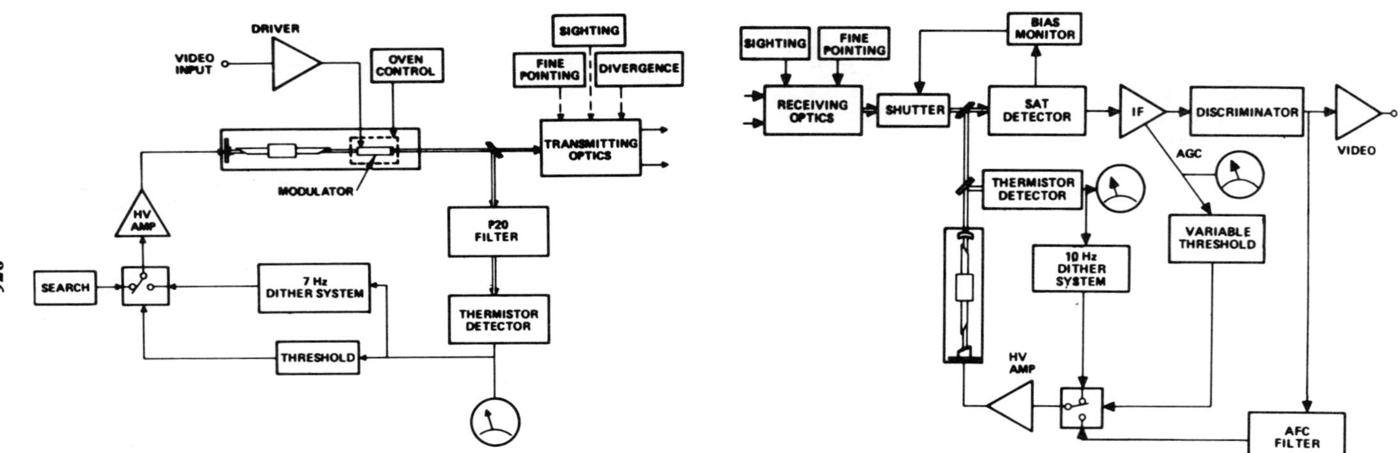

Fig. 10.10. Schematic of transmitter and receiver for 10.6-μm terrestrial communication link (from Nussmeier *et al.*, 1974).

The receiver schematic is also shown in Fig. 10.10. This system used an SAT-type A1 HgCdTe detector, which requires only cooling with liquid nitrogen. An automated system sensed the liquid nitrogen level in the Dewar cooling the detector and provided for automatic refilling. Incident radiation was collected by a telescope identical to that in the transmitter and combined with the local oscillator signal in a beam splitter before entering the detector. The local oscillator frequency is maintained at the center of the CO_2 $P(20)$ line when no signal is received by the dither system. Acquisition of a signal due to the transmitter results in the disabling of the dither system and a frequency-tracking control system maintains the local oscillator at 30 MHz above the incoming frequency.

The completed system was operated over a 4.1-mi test range and in semipermanent installations involving transmission over 3- and 20-mi paths. A summary of some operating data is given in Table 10.5. The high-frequency response limit given in Table 10.5 is that due to the discriminator in the receiver. The transmitter as a whole was reported to have a bandwidth >7 MHz. A downtime of 65 hr during the 1320-hr continuous run (95% reliability) was due mainly to weather conditions over the 3-mi path used for this measurement. Heavy fog and winds over 35 mph were responsible for breakdown of the communication link, although light to moderate rainfall and light snow produced no serious degradation in signal quality.

Forster *et al.* (1972) have made a comparative study of CO_2, Nd : YAG, and doubled Nd : YAG systems for an application involving satellite–satellite communications links. The high efficiency of the CO_2 laser and the

Table 10.5

Operating Parameters of Terrestrial 10.6-μm communications link[a]

Parameter	Response
Frequency response	86 Hz–4.2 MHz
Maximum digital bit rate	8.0 Mbit/sec
Operating margin	51 dB
Peak frequency deviation	2.1 MHz
Dewar hold time	50 hr
Operating temperature	0–45°C
Acquisition time	<5 min
Continuous run	1320 hr
Reliability during continuous run	95%

[a] From Nussmeier *et al.* (1974).

low quantum noise limit at 10 μm were found to make this system attractive in a link involving the transmission of digital bit rates of up to 1 Gbit/sec. However, problems involving Doppler tracking and heterodyne detection were anticipated.

This short survey has demonstrated that wideband communications links based on a carrier frequency of 10.6 μm are practical. Whether the CO_2 laser will develop as a strong candidate for commercial communications links depends on a variety of factors, some of which are technological and some economic. Certainly the next 10 years will see many astonishing developments in this and other areas involving the development and utilization of high-power CO_2 lasers.

Appendix A

Thermal Conductivity Data

Plots of K versus T are given for aluminum, copper, chromium, cobalt, gold, iron, lead, molybdenum, nickel, platinum, rhodium, silver, tantalum, tin, titanium, tungsten, uranium, vanadium, zinc, zirconium, Armco iron, 302, 303, and 304 stainless steel, aluminum oxide, fused quartz, magnesium oxide, and titanium dioxide. K is in units of W/cm°C.

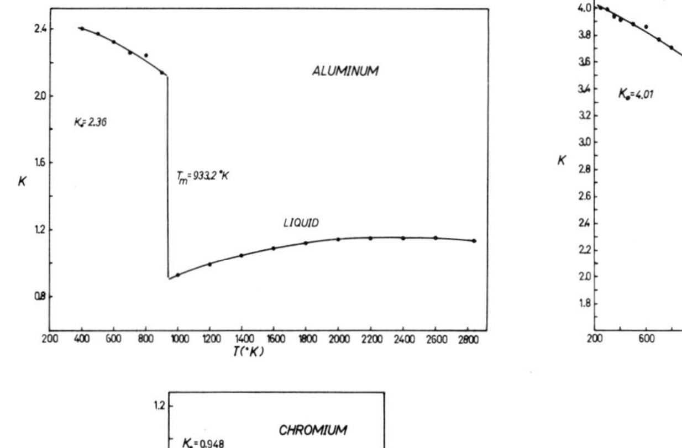

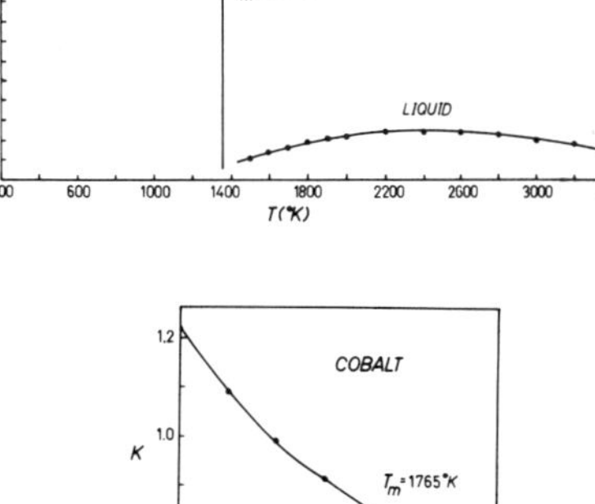

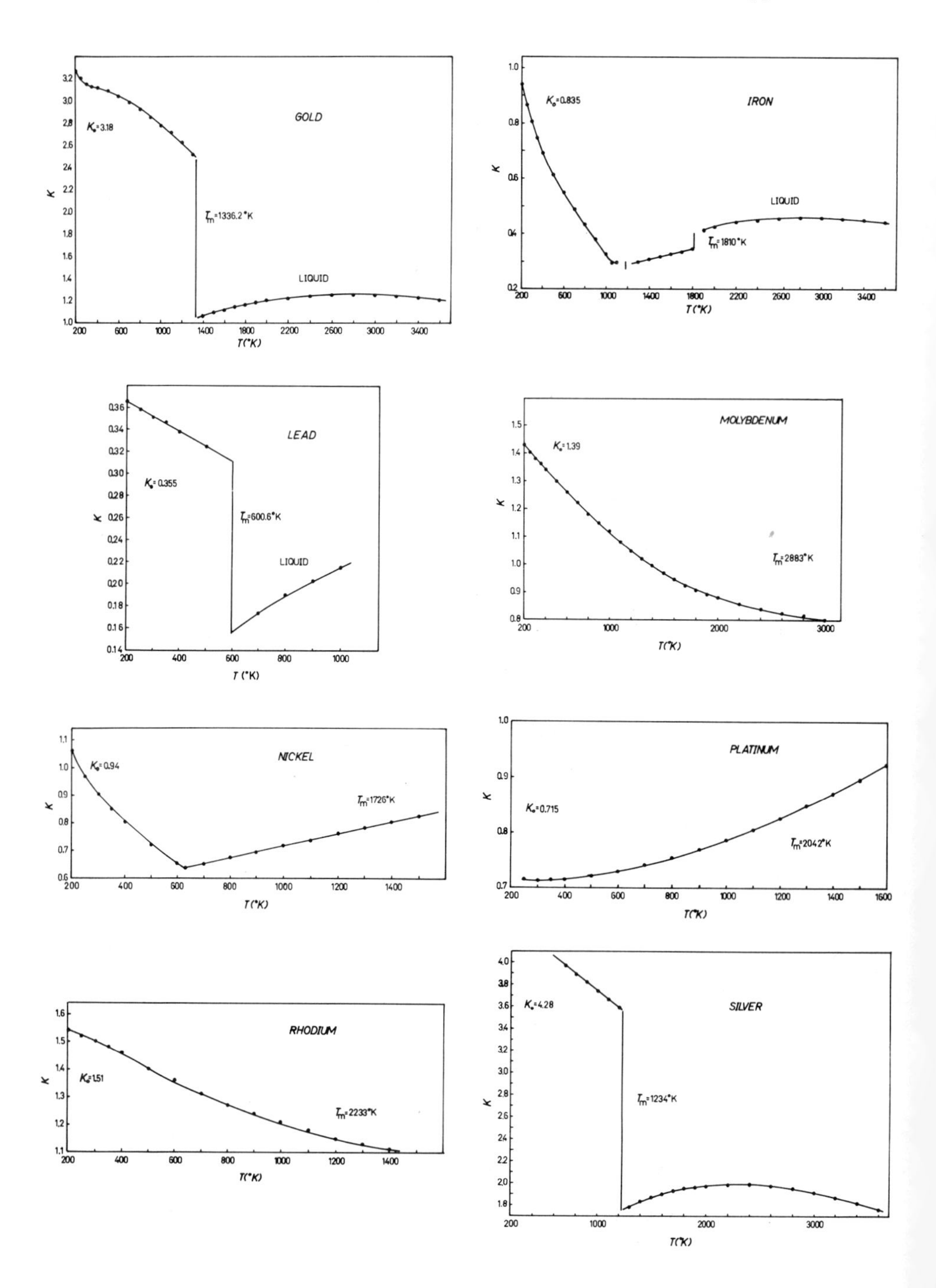
GOLD
K_e=3.18
T_m=1336.2°K
LIQUID
K
T(°K)
IRON
K_e=0.835
LIQUID
T_m=1810°K
LEAD
K_e=0.355
T_m=600.6°K
MOLYBDENUM
K_e=1.39
T_m=2883°K
NICKEL
K_e=0.94
T_m=1726°K
PLATINUM
K_e=0.715
T_m=2042°K
RHODIUM
K_e=1.51
T_m=2233°K
SILVER
K_e=4.28
T_m=1234°K

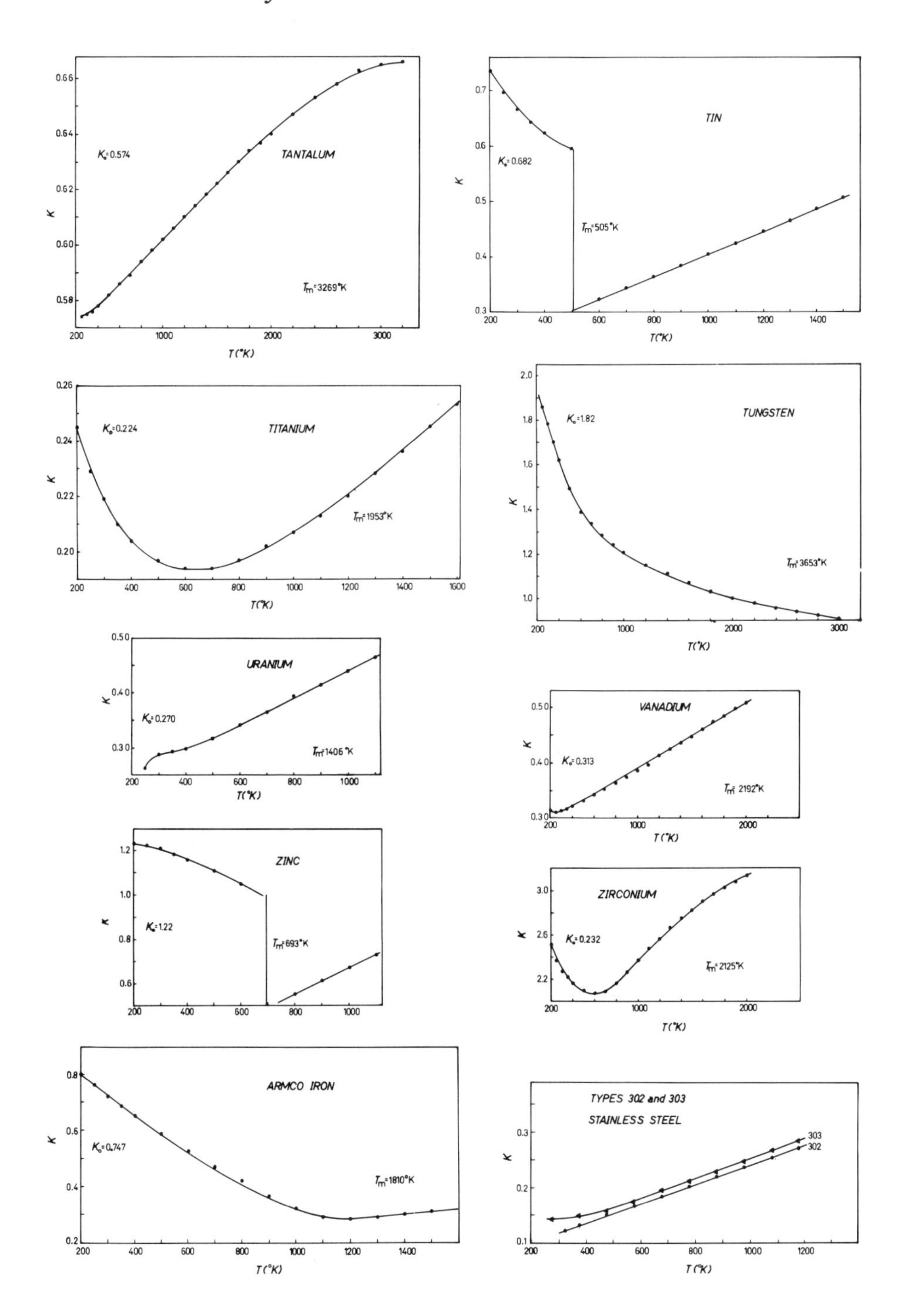
TANTALUM
K₀=0.574
Tm=3269°K
T(°K)
K
TIN
K₀=0.682
Tm=505°K
TITANIUM
K₀=0.224
Tm=1953°K
TUNGSTEN
K₀=1.82
Tm=3653°K
URANIUM
K₀=0.270
Tm=1406°K
VANADIUM
K₀=0.313
Tm=2192°K
ZINC
K₀=1.22
Tm=693°K
ZIRCONIUM
K₀=0.232
Tm=2125°K
ARMCO IRON
K₀=0.747
Tm=1810°K
TYPES 302 and 303
STAINLESS STEEL
303
302

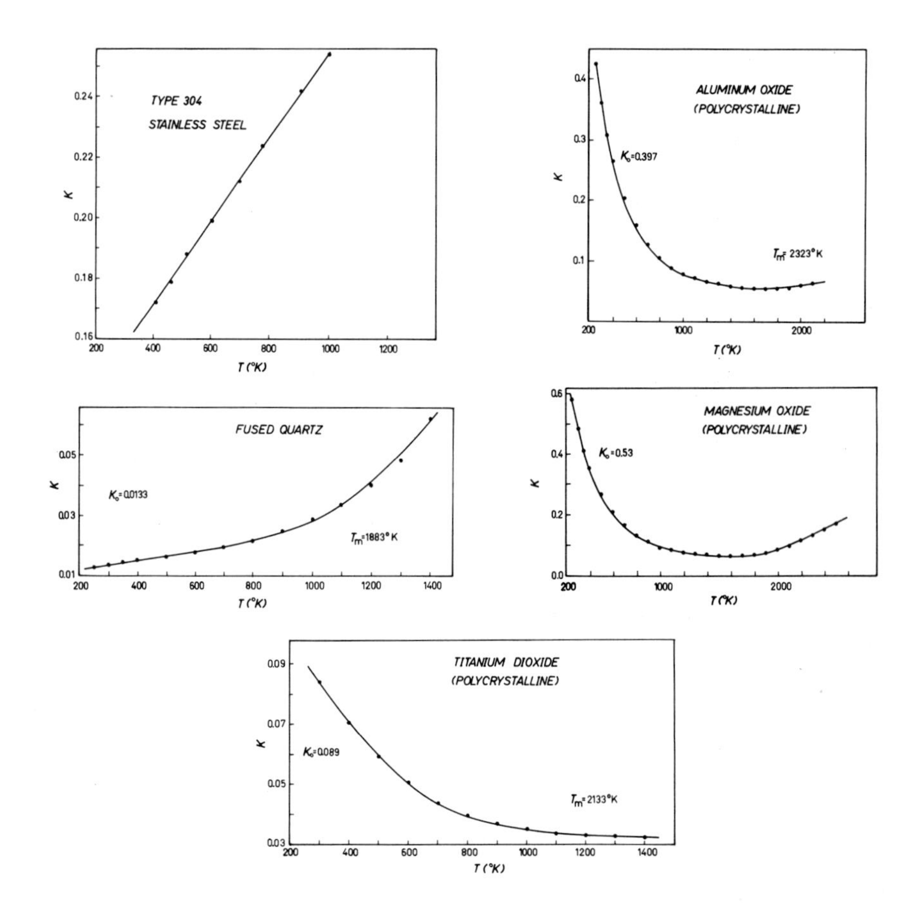
TYPE 304
STAINLESS STEEL
K
T (°K)
ALUMINUM OXIDE
(POLYCRYSTALLINE)
K₀=0.397
Tm= 2323°K
FUSED QUARTZ
K₀=0.0133
Tm=1883°K
MAGNESIUM OXIDE
(POLYCRYSTALLINE)
K₀=0.53
TITANIUM DIOXIDE
(POLYCRYSTALLINE)
K₀=0.089
Tm=2133°K

Appendix B

Heat Capacities

Plots of C_p versus T are given for aluminum, chromium, copper, gold, iron, lead, molybdenum, nickel, platinum, silver, tantalum, tin, titanium, tungsten, uranium, vanadium, zinc, zirconium, Armco iron, 304 stainless steel, aluminum oxide, magnesium oxide, fused quartz, and titanium dioxide. C_p is in units of J/g°C.

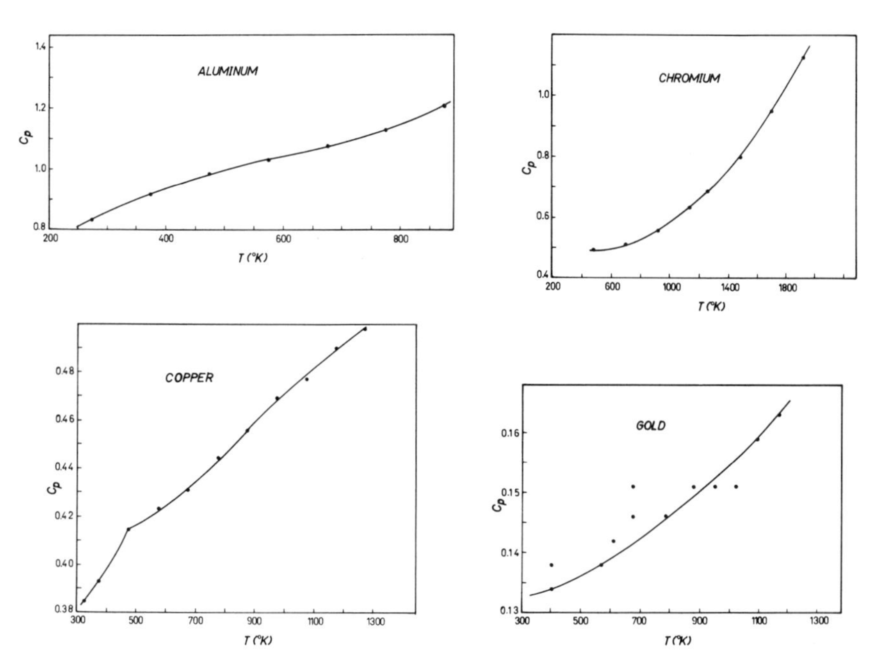

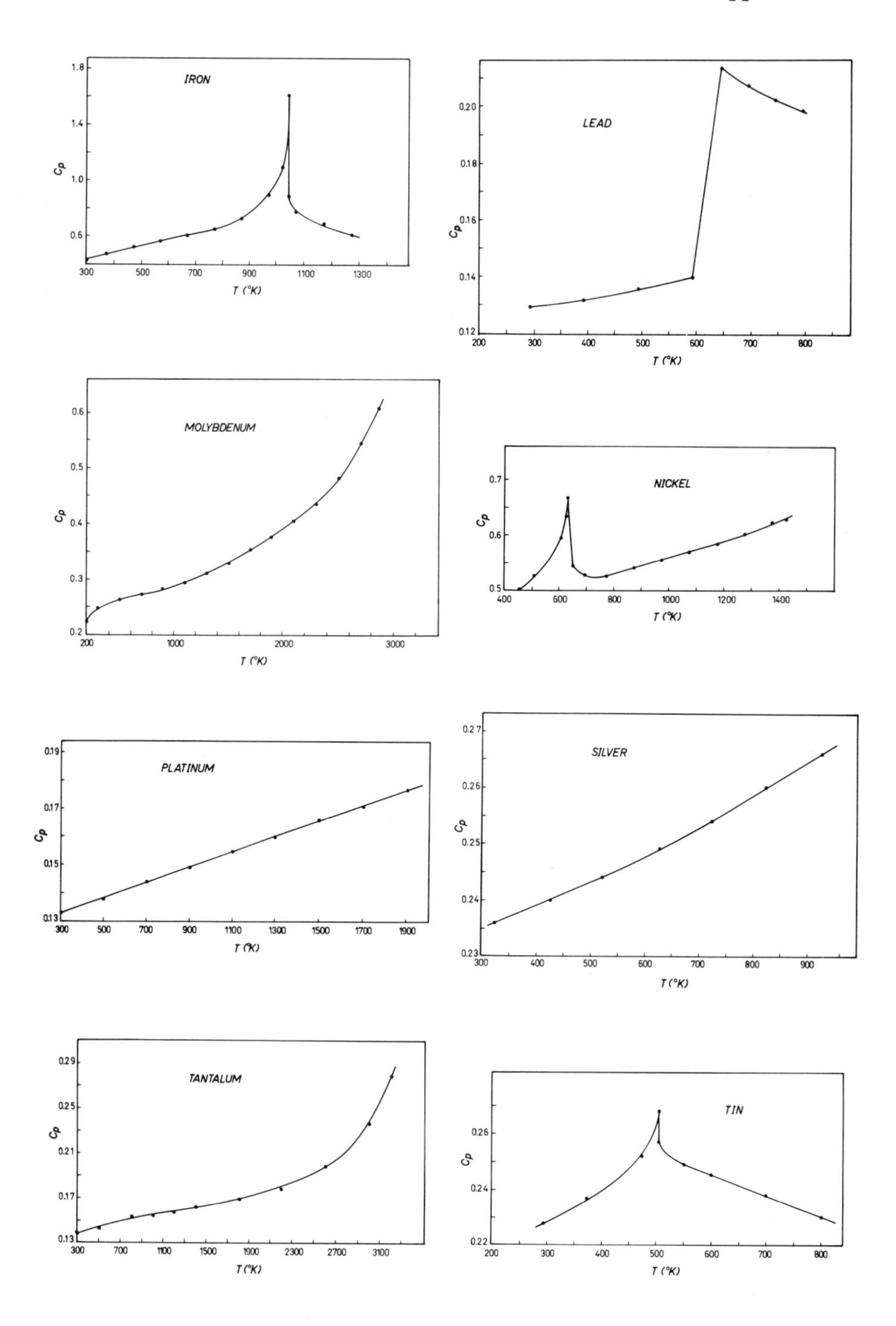
IRON
LEAD
MOLYBDENUM
NICKEL
PLATINUM
SILVER
TANTALUM
TIN
Cp
T (°K)

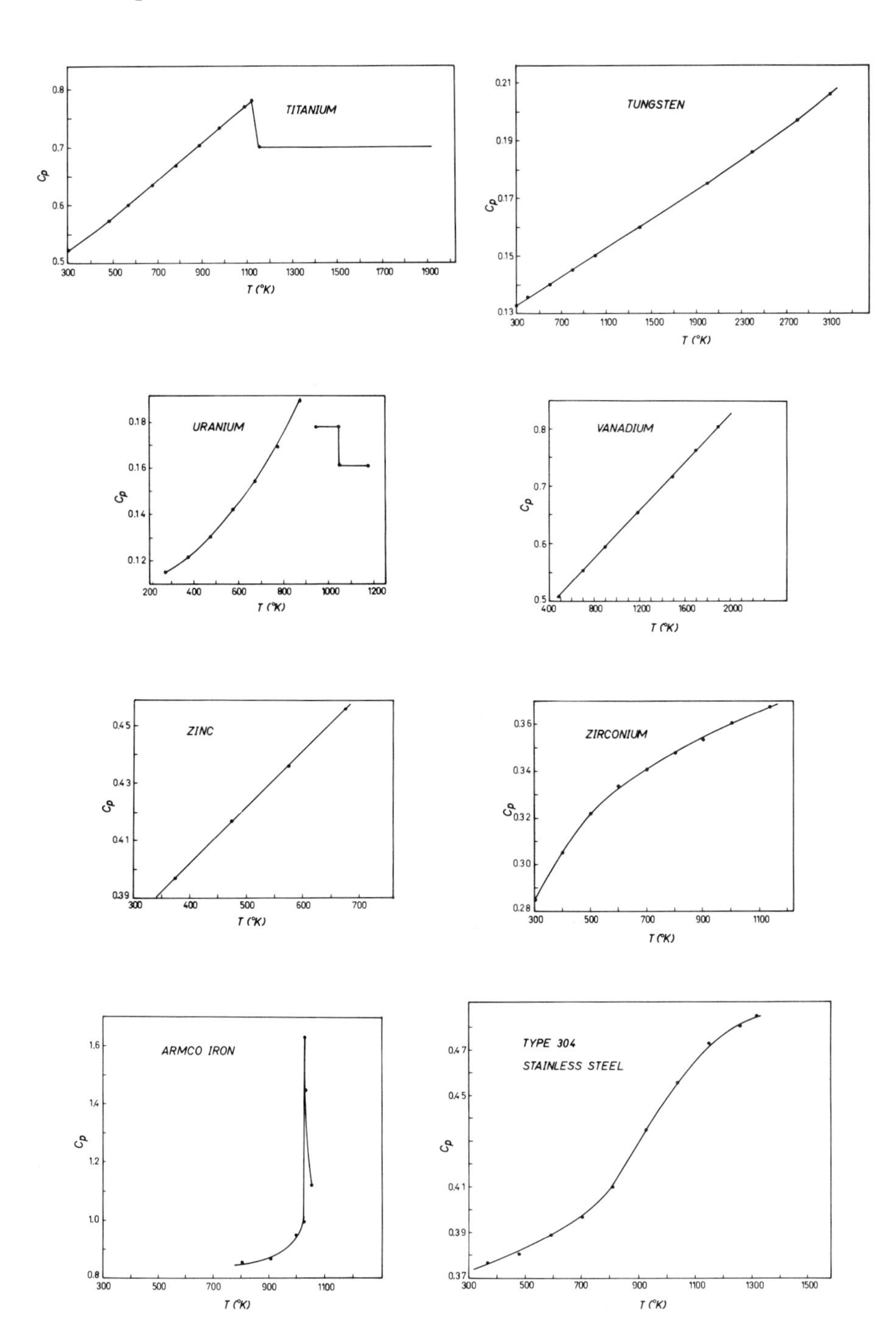
TITANIUM
C_p
T (°K)
TUNGSTEN
C_p
T (°K)
URANIUM
C_p
T (°K)
VANADIUM
C_p
T (°K)
ZINC
C_p
T (°K)
ZIRCONIUM
C_p
T (°K)
ARMCO IRON
C_p
T (°K)
TYPE 304
STAINLESS STEEL
C_p
T (°K)

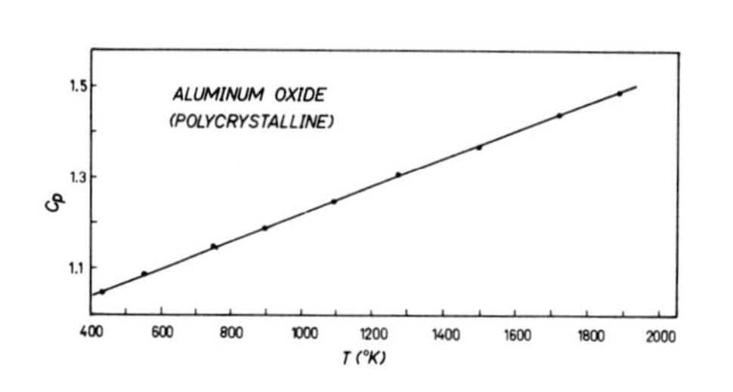
ALUMINUM OXIDE
(POLYCRYSTALLINE)
1.5
1.3
1.1
C_p
400
600
800
1000
1200
1400
1600
1800
2000
T (°K)

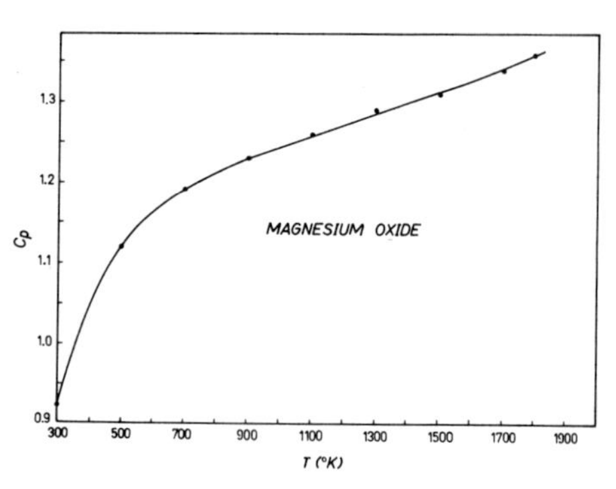
MAGNESIUM OXIDE
1.3
1.2
1.1
1.0
0.9
C_p
300
500
700
900
1100
1300
1500
1700
1900
T (°K)

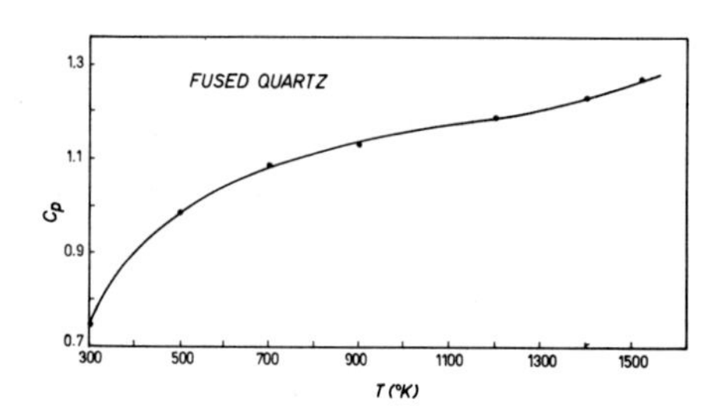
FUSED QUARTZ
1.3
1.1
0.9
0.7
C_p
300
500
700
900
1100
1300
1500
T (°K)

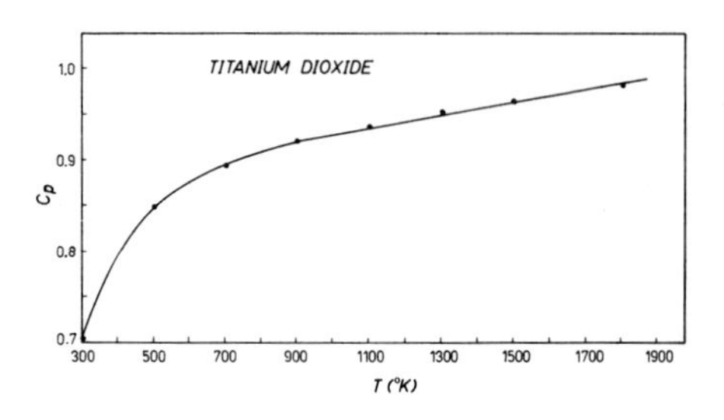
TITANIUM DIOXIDE
1.0
0.9
0.8
0.7
C_p
300
500
700
900
1100
1300
1500
1700
1900
T (°K)

Appendix C

Thermal Diffusivity Data

Plots of κ versus T are given for aluminum, chromium, copper, gold, iron, lead, molybdenum, nickel, platinum, silver, tantalum, titanium, tungsten, uranium, vanadium, zinc, zirconium, 304 stainless steel, aluminum oxide, magnesium oxide, fused quartz, and titanium dioxide. κ is in units of cm^2/sec.

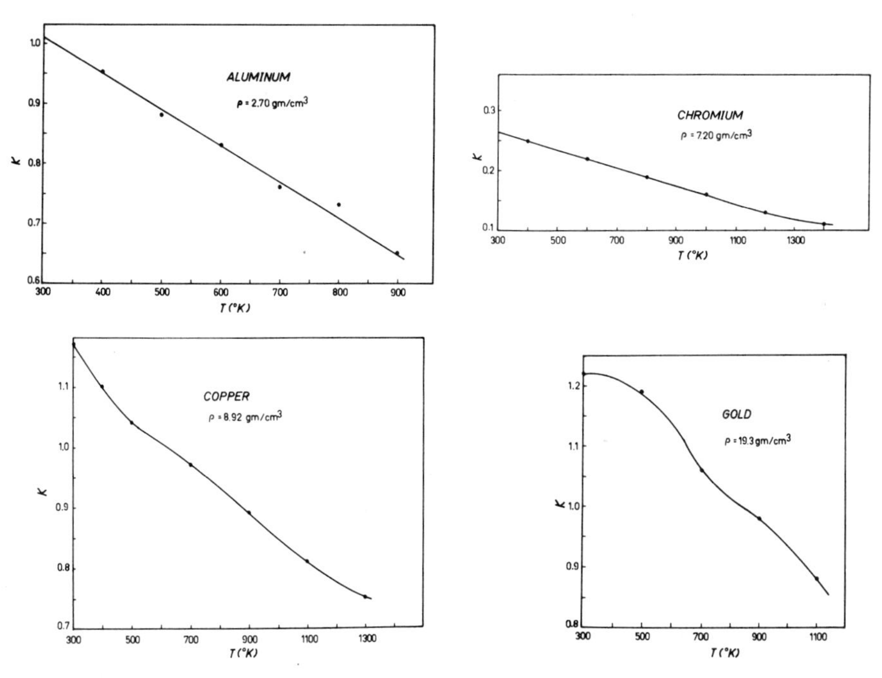

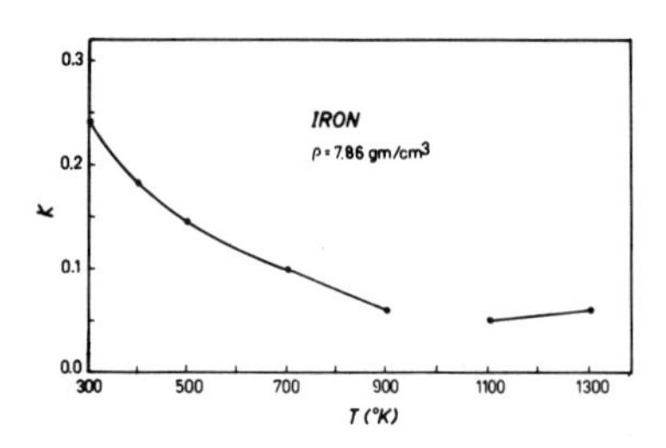
IRON
ρ = 7.86 gm/cm3
K
0.3
0.2
0.1
0.0
300
500
700
900
1100
1300
T (°K)

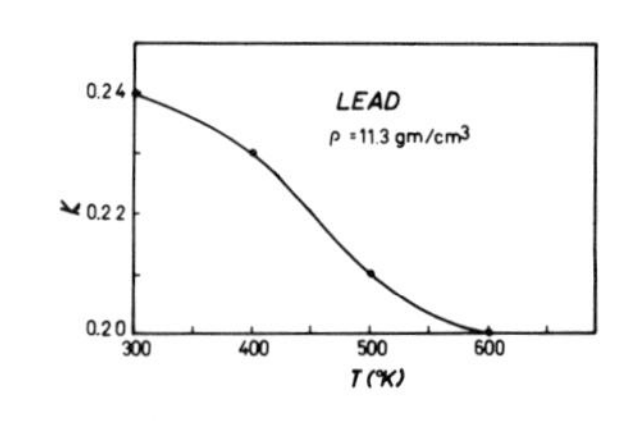
LEAD
ρ = 11.3 gm/cm3
K
0.24
0.22
0.20
300
400
500
600
T (°K)

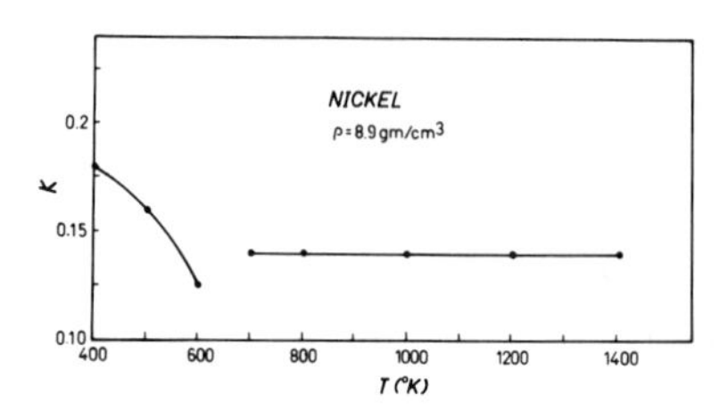
NICKEL
ρ = 8.9 gm/cm3
K
0.2
0.15
0.10
400
600
800
1000
1200
1400
T (°K)

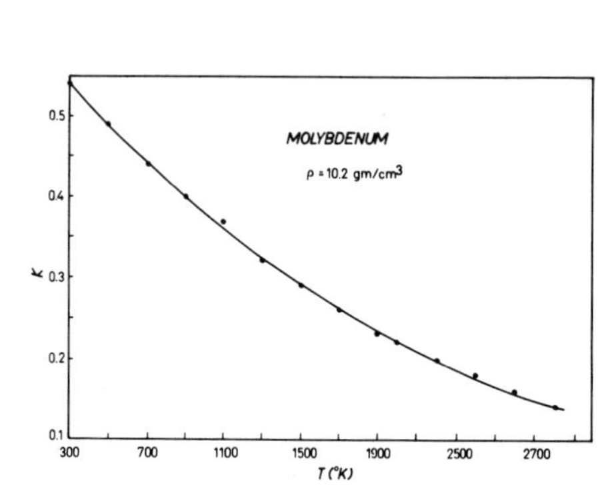
MOLYBDENUM
ρ = 10.2 gm/cm3
K
0.5
0.4
0.3
0.2
0.1
300
700
1100
1500
1900
2500
2700
T (°K)

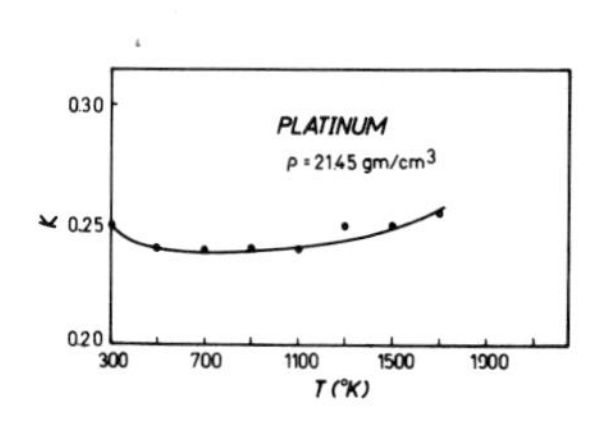
PLATINUM
ρ = 21.45 gm/cm3
K
0.30
0.25
0.20
300
700
1100
1500
1900
T (°K)

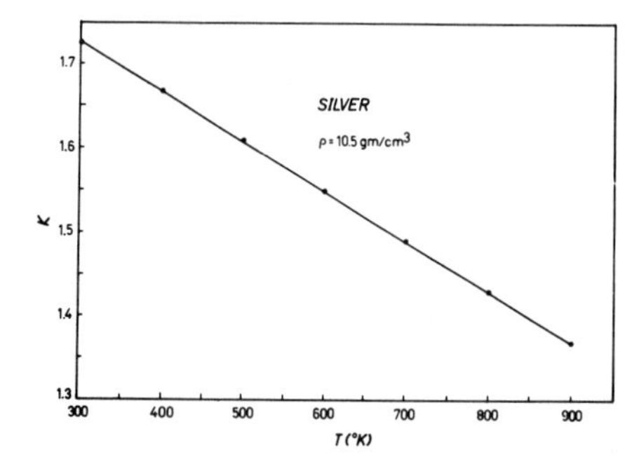
SILVER
ρ = 10.5 gm/cm3
K
1.7
1.6
1.5
1.4
1.3
300
400
500
600
700
800
900
T (°K)

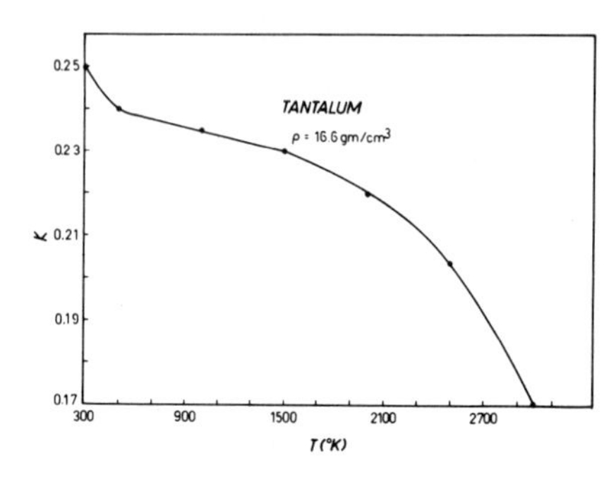
TANTALUM
ρ = 16.6 gm/cm3
K
0.25
0.23
0.21
0.19
0.17
300
900
1500
2100
2700
T (°K)

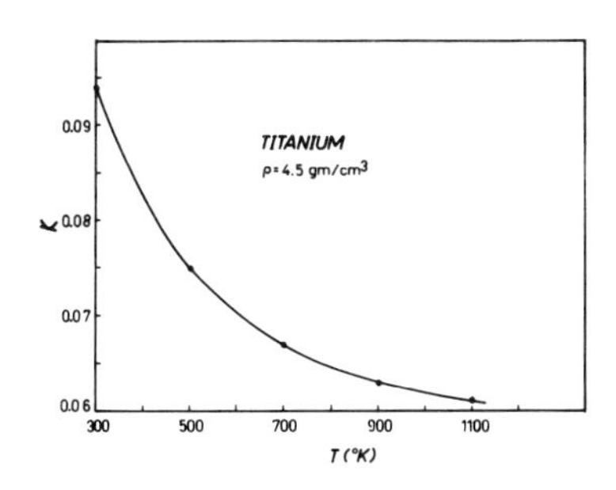
TITANIUM
ρ = 4.5 gm/cm³
κ
0.09
0.08
0.07
0.06
300
500
700
900
1100
T (°K)

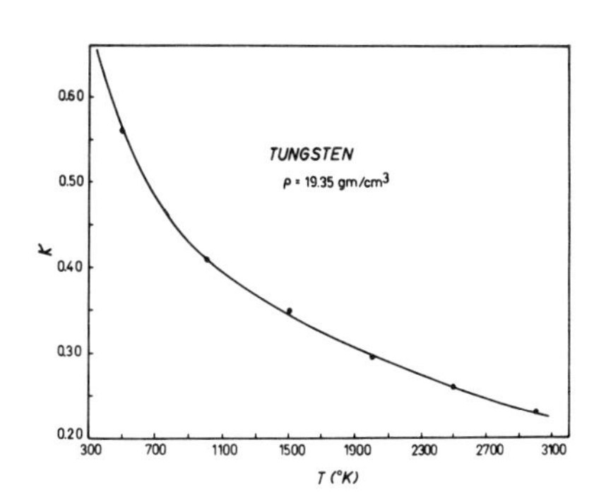
TUNGSTEN
ρ = 19.35 gm/cm³
κ
0.60
0.50
0.40
0.30
0.20
300
700
1100
1500
1900
2300
2700
3100
T (°K)

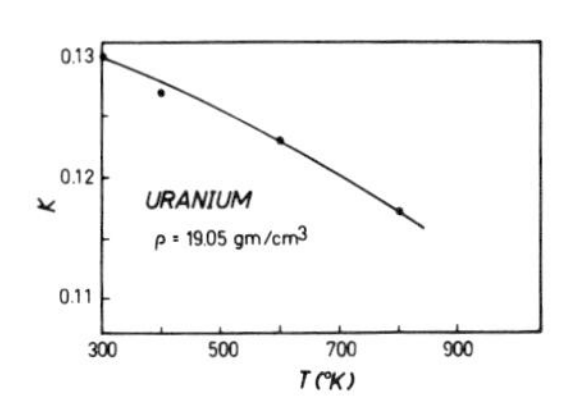
URANIUM
ρ = 19.05 gm/cm³
κ
0.13
0.12
0.11
300
500
700
900
T (°K)

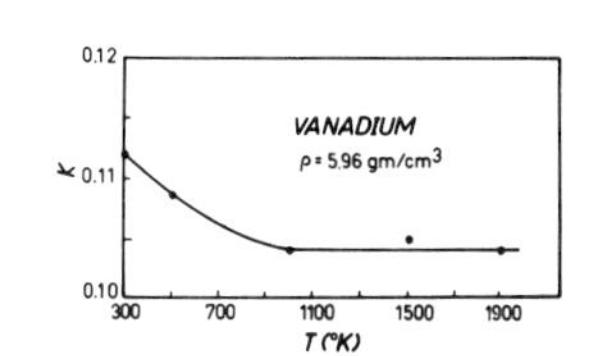
VANADIUM
ρ = 5.96 gm/cm³
κ
0.12
0.11
0.10
300
700
1100
1500
1900
T (°K)

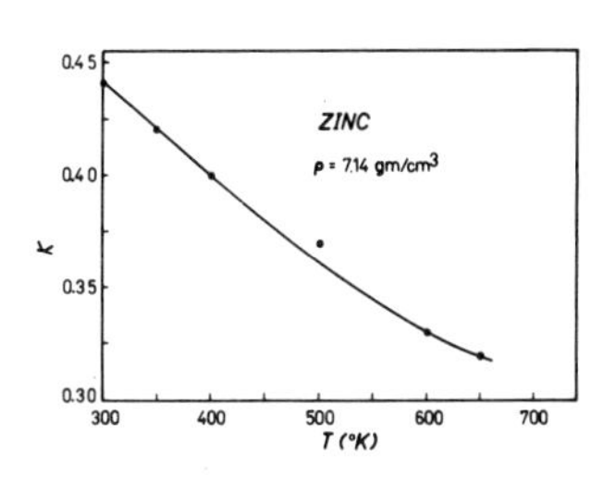
ZINC
ρ = 7.14 gm/cm³
κ
0.45
0.40
0.35
0.30
300
400
500
600
700
T (°K)

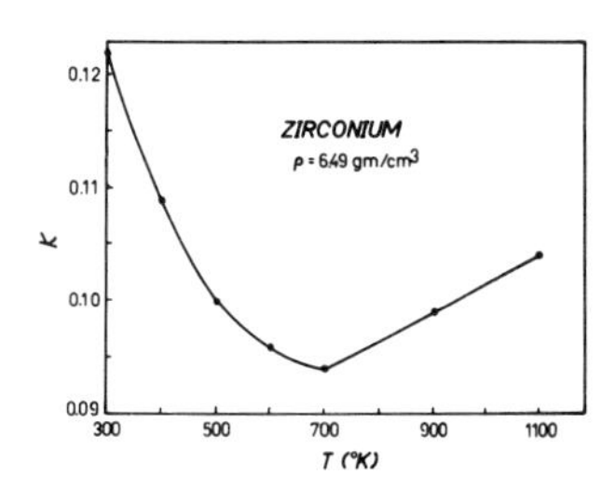
ZIRCONIUM
ρ = 6.49 gm/cm³
κ
0.12
0.11
0.10
0.09
300
500
700
900
1100
T (°K)

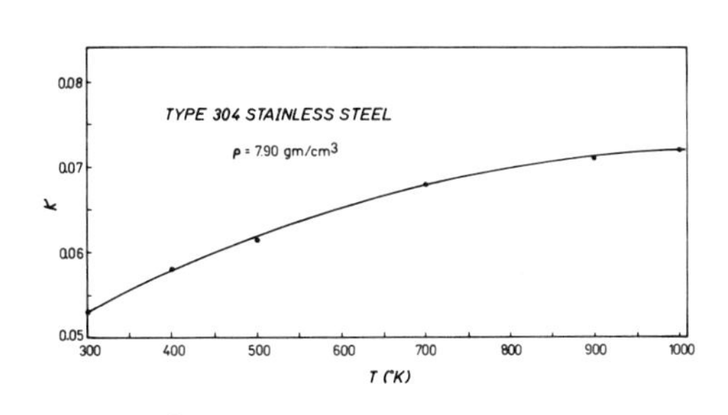
TYPE 304 STAINLESS STEEL
ρ = 7.90 gm/cm³
κ
0.08
0.07
0.06
0.05
300
400
500
600
700
800
900
1000
T (°K)

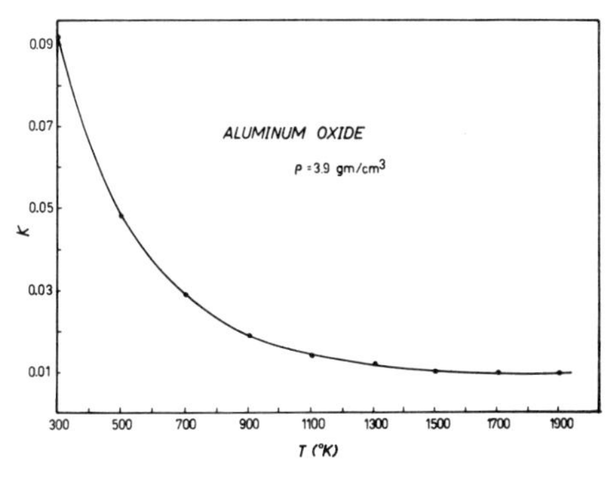
ALUMINUM OXIDE
ρ = 3.9 gm/cm³
κ
0.09
0.07
0.05
0.03
0.01
300
500
700
900
1100
1300
1500
1700
1900
T (°K)

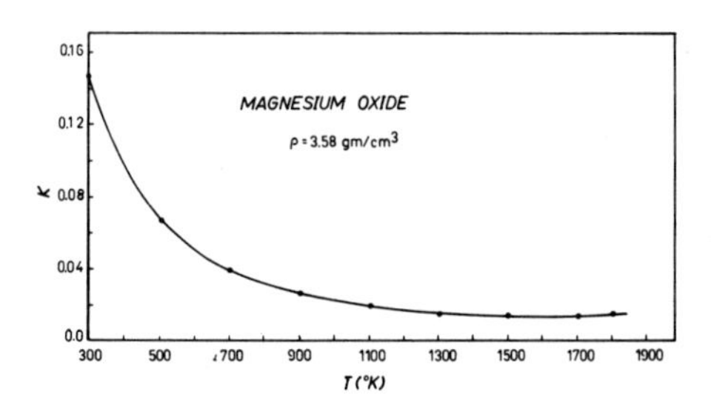
MAGNESIUM OXIDE
ρ = 3.58 gm/cm3
K
0.16
0.12
0.08
0.04
0.0
300
500
700
900
1100
1300
1500
1700
1900
T (°K)

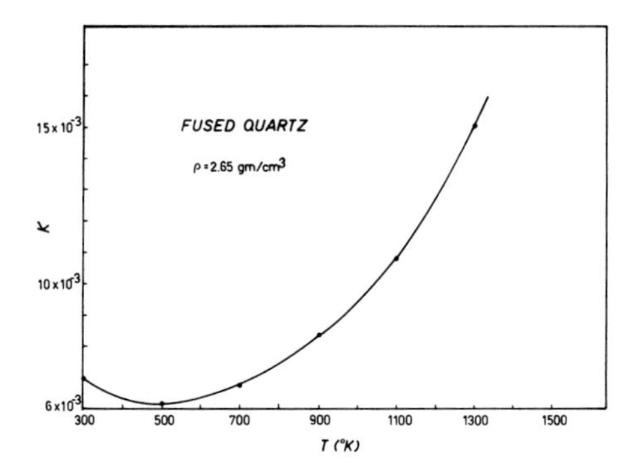
FUSED QUARTZ
ρ = 2.65 gm/cm3
K
15 x 10-3
10 x 10-3
6 x 10-3
300
500
700
900
1100
1300
1500
T (°K)

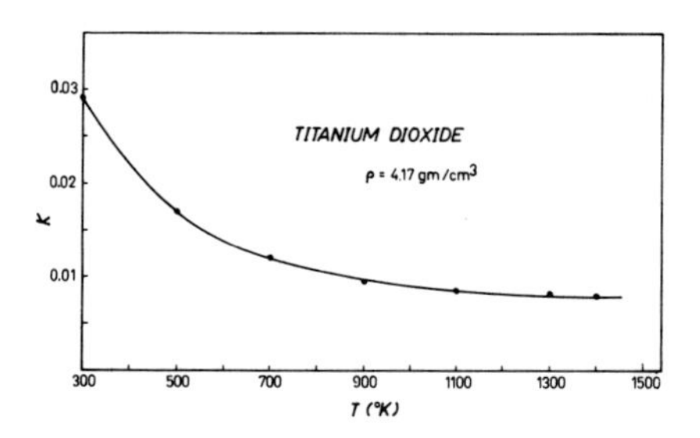
TITANIUM DIOXIDE
ρ = 4.17 gm/cm3
K
0.03
0.02
0.01
300
500
700
900
1100
1300
1500
T (°K)

References

Aboel Fotoh, M. O., and von Gutfeld, R. J. (1972). *J. Appl. Phys.* **43** (9), 3789.
Abrams, R. L. (1974). *Appl. Phys. Lett.* **25,** 304.
Abrams, R. L., and Bridges, W. B. (1973). *IEEE J. Quantum Electron.* **QE-9,** 940.
Abrams, R. L., and Gandrud, W. B. (1969). *IEEE J. Quantum Electron.* **QE-5,** 212.
Abrams, R. L., and Gandrud, W. B. (1970). *Appl. Phys. Lett.* **17,** 150.
Abrams, R. L., and Glass, A. M. (1969). *Appl. Phys. Lett.* **15,** 251.
Abrams, R. L., and Pinnow, D. A. (1971). *IEEE J. Quantum Electron.* **QE-7,** 135.
Abrams, R. L., and White, R. C., Jr. (1972). *IEEE J. Quantum Electron.* **QE-8,** 13.
Abrams, R. L., and Wood, O. R. (1971). *Appl. Phys. Lett.* **19,** 518.
Adams, M. D., and Tong, S. C. (1968). *Anal. Chem.* **40,** 1762.
Adams, M. J. (1968). *Brit. Welding Inst. Res. Bull.* **9,** 245.
Adelman, A. H. (1966). *J. Chem. Phys.* **45,** 3152.
Afanas'ev, Yu. V., Basov, N. G., Krokhin, O. N., Morachevskii, N. V., and Sklizkov, G. V. (1969). *Zh. Tekh. Fiz.* **39,** 894 [*English transl.: Sov. Phys.-Tech. Phys.* **14,** 669].
Agarbiceanu, I. I., Teodorescu, I., Popescu, I. M., and Dragamescu, V. (1969). *Rev. Roumaine Phys.* **14,** 309.
Aggarwal, R. L., Lax, B., Chase, C. E., Pidgeon, C. R., Limbert, D., and Brown, F. (1971). *Appl. Phys. Lett.* **18,** 383.
Ahlstrom, H. G., Inglesakis, G., Holzrichter, J. F., Kan, T., Jenson, J., and Kolb, A. C. (1972). *Appl. Phys. Lett.* **21,** 492.
Airey, J. R., and Smith, I. W. W. (1972). *J. Chem. Phys.* **57,** 1669.
Akhmanov, S. A., Krindach, D. P., Migulin, A. V., Sukhorukhov, A. P., and Khukhlov, R. V. (1968). *IEEE J. Quantum Electron.* **QE-4,** 568.
Akimov, A. I., and Mirkin, L. I. (1969). *Sov. Phys. Dokl.* **13,** 1162.

Alcock, A. J., and Walker, A. C. (1973). *Appl. Phys. Lett.* **23,** 467.
Alcock, A. J., and Walker, A. C. (1974). *Appl. Phys. Lett.* **25,** 299.
Alcock, A. J., Richardson, M. C., and Leopold, K. (1970). *Rev. Sci. Instrum.* **41,** 1028.
Alcock, A. J., Leopold, K., and Richardson, M. C. (1973). *Appl. Phys. Lett.* **23,** 562.
Alekseevskii, N. E., Zakosarenko, V. M., and Tsebro, V. I. (1970). *Pisma Zh. Eksper. Teor. Fiz.* **2,** 28 [*English transl.: JETP Lett.* **12,** 157].
Alekseevskii, N. E., Zakosarenko, V. M., and Tsebro, V. I. (1971). *Pisma Zh. Eksper. Teor. Fiz.* **3,** 292 [*English transl.: JETP Lett.* **13,** 412].
Alexander, J. C., and Nurmikko, A. V. (1973). *Opt. Commun.* **9,** 404.
Allen, L. (1968). *J. Phys. E* **1,** 794.
Allen, L., and Jones, D. G. C. (1967). "Principles of Gas Lasers." Butterworths, London.
Altschuler, S. J. (1973). Possible applications of laser isotope separation to nuclear and conventional technologies. Dow Chemical Co. Rep. RFP-2065.
Alwang, W. G., Cavanaugh, L. A., and Sammartino, E. (1969). *Weld. J.* (*Weld. Res. Suppl.*) **18,** 110.
Amat, G., and Pimbert, M. (1965). *J. Mol. Spectrosc.* **16,** 278.
Ambartzumian, R. V., and Letokhov, V. S. (1972). *Appl. Opt.* **11,** 354.
Ambartzumian, R. V., Letokhov, V. S., Makarov, G. N., and Puretskii, A. A. (1973). *Pisma Zh. Eksper. Teor. Fiz.* **17,** 91.
Ambartzumian, R. V., Letokhov, V. S., Ryabov, E., and Chekalin, N. V. (1974). *JETP Lett.* **20,** 273.
Ambartzumian, R. V., Gorokhov, Y. A., Letokhov, V. S., and Markarov, G. N. (1975). *JETP Lett.* **21,** 171.
Amodei, J. J., and Mezrick, R. S. (1969). *Appl. Phys. Lett.* **15,** 45.
Anderholm, N. C. (1970). *Appl. Phys. Lett.* **16,** 113.
Anderholm, N. C., and Boade, R. R. (1972). *J. Appl. Phys.* **43,** 434.
Anderson, J. E., and Jackson, J. E. (1965a). *Proc. Electron Laser Beam Symp., Penn. State Univ.* (A. B. El-Kareh, ed.), p. 17.
Anderson, J. E., and Jackson, J. E. (1965b). *Welding J.* **44,** 1018.
Andreev, S. I., Verzhikovskii, I. V., Dymshits, Yu. I., Kulikov, V. V., and Neverov, V. G. (1972). *Zh. Tekh. Fiz.* **42,** 893 [*English transl.: Sov. Phys.–Tech. Phys.* **17,** 705].
Anisimov, S. I., Bonch-Bruevich, A. M., El'yashevich, M. A., Imas, Ya. A., Pavlenko, N. A., and Romanov, G. S. (1967). *Sov. Phys.–Tech. Phys.* **11,** 945.
Apollonov, V. V., Barchukov, A. I., Konyukhov, V. K., and Prokhorov, A. M. (1972). *Pisma Zh. Eksper. Teor. Fiz.* **15,** 248 [*English transl.: JETP Lett.* **15,** 172].
Apollonov, V. V., Barchukov, A. I., and Prokhorov, A. M. (1974). *IEEE J. Quantum Electron.* **QE-10,** 505.
Arams, F., Sard, E., Peyton, B., and Pace, F. (1967). *IEEE J. Quantum Electron.* **QE-3,** 484.
Arata, Y., and Miyamoto, I. (1972). *Tech. Rep. Osaka Univ.* **22,** nos. 1027–1052, 77.
Ashkin, A. (1970). *Phys. Rev. Lett.* **24,** 156.
Ashkin, A. (1973). Isotope separation. German Patent 2,065,253 (Cl.B.036), 01 Feb.
Ashkin, A., and Dziedzic, J. M. (1972). *Appl. Phys. Lett.* **21,** 253.
Ashmarin, I. I., Bykovskii, Yu. A., Gridin, V. A., Elesin, V. F., Larkin, A. I., and Sipailo, I. P. (1971). *Kvantovaya Elektron.* (*Moscow*) **1,** 126.
Askar'yan, G. A., Rabinovich, M. S., Sauchenko, M. M., and Stepanov, V. K. (1967). *JETP Lett.* **5,** 121.
Asmus, J. F. (1971). *Rec. Symp. Electron, Ion, Laser Beam Technol., 11th,* p. 367. San Francisco Press, San Francisco.

Asmus, J. F., and Baker, F. S. (1969). *Rec. Symp. Electron, Ion, Laser Beam Technol., 10th* p. 241. San Francisco Press, San Francisco.
Astheimer, R. W., and Buckley, R. E. (1967). *Rev. Sci. Instrum.* **38,** 1764.
Aver'yanova, T. M., Mirkin, L. I., and Pilipetskii, N. F. (1966). *Zh. Prikl. Mekh. Tekh. Fiz.* No. 1, 781 [*English transl.: J. Appl. Mech. Tech. Phys.* **7,** 51].
Avotin, S. S., Krivchikova, E. P., Papirov, I. I., Stoev, P. I., and Tereshin, V. I. (1972). *Zh. Eksper. Teor. Fiz.* **62,** 288 [*English transl.: Sov. Phys-JETP* **35,** 155].
Baardsen, E. L., Schmatz, D. J., and Bisara, R. E. (1973). *Welding J.* **52,** 227.
Babenko, V. P., and Tychinskii, V. P. (1973). *Sov. J. Quantum Electron.* **2,** 399.
Bahun, C. J., and Engquist, R. D. (1963). *Proc. Nat. Electron. Conf.* **18,** 607.
Bailey, R. T., Cruikshank, F. R., and Jones, T. R. (1971). *Nature (London)* **234,** 92.
Bailey, R. T., Cruikshank, F. R., Farrell, J., Horne, D. S., North, A. M., Wilmot, P. B., and Win, T. (1974). *J. Chem. Phys.* **60,** 1699.
Baker, R. M. (1963). *Electronics* **36,** 36.
Baldwin, J. M. (1970). *Appl. Spectrosc.* **24,** 429.
Baldwin, J. M. (1973). *J. Appl. Phys.* **44,** 3362.
Ball, W. C., and Banas, C. M. (1974). Welding with a high power CO_2 laser. Nat. Aerosp. Eng. and Mfr. Meeting, San Diego, California.
Balochin, Y., Dupré, J., Pinson, P., and Meyer, C. (1972). *C.R. Acad. Sci.* **274,** 1322.
Ban, V. S., and Knox, B. E. (1969). *J. Chem. Phys.* **51,** 524.
Ban, V. S., and Knox, B. E. (1970a). *J. Chem. Phys.* **52,** 243.
Ban, V. S., and Knox, B. E. (1970b). *J. Chem. Phys.* **52,** 248.
Ban, V. S., and Kramer, D. A. (1970). *J. Mater. Sci.* **5,** 978.
Banas, C. M. (1971). UARL Rep. UAR 125 (June 1971). *IEEE Symp. Electron, Ion, Laser Beam Technol., 11th,* Boulder, Colorado. San Francisco Press, San Francisco.
Baranov, M. S., Metashop, L. A., and Geinrikhs, I. N. (1968a). *Svar. Proizvod.* No. 3, 13.
Baranov, M. S., Metashop, L. A., and Geinrikhs, I. N. (1968b). *Weld. Prod. GB* **15,** 23.
Barber, R. B., and Linn, D. L. (1969). *Rec. Symp. Electron, Ion, Laser Beam Technol., 10th* (L. Marton, ed.), p. 225. San Francisco Press, San Francisco.
Barber, T. L. (1969). *Rev. Sci. Instrum.* **40,** 1630.
Barchewitz, P., Dorbec, L., Farrenq, R., Truffert, A., and Vautier, P. (1965a). *C. R. Acad. Sci.* **260B,** 3581.
Barchewitz, P., Dorbec, L., Truffert, A., and Vautier, P. (1965b). *C. R. Acad. Sci.* **260B,** 5491.
Barger, R. L., and Hall, J. L. (1969). *Phys. Rev. Lett.* **22,** 4.
Barinov, V. V., and Sorokin, S. A. (1973). *Sov. J. Quantum Electron.* **3,** 89.
Barrett, C. S. (1952). "Structure of Metals, Crystallographic Methods, Principles and Data." McGraw Hill, New York.
Bartoli, F., Kruer, M., Esterowitz, L., and Allen, R. (1973). *J. Appl. Phys.* **44,** 3713.
Basov, N. G., and Oraevskii, A. N. (1963). *Sov. Phys.-JETP* **17,** 1171.
Basov, N. G., Krokhin, O. N., and Sklizkov, G. V. (1967). *Pisma Zh. Eksper. Teor. Fiz.* **6,** 683.
Basov, N. G., Boiko, V. A., Krokhin, O. N., Semenov, O. G., and Sklizkov, G. V. (1969a). *Sov. Phys.-Tech. Phys.* **13,** 1581.
Basov, N. G., Mikhailov, V. G., Oraevskii, A. N., and Shcheglov, V. A. (1969b). *Sov. Phys.-Tech. Phys.* **13,** 1630.
Basov, N. G., *et al.* (1971a). *Appl. Opt.* **10,** 1814.

Basov, N. G., *et al.* (1971b). *JETP Lett.* **13,** 352.
Basov, N. G., *et al.* (1971c). *JETP Lett.* **14,** 285.
Basov, N. G., *et al.* (1971d). *Sov. J. Quantum Electron.* **1,** 306.
Basov, N. G., *et al.* (1972). *JETP Lett.* **16,** 389.
Bastow, T. J. (1969). *Nature (London)* **222,** 1058.
Bastow, T. J., and Bowden, F. P. (1968). *Nature (London)* **218,** 150.
Bastow, T. J., Packer, M. E., and Gane, N. (1969). *Nature (London)* **222,** 5188, 27.
Batanov, V. A., Bunkin, F. V., Prokhorov, A. M., Fedorov, V. B., and Lebedev, P. N. (1970). *JETP Lett.* **11,** 113.
Baumhacker, H., Fill, E., and Schmid, W. (1973). *Phys. Lett.* **44A,** 3.
Bayer, E., and Schaack, G. (1969). *J. Sci. Instrum. (J. Phys. E) Ser. 2* **2** (2), 208.
Bazhin, H. M., Skubneuskaya, G. I., Sorokin, N. I., and Molin, Y. N. (1974). *JETP Lett.* **20,** 18.
Beatrice, E. S., and Glick, D. (1969). *Appl. Spectrosc.* **23,** 260.
Beatrice, E. S., Harding-Barlow, I., and Glick, D. (1969). *Appl. Spectrosc.* **23,** 257.
Beaulieu, A. J. (1970). *Appl. Phys. Lett.* **16,** 504.
Beaulieu, A. J. (1971). *Proc. IEEE* **59,** 667.
Bedair, S. M., and Smith, H. P. Jr. (1969). *J. Appl. Phys.* **40,** 4776.
Behrendt, R., Genzow, D., Herrmann, K. H., Hoerstel, W., Link, R., and Vogel, R. (1970). *Phys. Status Solidi A* **1,** k25.
Belanger, P. A., Tremblay, R., Boivin, J., and Otis, G. (1972). *Can. J. Phys.* **50,** 2753.
Bell, C. E., and Landt, J. A. (1967). *Appl. Phys. Lett.* **10,** 46.
Benanti, M. A., and Jacobs, H. (1972). *Proc. IEEE* **60,** 132.
Bennett, H. E. (1971). *In* "Damage in Laser Materials: 1971" (A. J. Glass and A. H. Guenther, eds.). NBS Spec. Publ. 356, p. 153.
Benoit, J. (1970). *Appl. Phys. Lett.* **16,** 482.
Berg, A. L., and Lood, D. E. (1968). *Solid State Electron.* **11,** 773.
Berger, P. J., and Smith, D. C. (1972). *Appl. Phys. Lett.* **21,** 167.
Bergman, J. G. Jr., McFee, J. H., and Crane, G. R. (1971). *Appl. Phys. Lett.* **18,** 203.
Berkowitz, J., and Chupka, W. A. (1964). *J. Chem. Phys.* **40,** 2735.
Bernal E. G., Levine, L. P., and Ready, J. F. (1966). *Rev. Sci. Instrum.* **37,** 938.
Bernhardt, A. F., Duerre, D. E., Simpson, J. R., and Wood, L. L. (1974). *Appl. Phys. Lett.* **25,** 617.
Bertie, J. G., and Whalley, E. (1967). *J. Chem. Phys.* **46,** 1271.
Beterov, I. M., Chebotayev, V. P., and Provorov, A. S. (1973). *Opt. Commun.* **7,** 410.
Beterov, I. M., Chebotayev, V. P., and Provorov, A. S. (1974). *IEEE J. Quantum Electron.* **QE-10,** 245.
Bettis, J. R., and Guenther, A. H. (1970). *IEEE J. Quantum Electron.* **QE-6,** 483.
Birnbaum, M., and Stocker, T. L. (1968). *J. Appl. Phys.* **39,** 6032.
Biscar, J. P. (1971). *J. Chromatogr.* **56,** 348.
Biscar, J. P., and Miknis, F. (1971). *J. Phys. Chem.* **75,** 2412.
Bishop, P. J., and Gibson, A. F. (1973). *Appl. Opt.* **12,** 2549.
Bishop, P. J., Gibson, A. F., and Kimmitt, M. F. (1973). *IEEE J. Quantum Electron.* **QE-9,** 1007.
Bisyarin, V. P., Bisyarina, I. P., and Sokolov, A. V. (1971a). *Radiotekh. Elektron. (USSR)* **16,** 1758 [*English transl.: Radio Eng. Electon. Phys.* **16,** (10), 1589].
Bisyarin, V. P., Bisyarina, I. P., Rubash, V. K., and Sokolov, A. U. (1971b). *Radiotekn. Elektron.* **16,** 1765 [*English transl.: Radio Eng. Electon. Phys.* **16,** 1594].
Bjorkholm, J. E., Ashkin, A., and Pearson, D. B. (1975). *Appl. Phys. Lett.* **27,** 534.

Blackburn, H., and Wright, H. C. (1970). *Infrared Phys.* **10**, 191.
Blackburn, W. H., Pelletier, Y. J. A., and Dennen, W. H. (1968). *Appl. Spectrosc.* **22**, 278.
Blaxell, D., Peterson, R., Malcolme-Lawes, D. J., and Wolfgang, R. (1972). *J. Chem. Soc. Chem. Commun.* **2**, 110.
Bliss, E. S., and Milam, D. (1972). *In* "Laser Induced Damage in Optical Materials" (A. J. Glass and A. H. Guenther, eds.). NBS Spec. Publ. 372, pp. 108–122.
Bloom, A. L. (1968). "Gas Lasers." Wiley, New York.
Bogdanov, S. V., Zubrinou, I. I., and Sheloput, D. V. (1971). *Izv. Akad. Nauk SSSR Ser. Fiz.* **35**, 1013.
Boling, N. L., and Dubé, G. (1973). *Appl. Phys. Lett.* **23**, 658.
Bonch-Bruevich, A. M., Kovalev, V. P., Romanov, G. S., Imas, Ya. A., and Libenson, M. N. (1968a). *Sov. Phys.–Tech. Phys.* **13**, 507.
Bonch-Bruevich, A. M., Imas, Ya. A., Romanov, G. S., Libenson, M. N., and Mal'tsev, L. N. (1968b). *Sov. Phys.–Tech. Phys.* **13**, (5), 640.
Bongers, P. F., and Zanmarchi, G. (1968). *Solid State Commun.* **6**, 291.
Boni, A. A., and Su, F. Y. (1973). *J. Appl. Phys.* **44**, 4086.
Boord, W. T., Pao, Y-H., Phelps, F. W., Jr., and Claspy, P. C. (1974). *IEEE J. Quantum Electron.* **QE-10**, 273.
Bordé, M. C., Henry, A., and Henry, M. L. (1966a). *C.R. Acad. Sci. Ser. B* **262**, 1389.
Bordé, M. C., Henry, A., and Henry, M. L. (1966b). *C.R. Acad. Sci. Ser. B* **263**, 619.
Boulanger, P., Heym, A., Mayer, J.-M., and Pietrzyk, Z. A. (1973). *J. Phys. E* **6**, 559.
Boyd, G. D., Bridges, T. J., and Burkhardt, E. G. (1968). *IEEE J. Quantum Electron.* **QE-4**, 515.
Boyd, G. D., Gandrud, W., and Buehler, E. (1971). *Appl. Phys. Lett.* **18**, 446.
Boyer, G., Huriet, J. R., and Lamouroux, B. (1970). *Opt. Laser Technol.* **2**, 196.
Bradley, L. P., and Davies, T. J. (1971). *IEEE J. Quantum Electron.* **QE-7**, 464.
Bradley, L. C., and Herrmann, J. (1974). *Appl. Opt.* **13**, 331.
Bradley, D. J., Higgins, J. R., Key, M. H., and Majumdar, S. (1969). *Opto-Electron.* **1**, 62.
Braginskii, V. B., Minakova, I. I., and Rudenko, V. N. (1967). *Sov. Phys.–Tech. Phys.* **12**, 753.
Bramson, M. A. (1968). "Infrared Radiation: A Handbook for Applications." Plenum Press, New York.
Brandenberg, W. M., Bailey, M. P., and Texeira, P. D. (1972). *IEEE J. Quantum Electron.* **QE-8**, 414.
Brandewie, R. A., and Davis, W. C. (1972). *Appl. Opt.* **11**, 1526.
Braun, L., and Breuer, D. R. (1969). *Solid State Technol.* **12**, 56.
Braunstein, A. I., and Braunstein, M. (1971). *J. Vac. Sci. Technol.* **8**, 412.
Braunstein, A. I., Wang, V., Braunstein, M., Rudisill, J. E., and Wade, G. (1973). "Laser Induced Damage in Optical Materials: 1973" (A. J. Glass and A. H. Guenther, eds.). NBS Spec. Publ. 387, pp. 151–156.
Breig, E. L. (1972). *J. Opt. Soc. Amer.* **62**, 518.
Brekhovskikh, V. F., Rykalin, N. N., and Uglov, A. A. (1970). *Sov. Phys.–Dokl.* **15**, 124.
Brewer, R. G., and Swalen, J. D. (1970). *J. Chem. Phys.* **52**, 2774.
Brewer, R. G., Kelly, M. J., and Javan, A. (1969). *Phys. Rev. Lett.* **23**, 559.
Bridges, T. J., and Burkhardt, E. G. (1967). *IEEE J. Quantum Electron.* **QE-3**, 168.
Bridges, T. J., and Cheo, P. K. (1969). *Appl. Phys. Lett.* **14**, 262.
Bridges, T. J., and Patel, C. K. N. (1965). *Appl. Phys. Lett.* **7**, 244.
Bridges, T. J., Chang, T. Y., and Cheo, P. K. (1968). *Appl. Phys. Lett.* **12**, 297.
Bridges, T. J., Burkhardt, E. G., and Smith, P. W. (1972). *Appl. Phys. Lett.* **20**, 403.

Brinkman, U., Hartig, W., Telle, H., and Walther, H. (1974). *Appl. Phys.* **5,** 109.
Brisbane, A. D., and Jackson, T. M. (1968). *Electron. Compon.* **9,** 73.
Britton, B. (1973). *Electron. Equip. News* **15,** 52.
Bronfin, B. R., Boedeker, L. R., and Cheyer, J. P. (1970). *Appl. Phys. Lett.* **16,** 214.
Brown, C. O. (1970). *Appl. Phys. Lett.* **17,** 388.
Brown, C. O., and Davis, J. W. (1972). *Appl. Phys. Lett.* **21,** 480.
Brown, F., Silver, E., Chase, C. E., Button, K. J., and Lax, B. (1972). *IEEE J. Quantum Electron.* **QE-8,** 499.
Brown, R. T. (1973). *IEEE J. Quantum Electron.* **QE-9,** 1120.
Bruce, F. M. (1947). *J. Inst. Elec. Eng.* **94,** 138.
Brueck, S. R. J., and Blum, F. A. (1972). *Phys. Rev. Lett.* **28,** 1458.
Brueck, S. R. J., and Mooradian, A. (1971). *Appl. Phys. Lett.* **18,** 229.
Brugger, K. (1972). *J. Appl. Phys.* **43,** 577.
Brunet, H. (1970). *IEEE J. Quantum Electron.* **QE-6,** 678.
Brunet, H., and Mabru, M. (1971). *C. R. Acad. Sci.* **272,** 232.
Brunet, H., and Mabru, M. (1972). *Appl. Phys. Lett.* **21,** 432.
Buczek, C. J., Freiberg, R. J., Chenansky, P. P., and Wayne, R. J. (1971). *Proc. IEEE* **59,** 659.
Buczek, C. J., Wayne, R. J., Chenansky, P. P., and Freiberg, R. J. (1970). *Appl. Phys. Lett.* **16,** 321.
Büchl, K., and Pfeiffer, H.-J. (1972). *Z. Angew. Phys.* **32,** 357.
Büchl, K., Hohla, K., Wienecke, R., and Wittowski, S. (1969). *Phys. Lett.* **26A,** 248.
Bukatyi, V. I., and Pogodayev, V. A. (1970). *Izv. Vyssh. Ucheb. Zaved. Fiz.* **1,** 141.
Bukatyi, V. I., and Pogodayev, V. A. (1972). *Laser-Unconventional Opt. J.* (*Sweden*) No. 40, 3.
Burkhardt, E. G., Bridges, T. J., and Smith, P. W. (1972). *Opt. Commun.* **6,** 193.
Buser, R. G., and Rhode, R. S. (1973). *Appl. Opt.* **12,** 205.
Bushnell, J. C., and McCloskey, D. J. (1968). *J. Appl. Phys.* **39,** 5541.
Caddes, D. E., Osterink, L. M., and Targ, R. (1968). *Appl. Phys. Lett.* **12,** 74.
Cady, W. G. (1946). "Piezoelectricity." McGraw Hill, New York.
Canavan, G. H., and Nielsen, P. E. (1973). *Appl. Phys. Lett.* **22,** 409.
Cape, J. A., and Lehman, G. W. (1963). *J. Appl. Phys.* **34,** 1909.
Carbone, R. J. (1967). *IEEE J. Quantum Electron.* **QE-3,** 373.
Carbone, R. J. (1968). *IEEE J. Quantum Electron.* **QE-4,** 102.
Carbone, R. J. (1969). *IEEE J. Quantum Electron.* **QE-5,** 48.
Carlson, C. O., Stone, E., Bernstein, H. L., Tomita, W. K., and Myers, W. C. (1966). *Science* **154,** 1550.
Carman, R., and Kelley, P. (1968). *Appl. Phys. Lett.* **12,** 241.
Carmichael, C. H. H., Garnsworthy, R. K., and Mathias, L. E. S. (1974). *Appl. Phys. Lett.* **24,** 608.
Carome, E. F., Clarke, N. A., and Moeller, C. E. (1964). *Appl. Phys. Lett.* **4,** 95.
Carome, E. F., Carreira, E. M., and Prochaska, C. J. (1967). *Appl. Phys. Lett.* **11,** 64.
Carr, J. F. (1972). *In* "Lasers in Industry" (S. S. Charschan, ed.). Van Nostrand-Reinhold, Princeton, New Jersey.
Carslaw, H. S., and Jaeger, J. C. (1959). "Conduction of Heat in Solids," 2nd ed. Oxford Univ. Press (Clarendon), London and New York.
Carswell, A. I., McQuillan, A. K., and McNeil, W. R. (1971). *Can. Aeronaut. Space J.* **17,** 419.
Carswell, A. I., Houston, J. D., McNeil, W. R., Pal, S. R., and Sizgoric, S. (1972). *Can. Aeronaut. Space J.* **18,** 335.

Caruso, A. (1971). *In* "Laser Interaction and Related Plasma Phenomena" (H. J. Schwarz and H. Hora, eds.), p. 289. Plenum Press, New York.
Cerrai, E., and Trucco, R. (1968). *Energ. Nucl. (Italy)* **15,** 581.
Cervay, R. R., and Perak, G. J. (1972). *Eng. Fract. Mech.* **4,** 991.
Chang, D. B., Drummond, J. E., and Hall, R. B. (1970). *J. Appl. Phys.* **41,** 4851.
Chang, T. Y. (1973). *Rev. Sci. Instrum.* **44,** 405.
Chang, T. Y., and Bridges, T. J. (1970). *Opt. Commun.* **1,** 423.
Chang, T. Y., and Wood, O. R. (1972a). *Appl. Phys. Lett.* **21,** 19.
Chang, T. Y., and Wood, O. R. (1972b). *IEEE J. Quantum Electron.* **QE-8,** 721.
Chang, T. Y., and Wood, O. R. (1973). *Appl. Phys. Lett.* **23,** 370.
Chang, T. Y., and Wood, O. R. (1974). *Appl. Phys. Lett.* **24,** 182.
Chang, T. Y., Bridges, T. J., and Burkhardt, E. G. (1970a). *Appl. Phys. Lett.* **17,** 249.
Chang, T. Y., Bridges, T. J., and Burkhardt, E. G. (1970b). *Appl. Phys. Lett.* **17,** 357.
Chang, W. S. C., and Loh, K. W. (1972). *IEEE J. Quantum Electron.* **QE-8,** 463.
Chen, D., Ready, J. F., and Bernal, G. (1968). *Laser Focus* **4,** 18.
Chen, H. L., Stephenson, J. C., and Moore, C. B. (1968). *Chem. Phys. Lett.* **2,** 593.
Chen, J. M., and Chang, C. C. (1972). *J. Appl. Phys.* **43,** 3884.
Cheo, P. K. (1971). "Lasers" (A. K. Levine and A. J. DeMaria, eds.), Dekker, New York.
Cheo, P. K., and Bass, C. D. (1971). *Appl. Phys. Lett.* **18,** 565.
Cheo, P. K., and Cooper, H. G. (1967). *IEEE J. Quantum Electron.* **QE-3,** 79.
Cheo, P. K., and Gilden, M. (1974). *Appl. Phys. Lett.* **25,** 272.
Cheo, P. K., Berak, J. M., Oshinsky, W., and Swindal, J. L. (1973). *Appl. Opt.* **12,** 500.
Chester, A. N., and Abrams, R. L. (1972). *Appl. Phys. Lett.* **21,** 576.
Christiansen, W. H., and Hertzberg, A. (1973). *Proc. IEEE* **61,** 1060.
Christensen, C. P., Freed, C., and Hans, H. A. (1969). *IEEE J. Quantum Electron.* **QE-5,** 276.
Chu, T. S., and Hogg, D. C. (1968). *Bell Syst. Tech. J.* **47,** 723.
Chun, M. K., and Rose, K. (1970). *J. Appl. Phys.* **41,** 614.
Clark, A. F., Moulder, J. C., and Reed, R. P. (1973). *Appl. Opt.* **12,** 1103.
Clark, J. H., Haas, Y., Houston, P. L., and Moore, C. B. (1975). *Chem. Phys. Lett.* **35,** 82.
Clark, W. M., Jr., and Lind, R. C. (1974). *Appl. Phys. Lett.* **25,** 284.
Claspy, P. C., and Pao, Y-H. (1971). *IEEE J. Quantum Electron.* **QE-7,** 512.
Cockayne, B., and Gasson, D. B. (1970). *J. Mater. Sci.* **5,** 837.
Cockayne, B., and Gasson, D. B. (1971). *J. Mater. Sci.* **6,** 126.
Cohen, C., Bordé, C., and Henry, L. (1967). *C.R. Acad. Sci., Ser. B* **265,** 267.
Cohen, M. I. (1967). *Bell Lab. Rec.* **45** (8), 247.
Cohen, M. I., and Epperson, J. P. (1968). *Advan. Electron. Electron Phys. Suppl. 4,* p. 139.
Cohen, M. I., Unger, B. A., and Milkosky, J. F. (1968). *Bell Syst. Tech. J.* **47,** 385.
Cohen, M. I., Mainwaring, F. J., and Melone, T. G. (1969). *Welding J.* **48,** 191.
Cohen-Solal, G., and Riant, Y. (1971). *Appl. Phys. Lett.* **19,** 436.
Cohn, D. B., and Ault, E. R. (1973). *Appl. Phys. Lett.* **22,** 138.
Colles, M. J., Dennis, R. B., Smith, J. W., and Webb, J. S. (1974). *Opt. Commun.* **10,** 145.
Collis, R. T. H. (1970). *Appl. Opt.* **9,** 1782.
Collis, R. T. H., and Uthe, E. E. (1972). *Opto-Electron.* **4,** 87.
Colwell, J. E., McClelland, J. D., Richardson, J. H., and Zehms, E. H. (1972). *Carbon* **10,** 352.
Condas, G. A. (1971). *IEEE J. Quantum Electron.* **QE-7,** 202.
Condas, G. A., and Brown, D. W. (1970). *Rev. Sci. Instrum.* **41,** 888.

Conti, R. J. (1969). *Welding J.* **48,** 800.
Contreras, B., and Gaddy, O. L. (1970). *Appl. Phys. Lett.* **17,** 450.
Contreras, B., and Gaddy, O. L. (1971). *Appl. Phys. Lett.* **18,** 277.
Cool, T. A. (1973). *IEEE J. Quantum Electron.* **QE-9,** 72.
Cool, T. A., and Shirley, J. A. (1969). *Appl. Phys. Lett.* **14,** 70.
Cool, T. A., and Stephens, R. R. (1969). *J. Chem. Phys.* **51,** 5175.
Cool, T. A., and Stephens, R. R. (1970a). *Appl. Phys. Lett.* **16,** 55.
Cool, T. A., and Stephens, R. R. (1970b). *J. Chem. Phys.* **52,** 3304.
Cool, T. A., Falk, T. J., and Stephens, R. R. (1969a). *Appl. Phys. Lett.* **15,** 318.
Cool, T. A., Stephens, R. R., and Falk, T. J. (1969b). *Int. J. Chem. Kinet.* **1,** 495.
Cool, T. A., Stephens, R. R., and Shirley, J. A. (1970a). *J. Appl. Phys.* **41,** 4038.
Cool, T. A., Shirley, J. A., and Stephens, R. R. (1970b). *Appl. Phys. Lett.* **17,** 278.
Cooper, J. (1962a). *Rev. Sci. Instrum.* **33,** 92.
Cooper, J. (1962b). *J. Sci. Instrum.* **39,** 467.
Corcoran, V. J., Cupp, R. E., Gallagher, J. J., and Smith, W. T. (1970). *Appl. Phys. Lett.* **16,** 316.
Courtoy, C. P. (1957). *Can. J. Phys.* **35,** 608.
Cowan, R. D. (1963). *J. Appl. Phys.* **34,** 926.
Crafer, R. C., Gibson, A. F., and Kimmitt, M. F. (1969a). Rate processes in the CO_2 laser. *Lasers Opto-Electron. Conf., IERE Conf. Proc.* No. 14, 238.
Crafer, R. C., Gibson, A. F., Kent, M. J., and Kimmitt, M. F. (1969b). *J. Phys. D.* **2,** 183.
Crank, J. (1957). *Quart. J. Mech. Appl. Math.* **10,** 220.
Crocker, A., and Lamberton, H. M. (1971). *Electron. Lett.* **7,** 272.
Dabby, F. W., and Paek, U.-C. (1972). *IEEE J. Quantum Elect.* **QE-8,** 106.
Daneu, V., Sokoloff, D., Sanchez, A., Javan, A. (1969). *Appl. Phys. Lett.* **15,** 398.
Danishevskii, A. M., Kastal'skii, A. A., Ryvkin, B. S., Yaroshetskii, I. D., and Ioffe, A. F. (1969). *JETP Lett.* **10,** 302.
Danishevskii, A. M., Kastalskii, A. A., Ryvkin, S. M., Yarashetskii, I. D. (1970). *Sov. Phys.–JETP* **31,** 292.
Daugherty, J. D., Pugh, E. R., and Douglas-Hamilton, D. H. (1972a). *Bull. Amer. Phys. Soc.* **17,** 399.
Dougherty, J. D., Pugh, E., House, D. A., and Douglas-Hamilton, D. (1972b). *Phys. Today* **25,** 18.
Davis, D. T., Smith, D. L., and Koval, J. S. (1972). *IEEE J. Quantum Electron.* **QE-8,** 846.
Davis, W. C., and Cathey, W. T., Jr. (1969). *Appl. Opt.* **8,** 715.
Davit, J. (1973). *In* "Laser Induced Damage in Optical Materials" (A. J. Glass and A. H. Guenther, eds.). NBS Spec. Publ. 387, p. 170.
Day, G. W., Gaddy, O. L., and Iversen, R. J. (1968). *Appl. Phys. Lett.* **13,** 289.
Day, G. W., Hamilton, C. A., Peterson, R. L., Phelan, R. L., Jr., and Mullen, L. O. (1974). *Appl. Phys. Lett.* **24,** 456.
deCremoux, B., and Leiba, E. (1969). *Proc. IEEE* **57,** 1674.
Deem, H. W., and Wood, W. D. (1962). *Rev. Sci.* **33,** 1107.
De Hemptinne, X. (1973). *Ann. Soc. Sci. Brux. I* **87,** 101.
DeJong, M., and Knapen, M. G. J. (1969). *Microelectron. Reliability* **8,** 89.
DeMaria, A. J. (1973). *Proc. IEEE* **61,** 731.
DeMaria, A. J., Cagosz, J. R., Heynan, H. A., Penny, A. W., and Wissin, G. (1966). *Appl. Phys. Lett.* **4,** 125.

Deming, J. L., Weber, J. H., and Tao, L. C. (1969). *Amer. Inst. Chem. Eng. J.* **15,** 501.
Demtröder, W. (1971). "Topics in Current Chemistry," No. 17. Springer-Verlag, Berlin.
Denes, L. J., and Farish, O. (1971). *Electron. Lett.* **7,** 337.
Dennis, J. H. (1967). *IEEE J. Quantum Electron.* **QE-3,** 416.
Derr, V. E., and Little, C. G. (1970). *Appl. Opt.* **9,** 1976.
DeSilets, C. S., and Patel, C. K. N. (1973). *Appl. Phys. Lett.* **22,** 543.
DeTemple, T. A., Plant, T. K., and Coleman, P. D. (1973). *Appl. Phys. Lett.* **22,** 644.
Deutsch, T. F. (1967). *Appl. Phys. Lett.* **10,** 234.
Deutsch, T. F. (1968). *Brit. J. Appl. Phys.* (*J. Phys. D*) *Ser. 2* **1,** 1711.
Deutsch, T. F. (1974). *Appl. Phys. Lett.* **25,** 109.
Deutsch, T. F., and Rudko, R. I. (1972). *Appl. Phys. Lett.* **20,** 423.
Deutsch, T. F., Horrigan, F. A., and Rudko, R. I. (1969). *Appl. Phys. Lett.* **15,** 88.
Dezenberg, G. J., Roy, E. L., and McKnight, W. B. (1972). *IEEE J. Quantum Electron.* **QE-8,** 58.
Diamond, J. J., and Dragoo, A. L. (1966). *Rev. Hautes Temp. Refract.* **3,** 273.
Dickson, L. D. (1970). *Appl. Opt.* **9,** 1854.
Dimmock, J. O., Hurwitz, C. E., and Reed, T. B. (1969). *Appl. Phys. Lett.* **14,** 49.
Dixon, R. W., and Chester, A. N. (1966). *Appl. Phys. Lett.* **9,** 190.
Doyle, W. M. (1970). *Laser Focus,* p. 34, July.
Dronov, A. P., D'yakov, A. S., Kudoyavtsev, E. M., and Sobolev, N. N. (1970). *JETP Lett.* **11,** 353.
Duley, W. W. (1967). *J. Sci. Instrum.* **44,** 629.
Duley, W. W., and Finnigan, P. J. (1973). *Amer. J. Phys.* **41,** 657.
Duley, W. W., and Gonsalves, J. N. (1972a). *Can. Res. Develop.*, Jan/Feb., 25.
Duley, W. W., and Gonsalves, J. N. (1972b). *Can. J. Phys.* **50,** 215.
Duley, W. W., and Gonsalves, J. N. (1974). *Opt. Laser Technol.* **6,** 78.
Duley, W. W., and Young, W. A. (1973). *J. Appl. Phys.* **44,** 4236.
Duley, W. W., and Young, W. A. (1974). *J. Phys. D* **7,** 987.
Duley, W. W., Hara, E. H., and Johnson, D. C. (1973). Unpublished work.
Dumanchin, R., and Rocca-Serra, J. (1969). *C.R. Acad. Sci.* **269,** 916.
Dumanchin, R., Michon, M., Farcy, J. C., Boudinet, G., and Rocca-Serra, J. (1972). *IEEE J. Quantum Electron.* **QE-8,** 163.
Duthler, C. J. (1974). *Appl. Phys. Lett.* **24,** 5.
Dyer, P. E., James, D. J., and Ramsden, S. A. (1972a). *J. Sci. Instrum.* **5,** 1162.
Dyer, P. E., James, D. J., and Ramsden, S. A. (1972b). *Opt. Commun.* **5,** 236.
Dzhidzhoev, M. S., Korolev, V. V., Markov, V. N., Platonenko, V. G., and Khokhlov, R. V. (1971). *JETP Lett.* **14,** 47.
Eärvolino, L. P., and Kennedy, J. R. (1966). *Weld. J. Suppl.* **45,** 127.
Eckbreth, A. C., and Davis, J. W. (1971). *Appl. Phys. Lett.* **19,** 101.
Eckbreth, A. C., and Davis, J. W. (1972). *IEEE J. Quantum Electron.* **QE-8,** 139.
Eckbreth, A. C., and Owen, F. S. (1972). *Rev. Sci. Instrum.* **43,** 995.
Eckbreth, A. C., Davis, J. W., and Pinsley, E. A. (1971). *Appl. Phys. Lett.* **18,** 73.
Eickhoff, K., and Gürs, K. (1969a). *J. Cryst. Growth* **6,** 21.
Eickhoff, K., and Gürs, K. (1969b). *J. Cryst. Growth* **6,** 21.
Eleccion, M. (1972). *IEEE Spectrum* **9,** 62.
Elliott, W. A., and Gagliano, F. P. (1972). *Appl. Phys. Lett.* **21,** 23.
Emmony, D. C., and Irving, J. (1969). *J. Phys. D* **2,** 1186.
Emmony, D. C., Howson, R. P., and Willis, L. J. (1973). *Appl. Phys. Lett.* **23,** 598.

Engel, A., Steffen, J., and Herziger, G. (1974). *Appl. Opt.* **13,** 269.
Epperson, J. P., Dyer, R. W., and Grzywa, J. C. (1966). *West. Elec. Eng.* **10,** 2.
Epstein, L. M., and Sun, K. H. (1966). *Nature* (*London*) **211,** 1173.
Ernest, J., Michon, M., and Debrie, J. (1966). *Phys. Lett.* **22,** 147.
Ertl, G., and Neumann, M. (1972). *Z. Naturforsch. A* **27A,** 1607.
Evans, R. G., and Thonemann, P. C. (1972). *Phys. Lett. A* **38,** 398.
Evenson, K. M., Wells, J. S., Matarrese, L. M., and Elwell, L. B. (1970a). *Appl. Phys. Lett.* **16,** 159.
Evenson, K. M., Wells, J. S., and Matarrese, L. M. (1970b). *Appl. Phys. Lett.* **16,** 251.
Ewing, C. E. (1972). *Ann. Rev. Phys. Chem.* **23,** 141.
Fairand, B. P., Wilcox, B. A., Gallagher, W. J., and Williams, D. N. (1972). *J. Appl. Phys.* **43,** 3893.
Fairbanks, R. H., and Adams, C. M. (1964). *Welding J.* **43,** 97s.
Fan, G. Y., and Greiner, J. H. (1968). *J. Appl. Phys.* **39,** 1216.
Fanter, D. L., Levy, R. L., and Wolf, C. J. (1972). *Anal. Chem.* **44,** 43.
Farmer, B. (1971). *Opt. Laser Technol.* **3,** 224.
Farrer, R. L., Jr., and Smith, D. F. (1972). Nucl. Div. Union Carbide Corp., Oak Ridge. Rep. 1972, K-L-3054 (Rev. 1).
Feiock, F. D., and Goodwin, L. K. (1972). *J. Appl. Phys.* **43,** 5061.
Feldman, B. J., and Figueira, J. F. (1974). *Appl. Phys. Lett.* **25,** 301.
Felici, N.-J. (1950). *Rev. Gen. Elec.* **59,** 479.
Felix, M. P., and Ellis, A. T. (1972). *Appl. Phys. Lett.* **21,** 532.
Fenner, N. C., and Daly, N. R. (1966). *Rev. Sci. Instrum.* **37,** 1068.
Fenstermacher, C. A., Nutter, M. J., Rink, J. P., and Boyer, K. (1971). *Bull. Amer. Phys. Soc.* **16,** 42.
Fenstermacher, C. A., Nutter, M. J., Leland, W. T., and Boyer, K. (1972). *Appl. Phys. Lett.* **20,** 56.
Ferguson, H. I. S., Mentall, J. E., and Nicholls, R. W. (1964). *Nature* (*London*) **204,** 1295.
Fermi, E. (1931). *Z. Phys.* **71,** 250.
Ferrar, C. M. (1969). *Appl. Opt.* **8,** 2356.
Fetterman, H. R., Schlossberg, H. R., and Waldman, J. (1972). *Opt. Commun.* **6,** 156.
Figueira, J. F. (1974). *Opt. Commun.* **11,** 220.
Figueira, J. F., Reichelt, W. H., Schappert, G. T., Stratton, T. F., and Fenstermacher, C. A. (1973). *Appl. Phys. Lett.* **22,** 216.
Figueira, J. F., and Sutphin, H. D. (1974). *Appl. Phys. Lett.* **25,** 661.
Finn, D., Groves, W. O., Hellwig, L. G., Craford, M. G., Chang, W. S. C., Chang, M. S., and Sopori, B. L. (1974). *Opt. Commun.* **11,** 201.
Fiorito, G., Gasparrini, G., and Svelto, F. (1973). *Appl. Phys. Lett.* **23,** 448.
Fleck, J. A., Jr. (1966). *J. Appl. Phys.* **37,** 188.
Fletcher, M. J. (1973). *Weld. Met. Fabr.* **41,** 336.
Flynn, J. B., and Schlickman, J. (1968). *Proc. IEEE* **56,** 322.
Folmer, O. F., Jr. (1971). *Anal. Chem.* **43,** 1057.
Folmer, O. F., Jr., and Azarraga, L. V. (1969). *J. Chromatogr. Sci.* **7,** 665.
Forster, D. C., Goodwin, F. E., and Bridges, W. B. (1972). *IEEE J. Quantum Electron.* **QE-8,** 263.
Fortin, R., Gravel, M., and Tremblay, R. (1971). *Can. J. Phys.* **49,** 1783.
Fortin, R., Rheault, F., Gilbert, J., Blanchard, M., and LaChambre, J.-L. (1973). *Can. J. Phys.* **51,** 414.
Foster, H. (1972). *Opt. Laser Technol.* **4,** 121.

Fourier, M., Redon, van Lerberghe, A., and Bordé, C. (1970). *C. R. Acad. Sci.* **270B**, 537.
Fox, A. G., and Li, T. (1963). *Proc. IEEE* **51**, 80.
Fox, J. A. (1974). *Appl. Phys. Lett.* **24**, 340.
Fox, J. A., and Barr, D. N. (1973a). *Appl. Phys. Lett.* **22**, 594.
Fox, J. A., and Barr, D. N. (1973b). *Appl. Opt.* **12**, 2547.
Fradin, D. W., and Bua, D. P. (1974). *Appl. Phys. Lett.* **24**, 555.
Fradin, D. W., and Yablonovitch, E. (1972). *In* "Laser Induced Damage in Optical Materials" (A. J. Glass and A. H. Guenther, eds.). NBS Spec. Publ. 372, pp. 27–39.
Frapard, C., Laures, P., Roulet, M., Ziegler, X., and Legay-Sommaire, N. (1966). *C. R. Acad. Sci.* **262B**, 1389.
Freed, C. (1968). *IEEE J. Quantum Electron.* **QE-4**, 404.
Freed, C., and Javan, A. (1970). *Appl. Phys. Lett.* **17**, 53.
Frenkel, L., Marantz, H., and Sullivan, T. (1971). *Phys. Rev. A* **3**, 1640.
Freund, S. M., and Ritter, J. J. (1975). *Chem. Phys. Lett.* **32**, 255.
Gagliano, F. P., and Paek, U. C. (1974). *Appl. Opt.* **13**, 274–279.
Gagliano, F. P., and Zaleckas, V. J. (1972). *In* "Lasers in Industry" (S. S. Charschan, ed.), p. 139. Van Nostrand-Reinhold, Princeton, New Jersey.
Gagliano, F. P., Lumley, R. M., and Watkins, L. S. (1969). *Proc. IEEE* **57**, 114.
Ganley, J. T., Harrison, F. B., and Leland, W. T. (1974). *J. Appl. Phys.* **45**, 4980.
Ganley, T., Verdeyan, J. T., and Miley, G. H. (1971). *Appl. Phys. Lett.* **18**, 568.
Garashchuk, V. P., and Molchan, I. V. (1969). *Avtomat. Svarka* **9**, 12.
Garashchuk, V. P., *et al.* (1969). *Avtomat. Svarka* **9**, 56.
Garnsworthy, R. K., Mathias, L. E. S., and Carmichael, C. H. H. (1971). *Appl. Phys. Lett.* **19**, 506.
Gasson, D. B., and Cockayne, B. (1970). *J. Mater. Sci.* **5**, 100.
Gauthier, R., Pinard, P., and Devoire, F. (1969). *Vide* **24**, 109.
Gaver, R. L., and Seguin, H. J. (1970). *Rev. Sci. Instrum.* **41**, (3), 427.
Gebhardt, F. G., and Smith, D. C. (1969). *Appl. Phys. Lett.* **14**, 52.
Gebhardt, F. G., and Smith, D. C. (1971). *IEEE J. Quantum Electron.* **QE-7**, 63.
Gebhardt, F. G., McCoy, J. H., and Smith, D. C. (1969). *IEEE J. Quantum Electron.* **QE-5**, 471.
Gelbwachs, J., and Hartwick, T. S. (1975). *IEEE J. Quantum Electron.* **QE-11**, 52.
Gelbwachs, J. A., Birnbaum, M., Tucker, A. W., and Fincher, C. L. (1972). *Opto-Electron.* **4**, 155.
Gerry, E. T. (1970). *IEEE Spectrum* **7**, 51.
Gibson, A. F., Kimmitt, M. F., and Walker, A. C. (1970). *Appl. Phys. Lett.* **17**, 75.
Gibson, A. F., Kimmitt, M. F., and Patel, B. S. (1971a). *J. Phys. D* **4**, 882.
Gibson, A. F., Kimmitt, M. F., and Rosito, C. A. (1971b). *Appl. Phys. Lett.* **18**, 546.
Gibson, A. F., Rosito, C. A., Raffo, C. A., and Kimmitt, M. F. (1972a). *Appl. Phys. Lett.* **21**, 356.
Gibson, A. F., Rosito, C. A., Raffo, C. A., and Kimmitt, M. F. (1972b). *J. Phys. D* **5**, 1800.
Gibson, A. F., Kimmitt, M. F., and Norris, B. (1974). *Appl. Phys. Lett.* **24**, 306.
Gilbert, J., and LaChambre, J.-L. (1971). *Appl. Phys. Lett.* **18**, 187.
Girard, A., and Beaulieu, A. J. (1974). *IEEE J. Quantum Electron.* **QE-10**, 521.
Glass, A. J. (1969). *Opto-Electron.* **1**, 174.
Glass, A. J., McFee, J. H., and Bergman, J. G., Jr. (1971). *J. Appl. Phys.* **42**, 5219.
Glass, A. M. (1968). *Appl. Phys. Lett.* **13**, 147.
Glass, A. M., and Negran, T. J. (1974). *Appl. Phys. Lett.* **24**, 81.

Glickler, S. L. (1971). *Appl. Opt.* **10,** 644.
Goldberg, L. S. (1970). *Appl. Phys. Lett.* **17,** 489.
Goldberg, M. W., and Yusek, R. (1970). *Appl. Phys. Lett.* **17,** 349.
Gonsalves, J. N. (1973). Ph.D. thesis, York Univ., Toronto.
Gonsalves, J. N., and Duley, W. W. (1971). *Can. J. Phys.* **49,** 1708.
Gonsalves, J. N., and Duley, W. W. (1972). *J. Appl. Phys.* **43,** 4684.
Gordon, E. I. (1966a). *IEEE J. Quantum Electron.* **QE-2,** 101.
Gordon, E. I. (1966b). *Proc. IEEE* **54,** 1391.
Grechikhin, L. I., and Min'ko, L. Ya. (1967). *Sov. Phys.–Tech. Phys.* **12,** 846.
Gregg, D. W., and Thomas, S. J. (1966). *J. Appl. Phys.* **37,** 2787.
Grigoriu, G., and Brinkschulte, H. (1973). *Phys. Lett.* **42A,** 347.
Groh, G. (1968). *J. Appl. Phys.* **39,** 5804.
Gross, R. W. F. (1969). *J. Chem. Phys.* **50,** 1889.
Guenot, R., and Racinet, J. (1967a). *Rev. Gen. Elec.* **76,** 1245.
Guenot, R., and Racinet, J. (1967b). *Brit. Weld. J.*, Aug., 427.
Guenther, A. H., and Bettis, J. R. (1967). *IEEE J. Quantum Electron.* **QE-3,** 11, 581.
Guenther, A. H., and Bettis, J. R. (1970). *In* "Laser Interaction and Related Plasma Phenomena" (H. Schwarz and H. Hora, eds.). Plenum Press, New York.
Guenther, A. H., and Bettis, J. R. (1971). *Proc. IEEE* **59,** 689.
Guenther, A. H., Bettis, J. R., Anderson, R. E., and Wick, R. V. (1970). *IEEE J. Quantum Electron.* **QE-6,** 492.
Guers, K. (1972). *Guer. Offen.* **2,** 232 (Cl. B Old, 13 July 1972).
Gunn, S. R. (1972). *Rev. Sci. Instrum.* **43,** 1523.
Guran, B. T., O'Brien, R. J., and Anderson, D. H. (1970). *Anal. Chem.* **42,** 115.
Hadni, A., Henninger, Y., Thomas, R., Vergnat, P., and Wyncke, B. (1965). *J. Phys.* **26,** 345.
Haesnner, F., and Seitz, W. (1971). *J. Mater. Sci.* **6,** 16.
Hake, R. D., Jr., and Phelps, A. V. (1967). *Phys. Rev.* **158,** 70.
Hall, D. R., and Pao, Y.-H. (1971). *Opt. Commun.* **4,** 264.
Hanna, D. C., Luther-Davies, B., Rutt, H. N., Smith, R. C., and Stanley, C. R. (1972). *IEEE J. Quantum Electron.* **QE-8,** 317.
Hansen, C. F., and Lee, G. (1972). *Astronaut. Aeronaut.* **10,** 74.
Hardway, G. A., and Callihan, C. C. (1968). *Solid State Technol.* **11,** 29.
Harrington, R. E. (1967). *J. Appl. Phys.* **38,** 3266.
Harris, A. L., Chen, M., and Bernstein, H. L. (1970). *Image Tech.* **12,** No. 3, 31.
Harris, N. W., O'Neill, F., and Whitney, W. T. (1974). *Appl. Phys. Lett.* **25,** 148.
Harrison, J. A. (1967). *Brit. J. Appl. Phys.* **18,** 1617.
Harry, J. E., and Lunau, F. W. (1972). *IEEE Trans. Ind. Appl.* **IA-8,** 418.
Hartman, B., and Kleman, B. (1966). *Can. J. Phys.* **44,** 1609.
Hartman, W. F., Forrestal, M. J., and Bushnell, J. C. (1972). *Trans. ASME Ser. E.* **39,** 119.
Hass, G., and Ransey, J. B. (1969). *Appl. Opt.* **8,** 1115.
Hattori, H., Umeno, M., Jimbo, T., Fujitani, O., and Miki, S. (1972). *Jap. J. Appl. Phys.* **11,** 1663.
Hayes, J. N. (1972). *Appl. Opt.* **11,** 455.
Hayes, J. N., Ulrich, P. B., and Aitken, A. H. (1972). *Appl. Opt.* **11,** 257.
Heard, H. G. (1968). "Laser Parameter Measurements Handbook." Wiley, New York.
Herrmann, K. H., and Vogel, R. (1972). *Proc. Intern. Conf. Phys. Semiconductors, 11th* (Polish Sci. Publ., Warsaw), p. 117.

Hertzberg, A., Christiansen, W. H., Johnston, E. W., and Ahlstrom, H. G. (1972). *AIAA J.* **10,** 394.
Herzberg, G. (1945). "Molecular Spectra and Molecular Structure," Vol. II, Infrared and Raman Spectra of Polyatomic Molecules. Van Nostrand-Reinhold, Princeton, New Jersey.
Herzberg, G. (1967). "Molecular Spectra and Molecular Structure," Vol. III, Electronic Spectra and Electronic Structure of Polyatomic Molecules. Van Nostrand-Reinhold, Princeton, New Jersey.
Herziger, G., Stemme, R., and Weber, H. (1973). *Z. Agnew. Math Phys.* **24,** 443.
Hess, M. S., and Milkosky, J. F. (1972). *J. Appl. Phys.* **43,** 4680.
Hettche, L. R., Schriempf, J. T., and Stegman, R. L. (1973). *J. Appl. Phys.* **44,** 4079.
Hidson, D. J., Makios, V., and Morrison, R. (1972). *Phys. Lett.* **40A,** 413.
Higuchi, T., Miyazawa, T., Yoshida, H., and Okuda, T. (1971). *Mitsubishi Denki Lab. Rep.* **45,** 1298.
Hill, A. E. (1968). *Appl. Phys. Lett.* **12,** 324.
Hill, A. E. (1970). *Appl. Phys. Lett.* **16,** 423.
Hill, A. E. (1971). *Appl. Phys. Lett.* **18,** 194.
Hinkley, E. D. (1970). *Appl. Phys. Lett.* **16,** 351.
Hinkley, E. D. (1971). *Phys. Rev. A* **3,** 833.
Hinkley, E. D. (1972). *Opto.-Electron.* **4,** 69.
Hinkley, E. D., and Kelley, P. L. (1971). *Science* **171,** 635.
Hoag, E., Pease, H., Staal, J., and Zar, J. (1974). *Appl. Opt.* **13,** 1959.
Hocker, L. O., Sokoloff, D. R., Daneu, V., Szoke, A., and Javan, A. (1968). *Appl. Phys. Lett.* **12,** 401.
Hokansen, J. L., and Unger, B. A. (1969). *J. Appl. Phys.* **40,** 3157.
Hongo, S., Panyakeow, S., Shirafuji, J., and Inuishi, Y. (1971). *Jap. J. Appl. Phys.* **10,** 717.
Horrigan, F., Klein, C., Rudko, R., and Wilson, D. (1969). *Microwaves* **8,** 68.
Horrocks, D. L., and Studier, M. H. (1965). *Anal. Chem.* **37,** 1782.
Hotz, D. F., and Austin, J. W. (1967). *Appl. Phys. Lett.* **11,** 60.
Howard, J. K., and Ross, R. F. (1972). *Thin Solid Films* **14,** 119.
Howe, J. A. (1963). *J. Chem. Phys.* **39,** 1362.
Howe, J. A. (1965). *Appl. Phys. Lett.* **7,** 21.
Howe, J. A., and McFarlane, R. A. (1966). *J. Mol. Spectrosc.* **19,** 224.
Huang, C.-C., Pao, Y.-H., Claspy, P. C., and Phelps, F. W., Jr. (1974). *IEEE J. Quantum Electron.* **QE-10,** 186.
Hulme, K. F., Jones, O., Davies, P. H., and Hobden, M. V. (1967). *Appl. Phys. Lett.* **10,** 133.
Hurle, I. R., and Hertzberg, A. (1965). *Phys. Fluids* **8,** 1601.
Inaba, H., and Ito, H. (1968). *IEEE J. Quantum Electron.* **QE-4,** 45.
Inaba, H., Kobayashi, T., Yamawaki, K., and Sugiyama, A. (1967). *Infrared Phys.* **7,** 145.
Inn, E. C. Y., Watanabe, K., and Zelikoff, M. (1953). *J. Chem. Phys.* **21,** 1648.
Inoue, E., Kokado, H., Shimizu, I., and Ootsuka, S. (1973). *Photogr. Sci. Eng.* **17,** 405.
Ippolitov, I. I. (1969). *Opt. Spectrosc.* **27,** 246.
Irving, W. M., and Pollack, J. B. (1968). *Icarus* **8,** 324.
Isenor, N. R., and Richardson, M. C. (1971). *Appl. Phys. Lett.* **18,** 224.
Ishizuka, T. (1973). *Anal. Chem.* **45,** 538.
Ivanovskii, G. F., and Varnakov, S. V. (1969). *Indust. Lab.* **35,** 1151.

Ivanovskii, G. F., Blyumkin, L. M., Varnakov, S. V., and Lisovskii, L. N. (1968). *Zavod. Lab.* **34,** 10.
Izatt, J. R., Caudle, G. F., and Bean, B. L. (1974). *Appl. Phys. Lett.* **25,** 446.
Jacob, J. H., Pugh, E. R., Daugherty, J. D., and Northam, D. B. (1973). *Rev. Sci. Instrum.* **44,** 471.
Jacobs, S. D. (1971). *Appl. Opt.* **10,** 2564.
Jacobs, S. D., Teegarden, K. J., and Ahrenkiel, R. K. (1974). *Appl. Opt.* **13,** 2313.
Jaeger, R., and Logan, W. (1973). *Opt. Spectrosc.* **Nov.** 40.
Javan, A., and Levine, J. S. (1972). *IEEE J. Quantum Electron.* **QE-8,** 827.
Jennings, D. A., and West, E. D. (1970). *Rev. Sci. Instrum.* **41,** 565.
Jensen, R. E., and Tobin, M. S. (1972). *IEEE J. Quantum Electron.* **QE-8,** 34.
Johns, T. W., and Nation, J. A. (1972). *Appl. Phys. Lett.* **20,** 495.
Johns, T. W., and Nation, J. A. (1973). *Rev. Sci. Instrum.* **44,** 169.
Johnson, B. C., Puthoff, H. E., Soo Hoo, J., and Sussman, S. S. (1971). *Appl. Phys. Lett.* **18,** 181.
Johnson, D. C. (1971). *IEEE J. Quantum Electron.* **QE-7,** 185.
Johnston, A. R., and Melville, R. D. S., Jr. (1971). *Appl. Phys. Lett.* **19,** 503.
Johnston, R. L., and O'Keefe, J. D. (1972). *Appl. Opt.* **11,** 2926.
Jones, E. D. (1971). *Appl. Phys. Lett.* **18,** 33.
Joy, W. K., Ladner, W. R., and Pritchard, E. (1968). *Nature* (*London*) **217,** 640.
Joy, W. K., Ladner, W. R., and Pritchard, E. (1970). *Fuel* **49,** 26.
Judd, O. P. (1973). *Appl. Phys. Lett.* **22,** 95.
Judd, O. P., and Wada, J. Y. (1974). *IEEE J. Quantum Electron.* **QE-10,** 12.
Jungling, K. C., and Gaddy, O. L. (1971). *IEEE J. Quantum Electron.* **QE-7,** 97.
Kafalas, P., and Ferdinand, A. P., Jr. (1973). *Appl. Opt.* **12,** 29.
Kafalas, P., and Herrmann, J. (1973). *Appl. Opt.* **12,** 772.
Kaldor, A., and Hastie, J. W. (1972). *Chem. Phys. Lett.* **16,** 328.
Kamibayashi, T., Yonemochi, S., and Miyakawa, T. (1973). *Appl. Phys. Lett.* **22,** 119.
Kaminow, I. P. (1968). *IEEE J. Quantum Electron.* **QE-4,** 23.
Kaminow, I. P., and Turner, E. H. (1966). *Proc. IEEE* **54,** 1374.
Kan, T., Stregack, J. A., and Watt, W. S. (1972). *Appl. Phys. Lett.* **20,** 137.
Kaplan, R. A. (1964). *Proc. Nat. Electron. Conf.* **20,** 929.
Karl, R. R., Jr., and Innes, K. K. (1975). *Chem. Phys. Lett.* **36,** 275.
Karlov, N. V. (1974). *Appl. Opt.* **13,** 301.
Karn, F. S., and Sharkey, A. G., Jr. (1968). *Fuel* **47,** 193.
Karn, F. S., and Singer, J. M. (1968). *Fuel* **47,** 235.
Karn, F. S., Friedel, R. A., and Sharkey, A. G., Jr. (1967). *Carbon* **5,** 25.
Karn, F. S., Friedel, R. A., and Sharkey, A. G., Jr. (1969). *Fuel* **48,** 297.
Karn, F. S., Friedel, R. A., and Sharkey, A. G., Jr. (1970). *Chem. Ind.* (*London*) **7,** 239.
Kato, T., and Yamaguchi, T. (1968). *NEC Res. Develop.* (*Jap.*) No. 12, 57.
Keilmann, F. (1970). *Appl. Opt.* **9,** 1319.
Kellock, H. A. (1969). *J. Phys. E* **2,** 377.
Kelly, M. J., Francke, R. E., and Field, M. S. (1970). *J. Chem. Phys.* **53,** 2979.
Kenemuth, J. R., Hogge, C. B., and Avizonis, P. V. (1970). *Appl. Phys. Lett.* **17,** 220.
Kerber, R. L., Cohen, N., and Emanuel, G. (1973). *IEEE J. Quantum Electron.* **QE-9,** 94.
Kerker, M. (1963). "Electromagnetic Scattering." Pergamon, Oxford.
Kiefer, J. E., and Yariv, A. (1969). *Appl. Phys. Lett.* **15,** 26.
Kiefer, J. E., Nussmeier, T. A., and Goodwin, F. E. (1972). *IEEE J. Quantum Electron.* **QE-8,** 173.

Kim, P. H., Taki, K., and Namba, S. (1971). *Record Symp. Electron, Ion Laser Beam Technol., 11th* p. 375.
Kimmitt, M. F., Tyte, D. C., and Wright, M. J. (1972). *J. Phys. E* **5**, 239.
Kleiman, H., and O'Neil, R. W. (1971). *J. Opt. Soc. Amer.* **61**, 12.
Klein, C. A., and Rudko, R. I. (1968). *Appl. Phys. Lett.* **13**, 129.
Kleinman, D. A., and Boyd, G. D. (1969). *J. Appl. Phys.* **40**, 546.
Kliwer, J. K. (1973). *J. Appl. Phys.* **44**, 490.
Klocke, H. (1969). *Spectrochim. Acta* **24B**, 263.
Knox, B. E. (1968). *Mater. Res. Bull.* **3**, 329.
Knox, B. E., and Ban, V. S. (1968). *Mater. Res. Bull.* **3**, 885.
Knox, B. E., Ban, V. S., and Schottmiller, J. (1968). *Mater. Res. Bull.* **3**, 337.
Kogelnik, H., and Bridges, T. J. (1967). *IEEE J. Quantum Electron.* **QE-3**, 95.
Kogelnik, H., and Li, T. (1966). *Appl. Opt.* **5**, 1550.
Kokodii, N. G., and Volitov, R. A. (1969). *Instrum. Exp. Tech.* No. 4, 1001.
Konyukhov, V. K., and Prokhorov, A. M. (1966). *JETP Lett.* **3**, 286.
Konyukhov, V. K., Matrosov, I. V., Prokhorov, A. M., Shalunov, D. T., and Shirokov, N. N. (1970). *JETP Lett.* **12**, 321.
Koren, G., Yacoby, Y., Lotem, H., Kosower, M., and Greenwald, G. (1973). *Appl. Phys. Lett.* **23**, 73.
Korinchikov, A. I., Panteleev, V. V., Putrenko, O. I., and Yankovskii, A. A. (1970). *Zh. Prikl. Spektrosk.* **12**, 819.
Kovacs, M. A., Flynn, G. W., and Javan, A. (1966). *Appl. Phys. Lett.* **8**, 62.
Kremenchugskii, L. S., Mal'nev, A. F., Stolyarov, V. M., and Shul'ga, A. Ya. (1969). *Instrum. Exp. Tech.* **4**, 997.
Kreuzer, L. B. (1971). *J. Appl. Phys.* **42**, 2934.
Kreuzer, L. B., and Patel, C. K. N. (1971). *Science* **173**, 45.
Kreuzer, L. B., Kenyon, N. D., and Patel, C. K. N. (1972). *Science* **177**, 347.
Krumme, J.-P., Verweel, J., Haberkamp, J., Tolksdorf, W., Bartels, G., and Espinosa, G. P. (1972). *Appl. Phys. Lett.* **20**, 451.
Krupke, W. F., and Sooy, W. R. (1969). *IEEE J. Quantum Electron.* **QE-5**, 575.
Kuehn, D. M. (1972). *Appl. Phys. Lett.* **21**, 112.
Kuehn, D. M., and Monson, D. J. (1970). *Appl. Phys. Lett.* **16**, 48.
Kuizenga, D. J., and Siegman, A. E. (1970a). *IEEE J. Quantum Electron.* **QE-6**, 694.
Kuizenga, D. J., and Siegman, A. E. (1970b). *IEEE J. Quantum Electron.* **QE-6**, 709.
Kuizenga, D. J., Phillion, D. W., Lund, T., and Siegman, A. E. (1973). *Opt. Commun.* **9**, 221.
Kulikov, I. S. (1967). Thermal Dissociation of Chemical Compounds. Israel Program for Scientific Translations, Jerusalem.
Kump, H. J., and Chang, P. T. (1966). *IBM J. Res. Develop.* **10**, 255.
Kuznetsov, V. A., and Shchuka, A. A. (1972). *Instrum. Exp. Tech.* **15**, 817.
LaChambre, J.-L. (1971). *Rev. Sci. Instrum.* **42**, 74.
LcChambre, J.-L., Rheault, F., and Gilbert, J. (1972). *Radio Electron. Eng.* **42**, 351.
Lacina, W. B., and Mann, M. M. (1972). *Appl. Phys. Lett.* **21**, 224.
Laflamme, A. K. (1970). *Rev. Sci. Instrum.* **41**, 1578.
Lamb, G. L., Jr., and Kinney, R. B. (1969). *J. Appl. Phys.* **40**, 416.
Lamb, W. E., Jr. (1964). *Phys. Rev.* **134**, A1429.
Lamberton, H. M., and Pearson, P. R. (1971). *Electron. Lett.* **7**, 141.
Landau, H. G. (1950). *Quart. Appl. Math.* **8**, 81.
Landman, A., Marantz, H., and Early, V. (1969). *Appl. Phys. Lett.* **15**, 357.

Landry, M. J. (1974). *Appl. Opt.* **13,** 63.
Laridjani, M., Ramachan, P., and Cahn, R. W. (1972). *J. Mater. Sci.* **7,** 627.
Latta, J. N. (1971). *Appl. Opt.* **10,** 609.
Laurent, V., and Kikindai, T. (1972). *Bull. Soc. Chim. Fr.* **4,** 1258.
Laures, P., and Ziegler, X. (1967). *J. Chim. Phys.* **64,** 100.
Laurie, K. A., and Hale, M. M. (1971). *IEEE J. Quantum Electron.* **QE-7,** 530.
Lavarini, B., Bettini, J. P., Brunet, H., and Michon, M. (1969). *C.R. Acad. Sci.* **269,** 1301.
Lebedev, V. K., and Granitsa, V. T. (1972). *Autom. Weld.* **25,** 63.
Lee, G., and Gowen, F. E. (1971). *Appl. Phys. Lett.* **18,** 237.
Lee, G., Gowen, F. E., and Hagen, J. R. (1972). *AIAA J.* **10,** 65.
Legay, F., and Legay-Sommaire, N. (1964). *C. R. Acad. Sci.* **259B,** 99.
Legay-Sommaire, N., Henry, L., and Legay, F. (1965). *C. R. Acad. Sci.* **260B,** 3339.
Leiba, E. (1969). *C. R. Acad. Sci. B* **268,** 31.
Leite, R. C. C., Moore, R. S., and Whinnery, J. R. (1964). *Appl. Phys. Lett.* **5,** 141.
Leite, R. C. C., Porto, S. P. S., and Damen, T. C. (1967). *Appl. Phys. Lett.* **10,** 100.
Lemaire, J., Houriez, J., Bellet, J., and Thibault, J. (1969). *C. R. Acad. Sci.* **268B,** 922.
Lencioni, D. E., and Lowder, J. E. (1974). *IEEE J. Quantum Electron.* **QE-10,** 235.
Leonard, D. A. (1965). *Appl. Phys. Lett.* **7,** 4.
Leonard, D. A. (1967). *IEEE J. Quantum Electron.* **QE-3,** 133.
Leone, S. R., and Moore, C. B. (1974). *Phys. Rev. Lett.* **33,** 269.
Letokhov, V. S. (1972). *Chem. Phys. Lett.* **15,** 221.
Letokhov, V. S. (1973). *Opt. Commun.* **7,** 59.
Levine, J. S., and Javan, A. (1972). *Phys. Lett.* **42A,** 173.
Levine, J. S., and Javan, A. (1973). *Appl. Phys. Lett.* **22,** 55.
Levine, L. P., Ready, J. F., and Bernal, E. G. (1967). *J. Appl. Phys.* **38,** 331.
Lin, T. P. (1967). *IBM J. Res. Develop.* **11,** 527.
Lind, R. C., Wada, J. Y., Dunning, G. J., and Clark, W. M., Jr. (1974). *IEEE J. Quantum Electron.* **QE-10,** 818.
Little, V. I., Key, P. Y., Wiltsher, R., and Rowley, D. M. (1971). *Nature (London) Phys. Sci.* **232,** 165.
Litvak, A. G. (1966). *JETP Lett.* **4,** 341.
Liu, Y. S. (1974). *Appl. Opt.* **13,** 2505.
Livingston, P. M. (1971). *Appl. Opt.* **10,** 426.
Lock, P. J. (1971). *Appl. Phys. Lett.* **19,** 390.
Locke, E. V. (1972). *Welding J.* **51,** 245s.
Locke, E. V., and Hella, R. A. (1974). *IEEE J. Quantum Electron.* **QE-10,** 179.
Locke, E. V., Hoag, E. D., and Hella, R. A. (1972). *IEEE J. Quantum Electron.* **QE-8,** 132.
Longfellow, J. (1970). *Rev. Sci. Instrum.* **41,** 1485.
Longfellow, J. (1971). *Amer. Ceram. Soc. Bull.* **50,** 251.
Longfellow, J. (1972). *In* "Lasers in Industry" (S. S. Charschan, ed.) p. 297. Van Nostrand-Reinhold, Princeton, New Jersey.
Longfellow, J. (1973). *Solid State Technol.* **16,** 45.
Lowder, J. E., and Pettingill, L. C. (1974). *Appl. Phys. Lett.* **24,** 204.
Lowder, J. E., Lencioni, D. E., Hilton, T. W., and Hull, R. J. (1973). *J. Appl. Phys.* **44,** 2759.
Lucy, R. F. (1972). *Appl. Opt.* **11,** 1329.
Lumley, R. M. (1969). *Amer. Ceram. Soc. Bull.* **48,** 850.
Lunau, F. W., and Paine, E. W. (1969). *Weld. Met. Fabric.*, Jan., 3.

Lunau, F. W., Paine, E. W., Richardson, M., and Wijetunge, M. D. S. P. (1969). *Opt. Technol.* **1,** 255.
Lydtin, H. (1972). *Int. Conf. Chem. Vapor Deposition, 3rd, Salt Lake City, April 24.*
Lyman, J. L., and Rockwood, S. D. (1976). *J. Appl. Phys.* **47,** 595.
Lyman, J. L., Jensen, R. J., Rink, J., Robinson, C. P., and Rockwood, S. D. (1975). *Appl. Phys. Lett.* **27,** 87.
Lyon, D. L. (1973). *IEEE J. Quantum Electron.* **QE-9,** 139.
Lyon, D. L., George, E. V., and Haus, H. A. (1970). *Appl. Phys. Lett.* **17,** 474.
McAvoy, N., Osmundson, J., and Schiffner, G. (1972). *Appl. Opt.* **11.** 473.
Maccomber, J. D. (1968). *IEEE J. Quantum Electron.* **QE-4,** 1.
McCoy, J. H., and Long, R. K. (1969). *Appl. Opt.* **8,** 834.
McCoy, J. H., Rensch, D. B., and Long, R. K. (1969). *Appl. Opt.* **8,** 1471.
McCubbin, T. K., Jr., and Mooney, T. R. (1968). *J. Quant. Spectrosc. Radiat. Transfer* **8,** 1255.
McFee, J. H., Bergman, J. G., Jr., and Crane, G. R. (1972). *Ferroelectrics* **3,** 305.
McGee, J. D., and Heilos, L. J. (1967). *IEEE J. Quantum Electron.* **QE-3,** 17.
McKenzie, R. L. (1970). *Appl. Phys. Lett.* **17,** 462.
McLean, E. A., Sica, L., and Glass, A. J. (1968). *Appl. Phys. Lett.* **13,** 369.
McLeary, R., and Gibbs, W. E. K. (1973). *IEEE J. Quantum Electron.* **QE-9,** 828.
McLeary, R., Beckwith, P. J., and Gibbs, W. E. K. (1974). *IEEE J. Quantum Electron.* **QE-10,** 649.
McMullen, J. D., Anderson, D. B., and Davis, R. L. (1974). *J. Appl. Phys.* **45,** 5084.
Madani, N., and Nichols, K. G. (1971). *Israel J. Technol.* **9,** 245.
Mallozzi, P. J., Epstein, H. M., Jung, R. G., Applebaum, D. C., Fairand, B. P., and Gallagher, W. J. (1973). *In* "Fundamental and Applied Laser Physics" (M. S. Feld, A. Javan, and N. A. Kurnit, eds.), p. 165. Wiley, New York.
Malz, D., Pohler, M., and Stanpendahl, G. (1973). *Phys. Status Solidi B* **58,** K35.
Manes, K. R., and Seguin, H. J. (1972). *J. Appl. Phys.* **43,** 5073.
Marcatili, E. A. J., and Schmeltzer, R. A. (1964). *Bell Syst. Tech. J.* **43,** 1783.
Marchenko, V. M., and Prokhorov, A. M. (1971). *JETP Lett.* **14,** 76.
Marcus, S. (1972). *Appl. Phys. Lett.* **21,** 18.
Marich, K. W., Carr, P. W., Treytl, W. J., and Glick, D. (1970). *Anal. Chem.* **42,** 1775.
Marine, J., and Motte, C. (1973). *Appl. Phys. Lett.* **23,** 450.
Marling, J. B. (1975). *Chem. Phys. Lett.* **34,** 84.
Maroloa, A. J. (1968). *IEEE J. Quantum Electron.* **QE-4,** 503.
Martin, A. J., Buck, R. H., Loasby, R. G., and Savage, J. (1968). *Thin Solid Films* **2,** 253.
Martin, J. M., Corcoran, V. J., and Smith, W. T. (1974). *IEEE J. Quantum Electron.* **QE-10,** 191.
Mason, W. P. (1966). "Crystal Physics of Interaction Processes." Academic Press, New York.
Masters, J. I. (1956). *J. Appl. Phys.* **27,** 477.
Masumura, R. A., and Achter, M. R. (1970). *Appl. Phys. Lett.* **16,** 395.
Matricon, M. (1951). *J. Phys.* **12,** 15.
Matyja, H., Giessen, B. C., and Grant, N. J. (1968). *J. Inst. Metals* **96,** 30.
Maydan, D. (1970). *J. Appl. Phys.* **41,** 1552.
Maydan, D. (1971). *Bell Syst. Tech. J.* **50,** 1761.
Mayer, L. (1958). *J. Appl. Phys.* **29,** 1454.
Mayer, S. W., Kwok, M. A., Gross, R. W. F., and Spencer, D. J. (1970). *Appl. Phys. Lett.* **17,** 516.

Mayerstr, R. (1972). *Int. Conf. Crystal Growth, 2nd, Freiburg, Breisgau, Germany, 21–23 Sept. 1972* p. 12 (Abstract only).
Measures, R. M., and Pilon, G. (1972). *Opto-Electron.* **4,** 141.
Megrue, G. H. (1967). *Science* **157,** 1555.
Melngailis, I., and Harman, T. C. (1968). *Appl. Phys. Lett.* **13,** 180.
Melngailis, I., and Tannenwald, P. E. (1969). *Proc. IEEE* **57,** 806.
Mentall, J. E., and Nicholls, R. W. (1967). *J. Chem. Phys.* **46,** 2881.
Menzies, R. T. (1971). *Appl. Opt.* **10,** 1532.
Menzies, R. T. (1972). *Opto-Electron.* **4,** 179.
Merchant, V., and Irwin, J. C. (1971). *Rev. Sci. Instrum.* **42,** 1437.
Metals and *Materials (GB)* (1973). **1,** 159.
Metz, S. A. (1973). *Appl. Phys. Lett.* **22,** 211.
Metz, S. A., and Smidt, F. A., Jr. (1971). *Appl. Phys. Lett.* **19,** 207.
Meyerhofer, D. (1968a). *IEEE J. Quantum Electron.* **QE-4,** 969.
Meyerhofer, D. (1968b). *IEEE J. Quantum Electron.* **QE-4,** 762.
Mezrich, R. S. (1969). *Appl. Phys. Lett.* **14,** 132.
Mezrich, R. S. (1970). *Appl. Opt.* **9,** 2275.
Michon, M., Guillet, H., LeGoff, D., and Raymond, S. (1969). *Rev. Sci. Instrum.* **40,** 263.
Miknis, F. P., and Biscar, J. P. (1971). *J. Phys. Chem.* **75,** 725.
Miller, C. H., and Osial, T. A. (1969). Status rep. on 250-W CO_2 laser for applications in the pulp and paper industry, *IEEE 1969 Annu. Pulp Paper Ind. Tech. Conf., Atlanta.*
Miller, K. J. (1966). *Weld. Eng.* **51,** 46.
Miller, K. J., and Nunnikhoven, J. D. (1965). *Welding J.* **44,** 480.
Mirkin, L. I. (1969). *Dokl. Akad. Nauk SSSR* **186,** 305 [*English transl.: Sov. Phys.-Dokl.* **14,** 494].
Mirkin, L. I. (1970). *Sov. Phys.–Dokl.* **14,** 1128.
Mirkin, L. I. (1973a). *Dokl. Akad. Nauk SSSR* **206,** 1339 [*English transl.: Sov. Phys.–Dokl.* **17,** 1026].
Mirkin, L. I. (1973b). *Izv. Vyssh. Ucheb. Zaved. Fiz.* **11,** 106.
Mirkin, L. I. (1973c). *Izv. Akad. Nauk SSSR Neorg. Mater.* **9,** 125 [*English transl.: Inorg. Mater.* **9,** 109].
Mirkin, L. I. (1973d). *Fiz. Khim. Obrab. Mater.* No. 1, 143.
Mirkin, L. I. (1973e). *Izv. Vyssh. Ucheb. Zaved. Fiz.* No. 2, 106.
Mirkin, L. I., and Pilipetskii, N. F. (1966). *Polym. Mech.* **2,** 384.
Miura, N., and Tanaka, S. (1968). *Appl. Phys. Lett.* **12,** 374.
Mocker, H. W. (1969). *Appl. Opt.* **8,** 677.
Mooradian, A., Brueck, S. R. J., and Blum, F. A. (1970). *Appl. Phys. Lett.* **17,** 481.
Moore, C. B. (1971). *Ann. Rev. Phys. Chem.* **22,** 387.
Moore, C. B. (1973). *Accounts Chem. Res.* **6,** 323.
Moore, C. B., Wood, R. E., Hu, B. L., and Yardley, J. T. (1967). *J. Chem. Phys.* **46,** 4222.
Moorhead, A. J. (1971). *Weld. J.* **50,** 97.
Moran, J. M. (1971a). *Appl. Opt.* **10,** 412.
Moran, J. M. (1971b). *Appl. Opt.* **10,** 1909.
Morrison, J. A., and Morgan, S. P. (1966). *Bell Syst. Tech. J.* **45,** 661.
Morrison, R. W., and Swail, C. (1972). *Phys. Lett.* **40A,** 375.
Moser, J. B., and Kruger, O. L. (1965). *J. Nucl. Mater.* **17,** 153.
Moser, J. B., and Kruger, O. L. (1967). *J. Appl. Phys.* **38,** 3215.
Müller, K.-H., and Nimtz, G. (1971). *Appl. Phys. Lett.* **19,** 373.

Müller, K.-H., Nimtz, G., and Selders, M. (1972). *Appl. Phys. Lett.* **20,** 322.
Mullaney, G. J., Christiansen, W. H., and Russell, D. A. (1968). *Appl. Phys. Lett.* **13,** 145.
Munjee, S. A., and Christiansen, W. H. (1973). *Appl. Opt.* **12,** 993.
Murabayashi, M., Takahashi, Y., and Mukaibo, T. (1970). *J. Nucl. Sci. Technol.* (*Jap.*) **7,** 312.
Murphy, R. J., and Ritter, G. J. (1966a). *Appl. Phys. Lett.* **9,** 272.
Murphy, R. J., and Ritter, G. J. (1966b). *Nature* (*London*) **210,** 191.
Muzii, L., Stagni, L., and Vitali, G. (1973). *Nuovo Cimento B Ser 2* **14B,** 173.
Nakada, Y., and Giles, M. A. (1971). *J. Amer. Ceram. Soc.* **54,** 354.
Nakatsuka, M., Yamabe, C., Yokoyama, M., and Yamanaka, C. (1972). *Jap. J. Appl. Phys.* **11,** 114.
Nakayama, S., and Kashiwabara, (1972). *Rev. Elec. Commun. Lab.* (*Jap.*) **20,** 145.
Nakayama, S., Saito, Y., and Takamoto, K. (1973). *Rev. Elec. Commun. Lab.* (*Jap.*) **21,** 63.
Namba, S., Kim, P. H., Kinoshita, N., and Arai, T. (1968). *Sci. Pap. Inst. Phys. Chem. Res.* (*Tokyo*) **62,** 8.
Namba, S., Kim, P. H., and Taki, K. (1969). *Record Symp. Electron Ion Laser Beam Technol., 10th* (L. Marton ed.), pp. 493–500. San Francisco Press, San Francisco, California.
Narasimha Rao, D. V. G. L. (1968). *J. Appl. Phys.* **39,** 4853.
Nasu, S., and Kikuchi, T. (1968). *J. Nucl. Sci. Technol.* **5,** 318.
Nebenzahl, I., and Szöke, A. (1974). *Appl. Phys. Lett.* **25,** 327.
Neill, A. H., Jr. (1971). *Nat. Bur. Std. Tech. News Bull.* **55,** 45.
Nelson, L. S. (1972). *Carbon* **10,** 356.
Nelson, L. S., and Richardson, N. L. (1972). *Mater. Res. Bull.* **7,** 971.
Nelson, L. S., Skaggs, S. R., and Richardson, N. L. (1970). *J. Amer. Ceram. Soc.* **53,** 115.
Nelson, L. S., Blander, M., Skaggs, S. R., and Keil, K. (1972a). *Earth Planet. Sci. Lett.* **14,** 338.
Nelson, L. S., Whittaker, A. G., and Tooper, B. (1972b). *High Temp. Sci.* **4,** 445.
Nelson, L. S., Richardson, N. L., Keil, K., and Skaggs, S. R. (1973). *High Temp. Sci.* **5,** 138.
Neuman, F. (1964). *Appl. Phys. Lett.* **4,** 167.
Nichols, D. B., and Brandenberg, W. M. (1972). *IEEE J. Quantum Electron.* **QE-8,** 718
Nighan, W. L. (1970). *Phys. Rev. A* **2,** 1989.
Nighan, W. L., and Wiegand, W. J. (1974). *Appl. Phys. Lett.* **25,** 633.
Nikolaev, N. N., and Koblova, M. M. (1971). *Kvantovaya Elektron. USSR* **1,** 57–64 [*English transl.: Sov. J. Quantum Electron.* **1,** 158].
Nikolov, N., Petrov, A. P., Dimitrov, G., and Dimov, D. (1970). *Mem. Soc. Roy. Sci. Liege Cail.* **19,** 267.
Nishihara, H., Inoue, T., and Koyama, J. (1974). *Appl. Phys. Lett.* **25,** 391.
Nowicki, R. (1971). *Electron. Lett.* **7,** 647.
Nurmikko, A. V. (1971). *IEEE J. Quantum Electron.* **QE-7,** 470.
Nurmikko, A. V., DeTemple, T. A., and Schwarz, S. E. (1971). *Appl. Phys. Lett.* **18,** 130.
Nussmeier, T. A., and Abrams, R. L. (1974). *Appl. Phys. Lett.* **25,** 615.
Nussmeier, T. A., Goodwin, F. E., and Zavin, J. E. (1974). *IEEE J. Quantum Electron.* **QE-10,** 230.
Oka, T. (1968). *J. Chem. Phys.* **48,** 4919.
Oka, T., and Shimizu, T. (1971). *Appl. Phys. Lett.* **19,** 88.
O'Keefe, J. D., and Skeen, C. H. (1972). *Appl. Phys. Lett.* **21,** 464.

Oliver, B. M. (1965). *Proc. IEEE* **53,** 436.

O'Neil, R. W., Carbone, R. J., Granek, H., and Kleiman, H. (1972). *Appl. Phys. Lett.* **20,** 461.

O'Neil, R. W., Kleiman, H., Marquet, L. C., Kilcline, C. W., and Northam, D. (1974). *Appl. Opt.* **13,** 314.

Otis, G, (1972), *Rev, Sci, Instrum,* **43,** 1621,

Otis, G., and Tremblay, R. (1971). *Opt. Commun.* **3,** 418.

Ozeki, T., and Saito, S. (1972). *IEEE J. Quantum Electron.* **QE-8,** 289.

Paek, U. C. (1974). *Appl. Opt.* **13,** 1383.

Paek, U. C., and Gagliano, F. P. (1972). *IEEE J. Quantum Electron.* **QE-8,** 112.

Paek, U. C., and Kestenbaum, A. (1973). *J. Appl. Phys.* **44,** 2260.

Palmer, A. J., and Asmus, J. F. (1970). *Appl. Opt.* **9,** 227.

Pan, Y.-L., Bernhardt, A. F., and Simpson, J. R. (1972). *Rev. Sci. Instrum.* **43,** 662.

Panarella, E., and Savic, P. (1968). *Can. J. Phys.* **46,** 183.

Panyakeow, S., Morisaki, H., Shirafuji, J., and Inuishi, Y. (1972a). *Tech. Rep. Osaka, Univ. (Jap.)* **22,** 563.

Panyakeow, S., Shirafuji, J., and Inuishi, Y. (1972b). *Appl. Phys. Lett.* **21,** 314.

Panyakeow, S., Tanigaki, Y., Shirafuji, J., and Inuishi, Y. (1972c). *J. Appl. Phys.* **43,** 4268.

Pappu, S. V., Kennedy, C., and Scully, M. O. (1972). *Appl. Opt.* **11,** 1879.

Parker, W. J., Jenkins, R. J., and Butler, C. P. (1961). *J. Appl. Phys.* **32,** 1679.

Patel, C. K. N. (1964a). *Phys. Rev. Lett.* **12,** 588.

Patel, C. K. N. (1964b). *Phys. Rev. Lett.* **13,** 617.

Patel, C. K. N. (1964c). *Phys. Rev.* **136,** A1187.

Patel, C. K. N. (1965). *Appl. Phys. Lett.* **7,** 15.

Patel, C. K. N. (1971a). *Appl. Phys. Lett.* **18,** 25.

Patel, C. K. N. (1971b). *Appl. Phys. Lett.* **19,** 400.

Patel, C. K. N. (1972). *Phys. Rev. Lett.* **28,** 649.

Patel, C. K. N. (1974). *Appl. Phys. Lett.* **25,** 112.

Patel, C. K. N., and Shaw, E. D. (1970). *Phys. Rev. Lett.* **24,** 451.

Patel, C. K. N., and Shaw, E. D. (1971). *Phys. Rev.* **B3,** 1279.

Patel, C. K. N., Tien, P. K., and McFee, J. H. (1965). *Appl. Phys. Lett.* **7,** 290.

Patel, C. K. N., Shaw, E. D., and Kerl, R. J. (1970). *Phys. Rev. Lett.* **25,** 8.

Patten, F. W., Garvey, R. M., and Haas, M. (1971). *Mater. Res. Bull.* **6,** 1321.

Pearson, P. R., and Lamberton, H. M. (1972). *IEEE J. Quantum Electron.* **QE-8,** 145.

Peercy, P. S., Jones, E. D., Bushnell, J. C., and Gobeli, G. W. (1970). *Appl. Phys. Lett.* **16,** 120.

Pendleton, W. K., and Guenther, A. H. (1965). *Rev. Sci. Instrum.* **36,** 1546.

Penner, S. S., and Sharma, O. P. (1966). *J. Appl. Phys.* **37,** 2304.

Peppers, N. A., Scribner, E. J., Alterton, L. E., Honey, R. C., Beatrice, E. S., Harding-Barlow, I., Rosan, R. C., and Glick, D. (1968). *Anal. Chem.* **40,** 1178.

Perceval, C. M. (1967). *J. Appl. Phys.* **38,** 5313.

Pert, G. J. (1973). *IEEE J. Quant. Electron.* **QE-9,** 435.

Peyton, B. J., DiNardo, A. J., Kanischak, G. M., Arams, F. R., Lange, R. A., and Sard, E. W. (1972). *IEEE J. Quantum Electron.* **QE-8,** 252.

Pfluger, A. R., and Maas, P. M. (1965). *Welding J.* **44,** 264.

Phelan, R. J., Jr., and Cook, A. R. (1973). *Appl. Opt.* **12,** 2494.

Phelan, R. J., Jr., Mahler, R. J., and Cook, A. R. (1971). *Appl. Phys. Lett.* **19,** 337.

Pirri, A. N. (1973). *Phys. Fluids* **16,** 1435.

Pirri, A. N., Schlier, R., and Northam, D. (1972). *Appl. Phys. Lett.* **21,** 79.

Poehler, T. O., and Walker, R. E. (1973). *Appl. Phys. Lett.* **22,** 282.
Poehler, T. O., Pirkle, J. C., Jr., and Walker, R. E. (1973). *IEEE J. Quantum Electron.* **QE-9,** 83.
Pogodaev, V. A., Kostin, V. V., Khmelevtsov, S. S., and Chistyakov, L. K. (1974). *Izv. Vyssh. Ucheb. Zaved. Fiz.* **3,** 56.
Polanyi, J. C. (1961). *J. Chem. Phys.* **34,** 347.
Polanyi, J. C. (1963). *J. Quantum Spectrosc. Radiative Transfer* **3,** 471.
Polanyi, F. G., and Tobias, I. (1968). "Lasers" (A. K. Levine, ed.). Dekker, New York.
Pollack, M. A. (1966). *Appl. Phys. Lett.* **8,** 237.
Poltavtsev, Yu. G., Zakharov, V. P., Protas, I. M., and Pozdnyakova, V. M. (1972). *Izv. Akad. Nauk SSSR Neorg. Mater.* **8,** 1535.
Posen, H., Bruce, J., Comer, J., and Armington, A. (1973). *In* "Laser Induced Damage in Optical Materials: 1973" (A. J. Glass, and A. H. Guenther, eds.). Nat. Bur. Std. Spec. Publ. 387, p. 181.
Poulsen, P. D. (1972). *Appl. Opt.* **11,** 949.
Pratt, W. K. (1969). "Laser Communication Systems." Wiley, New York.
Predicki, P., Mullendore, A. W., and Grant, N. J. (1965). *Trans. AIME* **233,** 1581.
Pressman, J. (1971). U.S. Patent 3558877.
Preston, J. S. (1971). *J. Phys. E* **4,** 969.
Preston, J. S. (1972). *J. Phys. E* **5,** 1014.
Pridmore-Brown, D. C. (1973). *Appl. Opt.* **12,** 2188.
Prokhorov, A. M., Batanov, V. A., Bunkin, F. V., and Fedorov, V. B. (1973). *IEEE J. Quantum Electron.* **QE-9,** 503.
Pugh, E. R., Wallace, J., Jacob, J. H., Northam, D. B., and Daugherty, J. D. (1974). *Appl. Opt.* **13,** 2512.
Putley, E. H. (1970). *In* "Semiconductors and Semimetals" (R. K. Willardson and A. C. Beer, eds.), Vol. 6. Academic Press, New York.
Putley, E. H. (1971). *Opt. Laser Technol.* **3,** 150.
Quel, E., and de Hemptinne, X. (1969). *Ann. Soc. Sci. Bruxelles* **83,** 262.
Quel, E., de Hemptinne, X., Fayt, A., and de Hemptinne, M. (1969). *Ann. Soc. Sci. Bruxelles I.* **83,** 388.
Rabinowitz, P., Keller, R., and LaTourrette, J. T. (1969). *Appl. Phys. Lett.* **14,** 376.
Raizer, Yu. P. (1967). *Sov. Phys.–JETP* **52,** 470.
Rampton, D. T., and Gandhi, O. P. (1972). *Appl. Phys. Lett.* **21,** 457.
Rasberry, S. D., Scribner, B. F., and Margoshes, M. (1967a). *Appl. Opt.* **6,** 81.
Rasberry, S. D., Scribner, B. F., and Margoshes, M. (1967b). *Appl. Opt.* **6,** 87.
Ready, J. F. (1963). *Appl. Phys. Lett.* **3,** 11.
Ready, J. F. (1965a). *J. Appl. Phys.* **36,** 462.
Ready, J. F. (1965b). *Phys. Rev.* **137,** A620.
Ready, J. F. (1971). "Effects of High Power Laser Radiation." Academic Press, New York.
Reichelt, W. H., and Stark, E. E., Jr. (1973). *In* "Laser Induced Damage in Optical Materials: 1973." NBS Spec. Publ. 387, p. 175.
Reichelt, W. H., Stark, E. E., Jr., and Stratton, T. F. (1974). *Opt. Commun.* **11,** 305.
Rheault, F., LaChambre, J.-L., Gilbert, J., Fortin, R., and Blanchard, M. (1972). *Can. J. Phys.* **50,** 1876.
Ribakovs, G., and Gundjian, A. A. (1974). *Appl. Phys. Lett.* **24,** 377.
Rich, J. W., Thompson, H. M., Treanor, C. E., and Daiber, J. W. (1971). *Appl. Phys. Lett.* **19,** 230.
Richards, F. A., and Walsh, D. (1969). *J. Phys. D* **2,** 663.

Richardson, M. C. (1974). *Opt. Commun.* **10,** 302.
Richardson, M. C., Alcock, A. J., Leopold, K., and Burtyn, P. (1973a). *IEEE J. Quantum Electron.* **QE-9,** 236.
Richardson, M. C., Leopold, K., and Alcock, A. J. (1973b). *IEEE J. Quantum Electron.* **QE-9,** 934.
Rigden, J. D., and Moeller, G. (1966). *IEEE J. Quantum Electron.* **QE-2,** 365.
Rinehart, E. A., Richardson, J. H., Johnson, D. C., and Hrubesh, L. W. (1976). *Appl. Phys. Lett.* **28,** 131.
Ristau, W. T., and Vanderborgh, N. E. (1970). *Anal. Chem.* **42,** 1848.
Ristau, W. T., and Vanderborgh, N. E. (1971). *Anal. Chem.* **43,** 702.
Ristau, W. T., and Vanderborgh, N. E. (1972). *Anal. Chem.* **44,** 359.
Ritter, G. J., and Murphy, R. J. (1970). *Proc. Intern. Congr. Electron Microscopy, 7th, Grenoble, France,* p. 331.
Roberts, T. G., Hutcheson, G. J., Ehrlich, J. J., Hales, W. L., and Barr, T. A. (1967). *IEEE J. Quantum Electron.* **QE-3,** 605.
Robinson, A. M. (1971). *IEEE J. Quantum Electron.* **QE-7,** 199.
Robinson, A. M., Bradette, C., and Kirkwood, E. (1971). *Rev. Sci. Instrum.* **42,** 1894.
Robinson, J. W., Woodward, C., and Barnes, H. M. (1968). *Anal. Chim. Acta* **43,** 119.
Röss, D. (1969). "Lasers, Light Amplifiers, and Oscillators." Academic Press, New York.
Rogowski, W. (1923). *Arch. Elektrotech.* **12,** 1.
Ronchi, L. (1972). *In* "Laser Handbook" (F. T. Arecchi and E. O. Shulz-Dubois, eds.). North-Holland Publ., Amsterdam.
Ronn, A. M. (1968). *J. Chem. Phys.* **48,** 511.
Ronn, A. M., and Lide, D. R., Jr. (1967). *J. Chem. Phys.* **47,** 3669.
Rosenthal, D. (1946). *Trans. Amer. Soc. Mech. Engrs.* **68,** 849.
Roundy, C. B., and Byer, R. L. (1972). *Appl. Phys. Lett.* **21,** 512.
Rudisill, J. E., Braunstein, M., and Braunstein, A. I. (1974). *Appl. Opt.* **13,** 2075.
Ruffler, C., and Gürs, K. (1972). *Opt. Laser Technol.* **4,** 265.
Rykalin, N. N., and Uglov, A. A. (1966). *Sov. Phys.–Dokl.* **10,** 1106.
Rykalin, N. N., and Uglov, A. A. (1971). *Teplofiz. Vys. Temp.* **9,** 575 [*English transl.: High Temp.* **9,** 522].
Rykalin, N. N., Uglov, A. A., and Makarov, N. I. (1967a). *Sov. Phys.–Dokl.* **11,** 632.
Rykalin, N. N., Uglov, A. A., and Makarov, N. I. (1967b). *Sov. Phys.–Dokl.* **12,** 636.
Rykalin, N. N., Uglov, A. A., and Makarov, N. I. (1967c). *Sov. Phys.–Dokl.* **12,** 644.
Saffir, A. J., Marich, K. W., and Orenburg, J. B. (1972). *Appl. Spectrosc.* **26,** 469.
Sakane, T. (1974). *Opt. Commun.* **12,** 21.
Samson, J. A. R., Padur, J. P., and Sharma, A. (1967). *J. Opt. Soc. Amer.* **57,** 966.
Sard, R., and Maydan, D. (1971). *J. Appl. Phys.* **42,** 5084.
Sarjeant, W. J., Kucerovsky, Z., Rumbold, D., and Brannen, E. (1971). *Rev. Sci. Instrum.* **42,** 1890.
Schaeffer, R., and Pearson, R. K. (1969). *J. Amer. Chem. Soc.* **91,** 2153.
Schatz, J. F., and Simmons, G. (1972a). *J. Appl. Phys.* **43,** 2586.
Schatz, J. F., and Simmons, G. (1972b). *J. Geophys. Res.* **77,** 6966.
Schmidt, A. J., and Greenhow, R. C. (1969). *J. Phys. E* **2,** 438.
Schmidt, A. O., Ham, I., and Hoshi, T. (1965). *Welding J. Suppl.* Nov., 481.
Schriempf, J. T. (1972a). *Rev. Sci. Instrum.* **43,** 781.
Schriempf, J. T. (1972b). *High Temp. High Pressures* **4,** 411.
Schriever, R. L. (1972). *Appl. Phys. Lett.* **20,** 354.
Schroth, H. (1972). *Z. Anal. Chem.* **261,** 21.

Schulz, G. J. (1964). *Phys. Rev.* **135,** A988.
Schwarz, F., and Poole, R. R. (1970). *Appl. Opt.* **9,** 1940.
Schwarz, H., and Tourtellote, H. A. (1969). *J. Vac. Sci. Technol.* **6,** 373.
Scott, B. F., and Stovell, J. E. (1968). *Opt. Technol.* **1,** 15.
Scott, R. H., Jackson, P. F. S., and Strasheim, A. (1971). *Nature (London)* **232,** 623.
Seguin, H. J., and Tulip, J. (1972). *Appl. Phys. Lett.* **21,** 414.
Seguin, H. J., Manes, K., and Tulip, J. (1972a). *Rev. Sci. Instrum.* **43,** 1134.
Seguin, H. J., Tulip, J., and White, B. (1972b). *Appl. Phys. Lett.* **20,** 436.
Seguin, H. J., Tulip, J., and McKen, D. (1973a). *Appl. Phys. Lett.* **23,** 344.
Seguin, H. J., Tulip, J., and McKen, D. (1973b). *Appl. Phys. Lett.* **23,** 527.
Seguin, H. J., Tulip, J., and McKen, D. C. (1974). *IEEE J. Quantum Electron.* **QE-10,** 311.
Séguin, J. N. (1972). Ph.D. thesis, York Univ.
Sharkey, A. G., Jr., Shultz, J. L., and Friedel, R. A. (1964). *Nature (London)* **202,** 968.
Shaulov, A., and Simhony, M. (1972). *Appl. Phys. Lett.* **20,** 6.
Shaw, E. D., and Patel, C. K. N. (1971). *Phys. Rev. Lett.* **18,** 215.
Shimazu, M., Suzaki, Y., Takatsuji, M., and Takami, K. (1967). *Jap. J. Appl. Phys.* **6,** 120.
Shimizu, F. (1969). *Appl. Phys. Lett.* **14,** 378.
Shimizu, F. (1970a). *Chem. Phys.* **52,** 3572.
Shimizu, F. (1970b). *J. Chem. Phys.* **53,** 1149.
Shimizu, T., and Oka, T. (1970a). *J. Chem. Phys.* **53,** 2536.
Shimizu, T., and Oka, T. (1970b). *Phys. Rev. A* **2,** 1177.
Shultz, J. L., and Sharkey, A. G., Jr. (1967). *Carbon* **5,** 57.
Siegman, A. E. (1965). *Proc. IEEE* **53,** 277.
Siegman, A. E. (1971). *Laser Focus* **7,** 42.
Siegman, A. E. (1974). *Appl. Opt.* **13,** 353.
Siegman, A. E., and Kuizenga, D. J. (1969). *Appl. Phys. Lett.* **14,** 181.
Siegman, A. E., and Miller, H. Y. (1970). *Appl. Opt.* **9,** 2729.
Siegrist, M., and Kneubühl, F. K. (1973). *Appl. Phys.* **2,** 43.
Siegrist, M., Kaech, G., and Kneubühl, F. K. (1973). *Appl. Phys.* **2,** 45.
Siekman, J. G. (1968). *Microelectron. Reliability* **7,** 305.
Siekman, J. G. (1969). *Microelectron. Reliability* **8,** 87.
Siekman, J. G., and Morijn, R. E. (1968a). *Phillips Res. Rep.* **23,** 367.
Siekman, J., and Morijn, R. (1968b). *Phillip Res. Rep.* **23,** 375.
Silverman, B. D. (1972). *J. Appl. Phys.* **43,** 5163.
Sinclair, D. C. (1970). *Appl. Opt.* **9,** 797.
Sinclair, D. C., and Cottrell, T. H. E. (1967). *Appl. Opt.* **6,** 845.
Skeen, C. H., and York, C. M. (1968). *Appl. Phys. Lett.* **12,** 369.
Skinner, D. R., and Whitcher, R. E. (1972). *J. Phys. E* **5,** 237.
Skolnik, L. H., Lipson, H. G., Bendow, B., and Schott, J. T. (1974). *Appl. Phys. Lett.* **25,** 442.
Skribanowitz, N., Herman, I. P., Osgood, R. M., Jr., Feld, M. S., and Javan, A. (1972a). *Appl. Phys. Lett.* **20,** 428.
Skribanowitz, N., Herman, I. P., and Feld, M. S. (1972b). *Appl. Phys. Lett.* **21,** 466.
Slusher, R. E., Patel, C. K. N., and Fleury, P. A. (1967). *Phys. Rev. Lett.* **18,** 77.
Smith, D. C. (1971). *Appl. Phys. Lett.* **19,** 405.
Smith, D. C., and Berger, P. J. (1971). *IEEE J. Quantum Electron.* **QE-7,** 172.
Smith, D. C., and Gebhardt, F. G. (1970). *Appl. Phys. Lett.* **16,** 275.

Smith, D. C., and McCoy, J. H. (1969). *Appl. Phys. Lett.* **15,** 282.
Smith, H. M., and Turner, A. F. (1965). *Appl. Opt.* **4,** 147.
Smith, J. L. (1973). *In* "Laser Induced Damage in Optical Materials: 1973" (A. J. Glass and A. H. Guenther, eds.). Nat. Bur. Std. Spec. Publ. 387, p. 103.
Smith, P. W. (1971). *Appl. Phys. Lett.* **19,** 132.
Smith, R. A., Jones, F. E., and Chasmar, R. P. (1968). "The Detection and Measurement of Infra-Red Radiation," 2nd ed. Oxford Univ. Press, Oxford.
Smith, R. C. (1972). *Appl. Phys. Lett.* **21,** 352.
Smith, R. L., Russell, T. W., Case, W. E., and Rasmussen, A. L. (1972). *IEEE Trans. Instrum. Measurement* **IM-21,** 434.
Smith, W. V. (1970). "Laser Applications." Artech House Inc., Dedham, Massachusetts.
Soref, R. A. (1966). *Electron Lett.* **2,** 410.
Sparks, M. (1971). *J. Appl. Phys.* **42,** 5029.
Speich, G. R., and Fisher, R. M. (1966). *Recryst. Grain Growth Textures, Pap. Seminar Amer. Soc. Metals,* p. 563.
Spinak, S., Barron, P. P., Karp, S., Hankin, R. B., and Meier, R. H. (1968). *Appl. Opt.* **7,** 17.
Spitz, H. Y. (1969). *Record Symp. Electron Laser Beam Technol., 10th, Gaithersberg, Maryland* p. 233.
Statz, H., Tang, C. L., and Koster, G. F. (1966). *J. Appl. Phys.* **37,** 4278.
Stearn, J. W. (1967). *J. Sci. Instrum.* **44,** 218.
Stegman, R. L., Schriempf, J. T., and Hettche, L. R. (1973). *J. Appl. Phys.* **44,** 3675.
Steinmetz, L. L. (1968). *Rev. Sci. Instrum.* **39,** 904.
Stephens, R. R., and Cool, T. A. (1972). *J. Chem. Phys.* **56,** 5863.
Stephenson, J. C., Finzi, J., and Moore, C. B. (1972). *J. Chem. Phys.* **56,** 5214.
Stern, F. (1973). *J. Appl. Phys.* **44,** 4204.
Steverding, B. (1970). *J. Phys. D* **3,** 358.
Steverding, B. (1971). *J. Phys. D* **4,** 787.
Stovell, J. E. (1967). *J. Sci. Instrum.* **44,** 1045.
Stoyanova, I. G., Timofeev, A. A., Antipova, A. V., Levadnyi, G. G., and Zelyanina, A. N. (1972). *Izv. Nauk SSSR Ser. Fiz.* **36,** 1973.
Stricker, J., and Rom, J. (1972). *Rev. Sci Instrum.* **43,** 1168.
Strickland, D. M., Bettis, J. R., and Guenther, A. H. (1973). *Rev. Sci. Instrum.* **44,** 1121.
Sueta, T., Matsushima, T., Nishimoto, T., and Makimoto, T. (1970). *Proc. IEEE* **58,** 1378.
Sukhorukov, A. P., Khokhlov, R. V., and Shumilov, E. N. (1971). *JETP Lett.* **14,** 161.
Sullivan, A. B. J., and Houldcroft, P. T. (1967). *Brit. Welding J.* **14,** 443.
Suminov, V. M., and Kuzin, B. G. (1972). *Russ. Eng. J.* **52,** 4.
Suzuki, I., and Suzuki, S. (1968). *Bull. Chem. Soc. Jap.* **41,** 2821.
Szoke, A., Daneu, V., Goldhar, J., and Kurmit, N. A. (1969). *Appl. Phys. Lett.* **15,** 376.
Tan, K. O., Makios, V., and Morrison, R. W. (1972). *Phys. Lett.* **38A,** 225.
Tandler, W. S. W. (1971). *Laser Focus* **7,** 24.
Taylor, R. E., and Cape, J. A. (1964). *Appl. Phys. Lett.* **5,** 212.
Taylor, R. L., and Bitterman, S. (1969). *Rev. Mod. Phys.* **41,** 26.
Tchernev, D. I., and Lewicki, G. (1968). *IEEE Trans. Magn.* **MAG-4,** 75.
Tencza, A. D., and Angelo, R. W. (1969). *Record Symp. Electron Ion Laser Beam Technol., 10th* (L. Marton, ed.), p. 259.
Thompson, H. M., Rehm, R. G., and Daiber, J. W. (1971). *J. Appl. Phys.* **42,** 310.
Thompson, S. A. (1970). *Elec. Eng.* **29,** 48.

Tiffany, W. B., Targ, R., and Foster, J. D. (1969). *Appl. Phys. Lett.* **15,** 91.
Tolmachev, A. V., and Kuz'michev, V. M. (1971). *JETP Lett.* **14,** 144.
Topol, L. E., and Happe, R. A. (1974). *J. Non-Crystalline Solids* **15,** 116.
Torrero, E. (1972). *Electronics* **20,** 44.
Touloukian, Y. S., and Ho, C. Y. (1970a). "Thermophysical Properties of Matter," Vol. 1, Thermal Conductivity, Metallic Elements and Alloys. Plenum Press, New York.
Touloukian, Y. S., and Ho, C. Y. (1970b). "Thermophysical Properties of Matter," Vol. 2, Thermal Conductivity, Nonmetallic Solids. Plenum Press, New York.
Treacy, E. B. (1968). *Proc. IEEE* **56,** 2053.
Treacy, E. B. (1969). *Appl. Opt.* **8,** 1107.
Treves, D., Hunt, R. P., and Dickey, B. (1969). *J. Appl. Phys.* **40,** 972.
Treytl, W. J., Marich, K. W., Orenburg, J. B., Carr, P. W., Miller, D. C., and Glick, D. (1971a). *Anal. Chem.* **43,** 1452.
Treytl, W. J., Orbenberg, J. B., Marich, K. W., and Glick, D. (1971b). *Appl. Spectrosc.* **25,** 376.
Tseng, D. Y. (1974). *Appl. Phys. Lett.* **24,** 134.
Tulip, J., and Seguin, H. (1971a). *Appl. Phys. Lett.* **19,** 263.
Tulip, J., and Seguin, H. (1971b). *J. Appl. Phys.* **42,** 3393.
Turgeon, M. F. (1971). *IEEE J. Quantum Electron.* **QE-7,** 495.
Twu, B.-L., and Schwarz, S. E. (1974). *Appl. Phys. Lett.* **25,** 595.
Tyte, D. C. (1970). *In* "Advances in Quantum Electronics" (D. W. Goodwin, ed.), Vol. 1. Academic Press, New York.
Tyte, D. C., and Wills, M. S. (1969). *Laser Opto-Electron. Conf., IERE Conf. Proc.* No. 14, p. 196.
Ujihara, K. (1968). *Proc. IEEE* **56,** 2090.
Ujihara, K., and Kamiyama, M. (1970). *IEEE J. Quantum Electron.* **QE-6,** 239.
Unger, B. A., and Cohen, M. I. (1968). *Electron. Components Conf., Washington, D.C.* p. 304.
Usikov, A. Ya., Kontorovich, V. N., Kaner, E. A., and Bliokh, P. V. (1972). *Ukri Fiz. Zh.* **17,** 1245.
Vallach, E., Zeevi, A., Greenfield, E., and Yatsiv, S. (1972). *Appl. Phys. Lett.* **20,** 395.
van de Hulst, H. C. (1957). "Light Scattering by Small Particles." Wiley, New York.
Vanderborgh, N. E., Ristau, W. T., and Coloff, S. (1971). *Record Symp. Electron Ion Laser Beam Technol., 11th* p. 403.
Vastola, F. J., and Pirone, A. J. (1968). *Advan. Mass. Spectrom.* **4,** 107.
Velichko, O. A., Garashchuk, V. P., and Moravskii, V. E. (1972). *Auto. Weld.* **25** (4), 75.
Vérié, C., and Sirieix, M. (1972). *IEEE J. Quantum Electron.* **QE-8,** 180.
Verreault, M., Otis, G., and Tremblay, R. (1974). *Opt. Commun.* **11,** 227.
Vlases, G. C., and Moeny, W. M. (1972). *J. Appl. Phys.* **43,** 1840.
Vlastaras, A. S. (1970). *J. Phys. Chem.* **74,** 2496.
Vogel, K., and Backlund, P. (1965). *J. Appl. Phys.* **36,** 3697.
Voronin, E. S., Divlekeev, M. I., Il'inskii, Yu. A., Solomatin, V. S., Badikov, V. V., and Godovikov, A. A. (1971). *Sov. J. Quantum Electron.* **1,** 115.
Voronkov, L. (1971). *Izmer. Tekh.* (*USSR*) **14,** 27 [*English transl.: Meas. Tech.* (*USA*) **14,** 1327].
Wallace, J., and Camac, M. (1970). *J. Opt. Soc. Amer.* **60,** 1587.
Wallace, R. W. (1970). *Appl. Phys. Lett.* **17,** 497.
Walsh, T. E. (1968). *1968 NEREM Record, Boston,* p. 162.

Wang, V., Braunstein, A., Braunstein, M., Rudisill, J. E., and Wada, J. Y. (1973a). *In* "Laser Induced Damage in Optical Materials: 1973" (A. J. Glass and A. H. Guenther, eds.). NBS Spec. Publ. 387, pp. 157–169.

Wang, V., Braunstein, A. I., and Wada, J. Y. (1973b). *In* "Laser Induced Damage in Optical Materials: 1973" (A. J. Glass and A. H. Guenther, eds.). NBS Spec. Publ. 387, pp. 183–193.

Waniek, R. W., and Jarmuz, P. J. (1968). *Appl. Phys. Lett.* **12,** 52.

Warlimont, H., Seitz, W., and Haessner, F. (1971). *Z. Metallk.* **62,** 896.

Warner, J. (1968a). *Appl. Phys. Lett.* **12,** 222.

Warner, J. (1968b). *Appl. Phys. Lett.* **13,** 360.

Watson, E., Jr., and Parrish, C. F. (1971). *J. Chem. Phys.* **54,** 1427.

Watt, D. A. (1966). *Brit. J. Appl. Phys.* **17,** 231.

Watt, W. S. (1971). *Appl. Phys. Lett.* **18,** 487.

Waynant, R. W., Cullom, J. H., Basil, J. T., and Baldwin, G. D. (1965). *Appl. Opt.* **4,** 1648.

Webb, M. S. W., and Cotterill, J. C. (1968). *Anal. Chim. Acta* **43,** 351.

Webster, J. M. (1970). *Metals Progr.* **98,** 59.

Weeks, R. W., and Duley, W. W. (1974). *J. Appl. Phys.* **10,** 4661.

Weick, W. W. (1972). *IEEE J. Quantum Electron.* **QE-8,** 126.

West, E. D., and Churney, K. L. (1970). *J. Appl. Phys.* **41,** 2705.

West, E. D., Case, W. E., Rasmussen, A. L., and Schmidt, L. B. (1972). *J. Res. Nat. Bur. Std.* **76A,** 13.

Whinnery, J. R., Miller, D. T., and Dabby, F. (1967). *IEEE J. Quantum Electron.* **QE-3,** 382.

White, R. M. (1963a). *J. Appl. Phys.* **34,** 2123.

White, R. M. (1963b). *J. Appl. Phys.* **34,** 3559.

Wiley, R. H., and Reich, E. (1970). *Ann. N.Y. Acad. Sci.* **168,** 610.

Wiley, R. H., and Veeravagu, P. (1968). *J. Phys. Chem.* **72,** 2417.

Williams, F. A. (1965). *Inst. J. Heat Mass Transfer* **8,** 575.

Willis, J. (1974). *Electron. Components* **16,** 35.

Wilson, J. R. (1969). *J. Phys. E* **2,** 215.

Winters, H. F., and Kay, E. (1967). *J. Appl. Phys.* **38,** 3928.

Winters, H. F., and Kay, E. (1972). *J. Appl. Phys.* **43,** 789.

Wisner, G. R., Foster, M. C., and Blaszuk, P. R. (1973). *Appl. Phys. Lett.* **22,** 14.

Witteman, W. J. (1965). *Phys. Lett.* **18,** 125.

Witteman, W. J. (1966a). *Phillips Res. Rep.* **21,** 73.

Witteman, W. J. (1966b). *IEEE J. Quantum Electron.* **QE-2,** 375.

Witteman, W. J. (1967a). *Appl. Phys. Lett.* **10,** 347.

Witteman, W. J. (1967b). *Phillips Tech. Rev.* **28,** 287.

Witteman, W. J. (1967c). *Appl. Phys. Lett.* **11,** 337.

Witteman, W. J. (1968). *IEEE J. Quantum Electron.* **QE-4,** 786.

Witteman, W. J. (1969). *IEEE J. Quantum Electron.* **QE-5,** 92.

Wood, A. D., Camac, M., and Gerry, E. T. (1971). *Appl. Opt.* **10,** 1877.

Wood, O. R. (1974). *Proc. IEEE* **62,** 355.

Wood, O. R., Abrams, R. L., and Bridges, T. J. (1970). *Appl. Phys. Lett.* **17,** 376.

Wood, O. R., Burkhardt, E. G., Pollack, M. A., and Bridges, T. J. (1971). *Appl. Phys. Lett.* **18,** 261.

Wood, R. A., Dennis, R. B., and Smith, J. W. (1972). *Opt. Commun.* **4,** 383.

Wu, C. C., Armstrong, R. W., and Lee, C. H. (1972). *J. Appl. Phys.* **43,** 821.

Yablonovitch, E., and Goldhar, J. (1974). *Appl. Phys. Lett.* **25,** 580.
Yamaka, E., Hayashi, T., and Matsumoto, M. (1971). *Infrared Phys.* **11,** 247.
Yang, L. C. (1974). *J. Appl. Phys.* **45,** 2601.
Yang, L. C., and Menichelli, V. J. (1971). *Appl. Phys. Lett.* **19,** 473.
Yarborough, J. M., Sussman, S. S., Puthoff, H. E., Pantel, R. H., and Johnson, B. C. (1969). *Appl. Phys. Lett.* **15,** 102.
Yariv, A. (1968). "Quantum Electronics." Wiley, New York.
Yariv, A., Mead, C. A., and Parker, J. V. (1966). *IEEE J. Quantum Electron.* **QE-2,** 243.
Yatsiv, S., Greenfield, E., Dothan-Deutsch, F., Chuchem, D., and Bin-Nun, E. (1971). *Appl. Phys. Lett.* **19,** 65.
Yatsiv, S., Greenfield, E., Dothan-Deutsch, F., and Chuchem, D. (1972). *IEEE J. Quantum Electron.* **QE-8,** 161.
Yeou Ta, (1938). *C.R. Acad. Sci.* **207,** 1042.
Yeung, E. S., and Moore, C. B. (1972). *Appl. Phys. Lett.* **21,** 109.
Yin, P. R. L., and Long, R. L. (1968). *Appl. Opt.* **7,** 1551.
Yogev, A., Loewenstein, R. M. J., and Amar, D. (1972). *J. Amer. Chem. Soc.* **94,** 1091.
Young, P. A. (1971). *Appl. Opt.* **10,** 638.
Young, W. A. (1973). Unpublished work.
Young, W. A., and Duley, W. W. (1974). Unpublished work.
Yurchak, R. P. (1971). *Teplofiz. Vys. Temp.* (*USSR*) **9,** 1304 [*English transl.: High Temp.* **9,** 1203].
Zakurenko, O. E., Valitov, R. A., Arzumanov, A. S., and Kuz'michev, V. M. (1971).
Zavitsanos, P. D. (1967). G. E. Rep. R67SD11.
Zavitsanos, P. D. (1968). *Carbon* **6,** 731.
Zavitsanos, P. D., and Sauer, W. E. (1968). *J. Electrochem. Soc.* **115,** 109.
Zelmanovich, I. L., and Shifrin, K. S. (1968). "Tables of Light Scattering," Vol. 3. Hydrometeorological Press, Leningrad.
Zhiryakov, B. M., Rykalin, N. N., Uglov, A. A., and Fanibo, A. K. (1971). *Zh. Tekh. Fiz.* (*USSR*) **41,** 1037 [*English transl.: Sov. Phys.-Tech. Phys.* **16,** 815].
Zuev, V. E., Sosnin, A. V., and Khmelevtsov, S. S. (1969). *Bull. Acad. Sci. Atmos. Oceanic Phys. Ser. U.S.* **5,** 4.
Zuev, V. E., Kuzikovskii, A. V., Pogodaev, V. A., Khmelevtsov, S. S., and Chistyakova, L. K. (1973). *Dokl. Akad. Nauk SSSR* **205,** 1069 *1972* [*English transl.: Sov. Phys.-Dokl.* **17,** 765].
Zukov, A. A., Kristal, M. A., Kokora, A. N., and Snezno, R. L. (1972). *Mem. Sci. Rev. Metall.* (*Fr.*) **69,** 211.

Index

A

B

C

D

E

Q

R

S

T

A 6
B 7
C 8
D 9
E 0
F 1
G 2
H 3
I 4
J 5

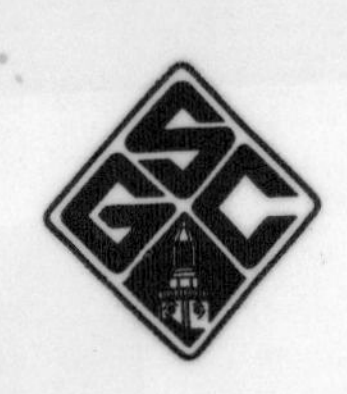